APPLICATION OF ENGINEERING PRINCIPLES AND PRACTICES IN BIOTECHNOLOGY

APPLICATION OF ENGINEERING PRINCIPLES AND PRACTICES IN BIOTECHNOLOGY

Edited by

Ann Rose Abraham, PhD

Leonardo Sepúlveda Torre, PhD

Tamara Tatrishvili, PhD

A. K. Haghi, PhD

AAP | APPLE ACADEMIC PRESS

First edition published 2025

Apple Academic Press Inc.
1265 Goldenrod Circle, NE,
Palm Bay, FL 32905 USA

760 Laurentian Drive, Unit 19,
Burlington, ON L7N 0A4, CANADA

CRC Press
2385 NW Executive Center Drive,
Suite 320, Boca Raton FL 33431

4 Park Square, Milton Park,
Abingdon, Oxon, OX14 4RN UK

Library and Archives Canada Cataloguing in Publication

Title: Application of engineering principles and practices in biotechnology / edited by Ann Rose Abraham, PhD, Leonardo Sepúlveda Torre, PhD, Tamara Tatrishvili, PhD, A.K. Haghi, PhD.
Names: Abraham, Ann Rose, editor. | Sepúlveda Torre, Leonardo, editor. | Tatrishvili, Tamara, editor. | Haghi, A. K., editor.
Description: First edition. | Includes bibliographical references and index.
Identifiers: Canadiana (print) 20240373073 | Canadiana (ebook) 2024037309X | ISBN 9781774915608 (hardcover) | ISBN 9781774915615 (softcover) | ISBN 9781003439929 (ebook)
Subjects: LCSH: Biotechnology. | LCSH: Bioengineering.
Classification: LCC TP248.2 .A67 2025 | DDC 660.6—dc23

Library of Congress Cataloging-in-Publication Data

CIP data on file with US Library of Congress

ISBN: 978-1-77491-560-8 (hbk)
ISBN: 978-1-77491-561-5 (pbk)
ISBN: 978-1-00343-992-9 (ebk)

About the Editors

Ann Rose Abraham, PhD
Assistant Professor, Sacred Heart College (Autonomous), Thevara, Kochi, Kerala, India

Ann Rose Abraham, PhD, is currently an Assistant Professor at the Department of Physics, Sacred Heart College (Autonomous), Thevara, Kochi, Kerala, India. She has expertise in the field of condensed matter physics, nanomagnetism, multiferroics and polymeric nanocomposites, and others. She has research experience at various reputed national institutes, including Bose Institute, Kolkata, India; SAHA Institute of Nuclear Physics, Kolkata, India; UGC-DAE CSR Centre, Kolkata, India; and she has collaborated with various international laboratories. She is a recipient of the Young Researcher Award in physics and Best Paper Awards—2020, 2021. She served as an Assistant Professor and Examiner at the Department of Basic Sciences, Amal Jyothi College of Engineering, under APJ Abdul Kalam Technological University, Kerala, India. Dr. Abraham is a frequent speaker at national and international conferences. She has a good number of publications to her credit in many peer-reviewed high impact journals of international repute. She has authored many book chapters and edited more than 10 books with Taylor and Francis, Elsevier, and others.

Leonardo Sepúlveda Torre, PhD
Professor, School of Chemistry at the Universidad Autónoma de Coahuila, Saltillo, Coahuila, México

Leonardo Sepúlveda Torre, PhD, is a full Professor at the School of Chemistry, Universidad Autónoma de Coahuila, Saltillo, Coahuila, México, where he is also a leader of the Bioprocesses and Microbial Biochemistry Group. His postgraduate studies were related to topics on Food Biotechnology in the Food Research Department of the UAdeC. In 2011, he visited the Institute of Biotechnology and Bioengineering at the University of Minho (Uminho), Braga, Portugal for research. He worked as a collaborator at the Center of Biological Engineering in Uminho, Braga, Portugal, with the link project "Biotechnologies for Regional Food Biodiversity in Latin America." He participated as author and coauthor in 35 scientific articles in indexed journals, one book, 24 book chapters and he holds two national patents.

Tamara Tatrishvili, PhD
Main Specialist, Office of the Academic Process Management, Ivane Javakhishvili Tbilisi State University (TSU); Director of the Institute of Macromolecular Chemistry and Polymeric Materials at TSU, Tbilisi, Georgia

Tamara Tatrishvili, PhD, is the Main Specialist in the Office of Academic Process Management (Faculty of Exact and Natural Sciences) at Ivane Javakhishvili Tbilisi State University, as well as Director of the Institute of Macromolecular Chemistry and Polymeric Materials at TSU, Tbilisi, Georgia; DAAD alumni; and a member of Georgian Chemical Society. Her research interests included polymer chemistry, polymeric materials, and chemistry of silicon-organic compounds. She is the executive editor of Journal of the Georgian Chemical Society. Dr. Tatrishvili is the author of more than 190 scientific publications, 12 books, and monographs.

A. K. Haghi, PhD
Professor Emeritus of Engineering Sciences and Senior Material Engineering Consultant, UK

A. K. Haghi, PhD, is a retired professor with over 250 academic research-oriented books as well as over 1000 research papers published in various journals and conference proceedings with over 3350 citations and h-index of 30, according to the Google Scholar database. He is currently a senior material engineering consultant in the UK. Professor A. K. Haghi has received several grants, consulted for several major corporations, and is a frequent speaker to national and international audiences. He is the Founder and former Editor-in-Chief of the *International Journal of Chemoinformatics and Chemical Engineering*, published by IGI Global as well as the *Polymers Research Journal*, published by Nova Science Publishers. Professor A. K. Haghi has acted as an editorial board member of many international journals. He has served as a member of the Canadian Research and Development Center of Sciences & Cultures and the Research Chemistry Centre, Coimbra, Portugal. He has supervised several PhD and MSc thesis at University of Guilan (UG) and cosupervised international doctoral projects. Professor Haghi holds a BSc in urban and environmental engineering from the University of North Carolina (USA), and holds two MSc degrees, one in mechanical engineering from North Carolina State University (USA) and the other one in applied mechanics, acoustics, and materials from the Université de Technologie de Compiègne (France). He was awarded a PhD in engineering sciences at Université de Franche-Comté (France).

Contents

Contributors

Cristobal N. Aguilar
Bioprocesses and Bioproducts Research Group. Food Research Department. Universidad Autónoma de Coahuila, Saltillo, México

H. Akhina
School of Energy Materials, Mahatma Gandhi University, Kottayam, Kerala, India

Maka Alexishvili
Department of Medical Chemistry, Tbilisi State Medical University, Tbilisi, Georgia

R. Arredondo-Valdés
Facultad de Ciencias Químicas, Universidad Autonoma de Coahuila, Saltillo, Coahuila, México

Mohammad Ashfaq
University Centre for Research and Development (UCRD), Chandigarh University, Gharaun, Mohali, Punjab, India
Department of Biotechnology, Chandigarh University, Gharaun, Mohali, Punjab, India

P. K. Binci
ICAR-Central Institute of Fisheries Technology, Cochin, Kerala, India

Namitha Binu
Pushpagiri Institute of Medical Sciences and Research Centre, Thiruvalla, Kerala, India

Rebeca Casique-Valdés
Instituto de Ciencias y Humanidades, Lic.Salvador González Lobo, Universidad Autónoma de Coahuila, México

Divya Chauhan
Department of Drinking Water and Sanitation, Ministry of Jal Shakti, Pandit Deendayal Antyodaya Bhawan, New Delhi, India

Yogesh B. Dalvi
Pushpagiri Institute of Medical Sciences and Research Centre, Thiruvalla, Kerala, India

Rajnandini Das
Department of Engineering Design IIT Madras, Chennai, India

M. Dávila-Medina
Facultad de Ciencias Químicas, Universidad Autonoma de Coahuila, Saltillo, Coahuila, México

Bankole Oluwatosin Emmanuel
Department of Chemical Sciences, Faculty of Science and Science Education, Anchor University, Ipaja, Lagos, Nigeria

J. D. García-García
Facultad de Ciencias Químicas, Universidad Autonoma de Coahuila, Saltillo, Coahuila, México

Bhaskar Gaonkar
Department of Chemistry and Biochemistry, Jain Deemed to-be University, Bengaluru, Karnataka, India

Sherin Sara George
Department of Pediatric and Preventive Dentistry, Pushpagiri College of Dental Sciences, Thiruvalla, Kerala, India

Subin P. George
Department of Engineering Design IIT Madras, Chennai, India

Manuchar Gvaramia
Faculty of Exact and Natural Sciences, Javakhishvili Tbilisi State University, Tbilisi, Georgia

Sherin Jacob
Faculty, School of Biosciences, MG University, Kottayam, Kerala, India

V. P. Jayachandran
Applied Biology Section, Department of Applied Sciences, University of Technology and Applied Sciences, Muscat, Sultanate of Oman

Shilpa Joy
Biotechnology, Sri Shakthi Institute of Engineering and Technology, Coimbatore, Tamil Nadu, India

Lali Kirvalidze
Faculty of Exact and Natural Sciences, Javakhishvili Tbilisi State University, Tbilisi, Georgia

Nino Kokiashvili
Faculty of Exact and Natural Sciences, Javakhishvili Tbilisi State University, Tbilisi, Georgia

Manoni Kurtanidze
Faculty of Exact and Natural Sciences, Javakhishvili Tbilisi State University, Tbilisi, Georgia

Nino Lominadze
Faculty of Exact and Natural Sciences, Javakhishvili Tbilisi State University, Tbilisi, Georgia

E. Martínez-Moreno
Facultad de Ciencias Químicas, Universidad Autonoma de Coahuila, Saltillo, Coahuila, México

Rekha Mirle
Department of Chemistry, School of Sciences, Jain University, Bangalore, Karnataka, India

Nikitha Mary Monson
Department of Physics, Catholicate College, Pathanamthitta, Kerala, India

Natela Okujava
Department of Neuromedicine, Tbilisi State Medical University, Tbilisi, Georgia

Tressia Alias Princy Paulose
Post Graduate and Research Department of Chemistry, Bishop Moore College, Mavelikara, Kerala, India

Preetha G. Prasad
Department of Chemistry, Kumbalathu Sankupillai Memorial Devaswom Board College, Sasthamcotta, Kerala, India

R. Ramos-González
Universidad Autonoma de Coahuila, Saltillo, Coahuila, México

Neha Kanwar Rawat
Materials Research Laboratory, Department of Chemistry, Jamia Millia Islamia, New Delhi, India

R. Roopashree
Department of Chemistry and Biochemistry, Jain Deemed to-be University, JC Road, Bengaluru, Karnataka, India

Marina Rukhadze
Faculty of Exact and Natural Sciences, Javakhishvili Tbilisi State University, Tbilisi, Georgia

Sergio René Sánchez-Peña
Dpto. Parasitología Agrícola, Universidad Autónoma Agraria Antonio Narro, México

A. Sáenz-Galindo
Facultad de Ciencias Químicas, Universidad Autonoma de Coahuila, Saltillo, Coahuila, México

Jose Sandoval
Departamento de Química Analítica, Facultad de Ciencias Químicas, Universidad Autónoma de Coahuila, Saltillo, México

Leonardo Sepúlveda-Torre
Dpto. Biotecnología, Facultad de Ciencias Químicas, Universidad Autónoma de Coahuila, México
Facultad de Ciencias Químicas, Universidad Autonoma de Coahuila, Saltillo, Coahuila, México

G. Subbulakshmi
Department of Chemistry, School of Sciences, Jain University, Bangalore, India
Department of Chemistry and Biochemistry, Jain Deemed to-be University, JC Road, Bengaluru, Karnataka, India

Anil Sukumaran
Department of Dentistry, Oral Health Institute, Hamad Medical Corporation, Doha, Qatar

V. Swarupa
Department of Chemistry and Biochemistry, Jain Deemed to-be University, JC Road, Bengaluru, Karnataka, India

Neetu Talreja
Faculty of Science and Technology, Department of Science, Alliance University, Bengaluru, Karnataka, India

Darieo Thankachan
Department of Materials Science and Engineering, National Taiwan University of Science and Technology, Taipei, Taiwan, Republic of China

Nebu George Thomas
Pushpagiri Research Centre, Tiruvalla, Kerala, India

George Thomas
Department of Physics, Catholicate College, Pathanamthitta, Kerala, India

P. H. Vaisakh
Post Graduate and Research Department of Chemistry, Bishop Moore College, Mavelikara, Kerala, India

Ruby Varghese
Department of Chemistry, School of Sciences, Jain University, Bangalore, India
Department of Chemistry and Biochemistry, Jain Deemed to-be University, Bengaluru, Karnataka, India
Pushpagiri Institute of Medical Sciences and Research Centre, Thiruvalla, Kerala, India

Sneha Sara Varghese
Post Graduate and Research Department of Chemistry, Bishop Moore College, Mavelikara, Kerala, India

Abbreviations

ALPase	alkaline phosphatase
ATR	attenuated total reflectance
BC	bacterial cellulose
BEA	beauvericin
BEAEs	beauvenniatins
BEVS	baculovirus expression system
B-MBG	boron-containing mesoporous bioactive glass
BMPs	bone morphogenetic proteins
BTE	bone tissue engineering
CAP	cellulose acetate phthalate
CB-NMs	carbon-based-NMs
CCF	commercial cotton fibres
CFB	coir fiber cement board
CFU	colony-forming units
CHP	cholesterol-bearing pullulan
CHR	compact highrise
CLR	compact lowrise
CMR	compact midrise zone
CNF	carbon nanofiber
CNTs	carbon nanotubes
COF	covalent organic framework
CR	Congo red
Cs	capacitance
CSP	corn starch polymers
CT	computer tomography
CuO	copper oxide
CVD	chemical vapor deposition
DNA	deoxyribonucleic acid
DSSC	dye-sensitized solar cells
DWCNT	double-walled nanotubes
EBT	Eriochrome Black T

ECM	extracellular matrix
EDA	ethylenediamine
EHDP	electrohydrodynamic printing
ELISA	enzyme-linked immunosorbent assay
ENNs	enniatins
EPA	Environmental Protection Agency
EPF	entomopathogenic fungi
EPN	entomopathogenic nematodes
EVs	entomopathogenic viruses
FTIR	Fourier transform infra-red spectroscopy
GAGs	glucosaminoglycans
GO	graphene oxide
GSTs	glutathione S-transferases
HA	hydroxyapatite
HAp	hydroxyapatite
HI	heavy Industry
HME	hereditary multiple exostoses
HPC	hierarchical porous carbon
HRP	horseradish peroxidase
HS-SPME	headspace solid-phase microextraction
HUS	hemolytic-uremic syndrome
IGF-1	insulin-like growth factor-1
Ihh	Indian hedgehog
IJs	infective juveniles
LB	*Lactobacillus*
LC-MS	liquid chromatography–mass spectrometry
LCZ	local climate zones
LIBs	lithium-ion batteries
LLR	large lowrise
LWLR	lightweight lowrise
MAE	mean absolute error
MB	methylene blue
MBR	membrane bioreactor
M-CSF	macrophage colony-stimulating factor
MDR	multidrug resistance
MeCS	methacrylated CS
MFO	mixed function oxidases

MOF	metal-organic framework
MONP	metal oxide nanoparticle
MPC	methacryloyloxyethyl phosphorylcholine
MPNs	metal–phenolic networks
MRE	mean relative error
MSMC	magnetostrictive microcantilever
MSPR	multichannel surface plasmon resonance
MWCNT	multi-walled carbon nanotubes
NFRC	natural fiber-reinforced composites
NF-κB	nuclear factor-kappa B
nHA	nano-hydroxyapatite
NMs	nanomaterials
NRPS	nonribosomal peptide synthesis
NS	not specific
OAKs	oligomers of acylated lysines
OB	occlusion bodies
OHR	open highrise
OLR	open lowrise
OMR	open midrise
PAA	polyacrylic acid
PAN	polyacrylonitrile
PCL	polycaprolactone
PEG	polyethylene glycol
PEI	polyethylenimine
PEP	percent error in peak
PGA	poly(glycolic acid)
PHAs	polyhydroxyalkanoates
PHB	polyhydroxy butyrate
PKS	polyketide synthesis
PLA	poly(lactic acid)
PLGA	poly (D, L-lactide-co-glycolide)
PM-PI	polymeric micelles in the porous implant
PS	polystyrene
PVA	polyvinyl alcohol
RANK	receptor activator of NF-κB
RGO	reduced graphene oxide
rGO	reduced oxides of graphene

RhB	rhodamine B
Risp	risperidone
RMSE	root mean squared error
RNA	ribonucleic acid
RPS	ribosomal peptide synthesis
RTE	ready-to-eat
SB	sparsely built
SDS	sodium dodecyl sulfate
SEB	simultaneous enrichment broth
SELEX	systematic evolution of ligands through exponential enrichment
SEM	scanning electron microscope
SIBs	sodium–ion batteries
SiNPs	silicon nanoparticles
SPR	surface plasmon resonance
SWCNT	single-walled carbon nanotube
TMV	tobacco mosaic virus
TRAP	tartrate-resistant acid phosphatase
Trx	thioredoxin
TSC	tamarind seed-based carbon
UHI	urban heat island
UNEP	United Nations Environment Program
VOC	volatile organic carbon
ZIF-8	zeolite-imidazole frameworks-8
ZMO	zinc–manganese oxide
ZnO	zinc oxide

Preface

Biotechnology engineering is a part of applied engineering science and is an emerging discipline that combines both biological science and technology for development in the medical, agriculture, and bioresearch. Therefore, as the name suggests, "biotechnology engineering" is simply an engineering discipline with a combination of biology and technology that is concerned with the study of biological systems. This book clearly reflects the multidisciplinary nature of "biotechnology engineering" goals and provides a firm foundation in the science and engineering of biological processes. It is a research-oriented reference book to help equip practitioners in biotechnology and bioengineering with a highly technical career path. The book discusses the combination of both engineering and science of biological processes from wastewater treatment to tissue engineering.

The first part of this book discusses experimental and theoretical solutions for environmental pollution. The second part covers frontiers in bioengineering and biotechnology. Part 3 illustrates the use of biotechnology and bio-based routes to sustainable composites, and finally, case studies with detailed information are presented in Part 4.

PART I

SOLUTIONS FOR ENVIRONMENTAL POLLUTION

CHAPTER 1

Novel Approach of Interfacing Organic-Inorganic Hybrid Materials in Biological Systems for Effective Wastewater Treatment

REKHA MIRLE, RUBY VARGHESE, and G. SUBBULAKSHMI

Department of Chemistry, School of Sciences, Jain University, Bangalore, India

ABSTRACT

Water, a valuable and inadequate resource on earth, plays crucial role in ecological processes. Due to various industrial processes, agricultural activities, and population explosion, toxic chemicals are released that contaminates the water resources drastically. These pollutants cause imbalance in human health and ecological systems; hence, it is necessary to address this issue globally. The prevailing physical, chemical, and biological methods of wastewater treatment are neither eco-friendly nor cost-effective; under this condition, removal of pollutants from water demands alternative eco-friendly technologies. Till date, nanotechnology and biological sciences has brought great revolution in treating wastewater. In this chapter, we provide a critical overview of recent developments in the materials and synthetic strategies of nanobiohybrids. The synthesis of nanobiohybrids are carried at multimilligram scale using liquid enzyme and water at room temperature without use of any special apparatus. Bio polymers are also the most exploited material for nanobiohybrids synthesis and monitors biological properties in living systems. Nanobiohybrids are an alternative to other methods, which comprises interfacing of organic-inorganic hybrid materials in biological systems that enable new bioaugmentation functions that assures

Application of Engineering Principles and Practices in Biotechnology.
Ann Rose Abraham, Leonardo Sepúlveda Torre, Tamara Tatrishvili, and A. K. Haghi (Eds.)

wide applications across many fields of science, including wastewater treatment. Nanobiohybrids perform dual role as metal nanoparticles and enzyme catalysis that makes them a very powerful tool in degradation of water pollutants and environmental pollution control. Bio-nanomaterials has other potential applications as numerous catalysts for a chemical domino reaction, avoids aggregation of nanoparticles which generates very impressive heterogeneous materials, easy recovery, high degree of recyclability, good stereo selectivity, studies antimicrobial activity and stability, which are discussed in detail.

1.1 INTRODUCTION

Water being an essential solvent, its supply for industrial activities is very much essential. Major quantities of water are required to carry out various process needs, and for drinking and sanitary purposes (https://www.watertechnologies.com/handbook/handbook-industrial-water-treatment). Water gets contaminated by the substances that comes in contact with it, so its availability is in impure state. Almost all natural substances are soluble in water and hence water is entitled as "universal solvent." This solubility property of water causes major damage to industrial equipment such as corrosion reaction, scale formation on surfaces, etc. Some impurities are water soluble and forms clear solutions whereas few particles are suspended, which imparts visible turbidity to the solution (Ghernaout et al., 2011). Due to increased population, various impurities such as sewage water discharges, domestic wastes, industrial wastes, and agricultural wastes are contaminating different sources of water. The contaminants include pathogenic organisms, toxic substances like oil, pesticides, and metals, and organic and inorganic pollutants. In the current scenario, measures need to be taken to avoid disposal of pollutants to water sources and to treat wastewater.

Toxic chemicals of wastewater are causing major health hazard for both marine and terrestrial ecosystems. Although various studies have been done on nanomaterials, but some nanoparticles are now frequently used for wastewater treatment. Currently, intensive research study on exploiting nanoparticles for wastewater treatment is under evolution and it is crucial to explore most recent advancements in nanomaterials for sustainable treatment of wastewater (Palani et al., 2021). The wastewater treatment aims to reduce contaminants from wastewater and can be reused safely for various purposes. Based on the type and extent of contaminants, numerous processes can be employed to treat wastewater. It includes physical, chemical, and biological processes. Water being a vital and most valuable natural resource, its conservation for next generation is very essential. The treated water should not cause any negative impact on environment (Massoud et al., 2009). Survey of literature exposes on innumerable wastewater treatment methods. But the prevailing physical, chemical, and biological methods are neither eco-friendly nor cost-effective; under these conditions, removal of pollutants from water demands alternative eco-friendly technologies (Fig. 1.1). Till date, nanotechnology and biological sciences has brought great revolution in treating wastewater.

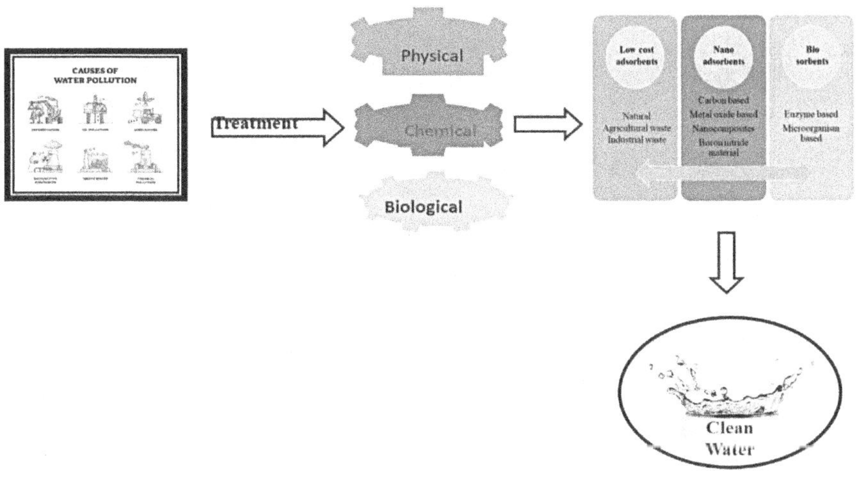

FIGURE 1.1 Eco-friendly technologies in wastewater treatment.

Evolution through millions of years has lead biological species to achieve many of their biofunctionalities; even though, given the notable diversity in structure and composition of advanced synthetic materials, the integrated approach of functional synthetic materials with biological systems are more rapid, effective, and reasonable alternative than natural evolution for the design and fabrication of nanobiohybrids.

Remarkable effort had been made in the past to design nanobiohybrid systems which comprise of amalgamated materials that have both synthetic component and biologically derived constituent. The biological constituent ranges from refined biomolecules such as proteins and DNA (Ahmed et al., 2022) to composite life systems which includes living cells, organisms, and tissues (Liang et al., 2016; Richardson et al., 2018) while the synthetic constituent includes inorganic materials like $CaCO_3$, SiO_2, Au, and iron oxide (Lauth et al., 2017; Setyawati et al., 2015), organic materials such as polymers and lipids (Niu et al., 2017; Lynge et al., 2011), or hybrid materials (Su et al., 2016; Lykourinou et al., 2011) as metal-organic frameworks (MOFs) and metal-phenolic networks (MPNs). Finally, biofunctionality aspects depend on the selection of both living and non-living constituents (Fig. 1.2).

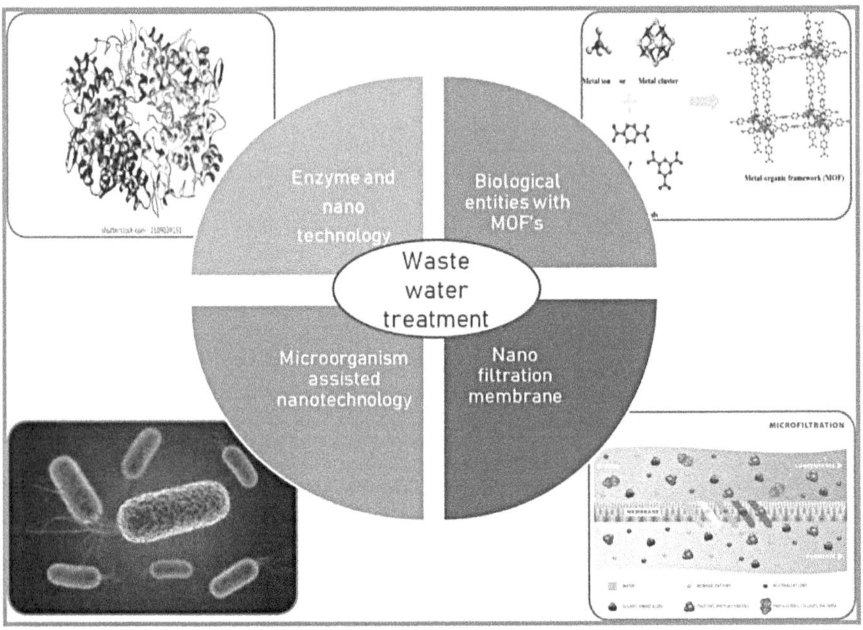

FIGURE 1.2 Interfacing functional nanomaterials with biological systems for the effective removal of contaminants from polluted water.

In this chapter, recent developments in the materials and synthetic strategies of nanobiohybrids are critically discussed. The synthesis of nanobiohybrids is carried out at room temperature using liquid enzyme and water at multimilligram scale by simple apparatus. Biopolymers are the most exploited material for nanobiobybrids synthesis and monitors biotic features in living systems. Nanobiohybrids is an alternative to other methods which comprises interfacing of organic-inorganic hybrid materials in biological systems that enable new bioaugmentation functions that assures wide applications across many fields of science including wastewater treatment. Nanobiohybrids perform dual role as metal nanoparticles and enzyme catalysis that makes them a very powerful tool in degradation of water pollutants and environmental pollution control. Bio-nanomaterials has other potential applications as numerous catalysts for a chemical domino reaction, avoids aggregation of nanoparticles, generates very notable multifarious materials, simple and incredible revival, good stereo selectivity, and studies antimicrobial activity and its stability are discussed in detail.

1.2 NANOBIOHYBRIDS AS AN EFFECTIVE TOOL FOR WASTEWATER TREATMENT

Nanobiohybrids is the latest enlivening topic of exploration emerged as the frontier between material fabrication and ecological science. The integration among nanoscience and nanotechnology also brought huge reformation in the field of science; especially the synthesis of metal nanoparticles being a crucial part in the study of antimicrobial properties, as catalyst in synthesis of chemicals and biomedicine. Presently, enormous innovative and efficient protocols for the nanoparticle synthesis using enzymes as catalyst have been reported. Literature survey reveals that enzyme catalysis is an alternative greener methodology over other various approaches—that too under harsh conditions. Recent advances focuses on green technology for the production of metal nanoparticles and examined the function of enzymes in the course of nanoparticle formation and its consequence on the functionality of nanomaterials. This innovative metal-enzyme nanoparticle serves as heterogeneous catalysts in synthetic chemistry and explored their capability as antimicrobial and eco-friendly sustainable agents. A biological entity in the synthesis of nanoparticles helps in controlling particle size, shape, and also restricts accumulation glitches (Banerjee et al., 2013; Chinnadayyala et al., 2015).

Selection of biological entities plays an important role in green synthetic strategy, which depends on usage of microorganisms (Vetchinkina et al., 2017; Gonzalez-Moragas et al., 2017; Patil and Kim, 2018; Carballares et al., 2022). Nanoparticles of various metals (Ag, Au, Cd, Pt, Fe, and Zn) are structured under moderate conditions by prokaryotic or eukaryotic microorganisms. These microorganisms have the ability to secrete huge amount of enzymes, which contribute in reduction of metal ions (Zhang et al., 2011). Nanoparticles of distinct sizes are due to assorted blends of proteins and enzymes utilized in synthetic pathway and hence control, localization, and morphology of nanoparticles depends on microorganism species (Boroum and Moghaddam et al., 2015).

Recently, the heterogeneous enzyme–metal nanobiohybrids are fabricated with various enzymes and its proficiency lets the synthesis of biohybrid materials in multimilligrams range. These fabricated nanobiohybrids has wide practical applications in various areas of research.

Due to rapid industrialization and population explosion, various types of pollutants are contaminating freshwater resources, which may possibly jeopardize and degrade the proficiency of existing water purification techniques. Also, these water-purification methods require expensive specialized chemicals and generate various hazardous chemical wastes. To overcome these issues, highly precise and effectual enzyme biocatalysts are preferred to deal with pollutant substrates (Nelson et al., 2008). These enzymes act as greener catalysts, which works efficiently even under mild reactions conditions, on wide range of substrates with less reaction time (Ali et al., 2014; Subrizi et al., 2014; Siddique et al., 1993). But, these free enzymes are having poor stability and sensitivity due to mechanical strains (Brena et al., 2013; Feng and Ji, 2011). Hence, ability and stability of enzymes can be enhanced by enzyme immobilization on the surface, which increases catalytic activity, mechanical stability, operates on broad range of temperature, and pH under harsh conditions compared to free enzymes (Brena et al., 2013; Feng and Ji, 2011; Asuri et al., 2006a). These enzyme catalyst are used for numerous applications as its recovery is simple upon immobilization than to its free state (Subrizi et al., 2014); hence, water-purification technique by this enzyme catalysis is proven to be a stable and economically viable method. Research studies has employed immobilized enzymes such as tyrosinase (Subrizi et al., 2014), horseradish peroxidase (HRP) (Lee et al., 2006), lactase (Liu et al., 2006), and glucose oxidase (Guiseppi-Elie et al., 2002) on CNTs. Undesirably, these hybrids will only sense and detect water pollutants instead of eradicating them from composite wastewater medium. In near future, there is a wide opportunity for developing and enhancing nanobiohybrid as catalyst and it will be a promising tool suitable to eliminate pollutants from the different water sources. In this chapter, we briefly discussed the possible ways of synthesizing nanobiohybrids, its diverse applications in the removal of water pollutants, and parallel concentration of water pollutants can be detected and analyzed efficiently.

1.3 APPLICATIONS OF METAL NANOPARTICLES BIOHYBRIDS IN VARIOUS FIELD OF RESEARCH

1.3.1 DUAL ACTIVITY OF NANOBIOHYBRIDS IN SYNTHETIC CASCADE PROCESS

Nanobiohybrids are used as catalysts in multiple chemical cascade reaction (Filice et al., 2013, O'Brien et al., 2018). It is one of the potential tools in modern organic chemistry due to its dual activity (enzyme catalysis and metal nanoparticles in one).For instance, in a domino reaction, at room temperature heterogeneous nanobiohybrid executes dual action, that is, hydrolytic activity of the enzyme and the reducing activity of the metal to transmute p-nitrophenyl propionate in p-aminophenol in water (Filice et al., 2013, O'Brien et al., 2018; San et al., 2016). These twofold action of nano-biohybrids makes them a very potential tool in modern synthetic strategies.

1.3.2 APPLICATIONS OF METAL NANOPARTICLES IN SYNTHETIC REACTIONS

Transition metal nanoparticles catalyze (Dodekatos et al., 2018) numerous ranges of reactions and hence extend huge relevance of these nanobiohybrids in synthetic chemistry. Certain unique nanobiohybrids such as Pd and Pt nanoparticles hybrids were effectively considered as catalysts for a group discrete chemical reactions (Filice et al., 2013, O'Brien et al., 2018; San et al., 2016; Lopez-Tejedor et al., 2018) like oxidation, reduction, C-C bond formation, etc. It is worthwhile to achieve variety of molecules such as aromatic aldehydes, biaryls, etc., stimulating as platform molecule in the production of pharmaceutical stuffs. It also leads for the fabrication of immense range of molecules, natural products, and polymers (Mpungose et al., 2018).

1.3.3 CNTs-BASED NANOBIOHYBRID FOR WATER PURIFICATIONS

Organic water pollutants can be broken down into its constituents by CNT-based nanobiohybrid. These acts as a catalyst for detecting, analyzing, and decomposing of several pollutants from water. This was developed by immobilizing enzymes on CNTs by three main approaches like physisorption and covalent bonding, cross-linking, and entrapment or encapsulation (Hwang and Gu, 2013).

During physisorption, uncontrolled adsorption of enzymes on CNTs occurs due to hydrophobic and electrostatic interactions between CNTs and enzyme (Gao and Kyratzis, 2008; Nepal and Geckeler, 2006). Covalent bonding of enzymes with CNT induces reaction between carboxylic acid group and free amine groups on the protein surface produced due to oxidation of CNTs and subsequent reactions (Asuri et al., 2006b; Huang et al., 2002; Jiang et al., 2004). Many crosslinking polymers like chitosan and poly (diallyl dimethyl ammonium chloride) are spent to immobilize enzymes on CNTs (Subrizi et al., 2014; Lawrence et al., 2005). Thirdly, enzyme encapsulation is done layer-by-layer manner for immobilizing enzyme. This allows the smearing of enzyme films on CNTs layer-by-layer (Feng and Ji, 2011).

Some advantages of nanobiohybrids over conventional oxidation of water pollutants:

i. Nanobiohybrids are utilized for purification of water wherein no other chemical degradation of pollutants is possible.
ii. These nanobiohybrids provide good material stability, high catalytic action, and can perform over a range of temperature and pH under rigid conditions (Brena et al., 2013; Asuri et al., 2006b). These nanobiohybrids can be regenerated and reused for numerous purification cycle (Subrizi et al., 2014) and hence proved to be economical.
iii. It paves way for the surplus production of commercially significant chemicals or platform chemicals from refractory organic pollutants of water.
iv. Therefore, the dual performance of nanobiohybrids lies in the reduction of total water impurities and consecutively increases its commercial viability (Das et al., 2016).

1.3.4 APPLICATION OF NANOBIOHYBRIDS AS ENVIRONMENTAL AND ANTIMICROBIAL AGENTS

Nanobiohybrids exhibits synthetic capability and literature survey reveals its application of the metal nanoparticle biohybrids on many essential domains like ecological remediation or as antimicrobial agent (Ahmed et al., 2018; Tao et al., 2018). Globally, contamination of drinking water and wastewater are caused by organic pollutants which is increasing day-by-day, so these pollutants are removed by environmental bioremediation technique (Sousa et al., 2018). Nanobiohybrids containing AgNps are successively synthesized for the complete degradation of various dyes (Ahmed et al., 2018). These AgNP's nanobiohybrids incorporating agalactosidase are actual competent catalyst for the dwindling of industrial dyes. Also, recent studies show that oxidative dwindling of p-aminophenol in water was effectively catalyzed by super paramagnetic material such as iron nanobiohybrids (Benavente et al., 1970). Metal nanoparticles biohybrids are proven to give excellent results in refinement of wastewater from deadly bisphenol-A (Das et al., 2016). Antimicrobial activity against cluster of pathogenic microorganisms (Ahmed et al., 2018) are demonstrated by bionanohybrids of AgNPs from keratinase and silver nanoparticles from galactosidase.

Literature review provides an indepth knowledge of nanotechnology as an emerging science in wastewater treatment. Depending on the class of contaminants present, different forms of nanomaterials are utilized to get desired efficacy. Carbon-based materials, single-walled and multiple–walled CNTs, organic and inorganic frameworks, and metal and metal oxide-based nanoparticles are used for wastewater treatment. Even graphene-based nanoparticles, their oxides (GO), and reduced oxides of graphene (rGO) achieve remarkable applicability for treating wastewater (Bhat et al., 2022).

1.4 STRUCTURING OF NANOBIOHYBRIDS VIA DIVERSE STRATEGICAL APPROACH FOR WASTEWATER TREATMENT

1.4.1 BIOPOLYMERS-BASED NANOCOMPOSITES

Naturally abundant polymers present in biological system like proteins, nucleic acids, and polysaccharides are considered as a main source of bio-based materials. Biopolymers due to its remarkable properties of biocompatibility and biodegradability offer instigating functional properties that pave way for its wide range of enriched applications in the field of catalysis, environmental remediation, bioplastics, sensors, and biomedical purposes. Also, these biopolymers are blended with inorganic nanoparticles such as oxides, metal oxides, silicates, phosphates, etc., to form bio nanocomposites with enhanced mechanized and thermal properties. These well-designed biohybrid nanostructures can be synthesized by bottom-up approach, wherein physical and chemical interfaces occurs at nanoscale between biopolymers and inorganic materials.

Employing numerous bottom-up approaches such as grafting processes, in-situ methods, solvent casting, layer-by-layer, intercalation, etc., results in bionanocomposite material with varying properties and functionalities. In the forthcoming years, various innovative strategies of fabricating these bionanocomposites in engineering materials and components play a pivotal role (Alcântara et al., 2020). Many review of literature focuses on biopolymers and composites used as a main source of adsorbent material for the removal of various impurities from the environment. These adsorption processes are proven to be better techniques to remove pollutants as it is cost-effective and easy-to-use compared to other traditional methods such a precipitation method, ion exchange processes, etc. Plenty of effort in this direction has made to develop efficient, more stable, and cost-effective adsorbents to be employed in batch-scale remediation process (Yaashikaa et al., 2017). As these biopolymer composites are good adsorbent, they are suitable for adsorbing water pollutants, thus reducing the cost of remediation procedure (Foroutan et al., 2020). Prominent properties exhibited by biopolymer composites like enhanced durability and operating ability provides large surface area and high functionality which assists to remove the pollutants from the environment through surface phenomenon (Udayakumar et al., 2021). Recently, biopolymer-based composites such as hydrogel and hydroxyapatite are used to remove heavy metals and dyes from contaminated water (Yaashikaa et al., 2022). The inherent properties and its sustainable nature of biopolymer composites allowed them to use in membrane-based remedial methods (Aji et al., 2020). Some of the most common polymers such as chitin, chitosan, alginate, and carrageenan are widely used in membrane modification and, hence, biopolymer-based membranes have wide prospects in the adsorption of contaminants (Russo et al., 2021). Recent studies have ascertained the role of carbohydrate polymer composites in removal of contaminants via adsorption. Other than its application in treating wastewater, a biopolymer composite exhibits wide range of applications in cosmetic segment and industrial domain.

1.4.2 ORGANIC-INORGANIC HYBRID MATERIAL IN BIOLOGICAL SYSTEMS EXHIBITS BIOAUGMENTATION FUNCTIONS—EFFECTIVE TOOL FOR WASTEWATER TREATMENT

Adsorption forms a renowned segregation technique and accepted as one of the reasonable and competent methods for controlling water pollution. There are numerous quantity of adsorbents such as activated charcoal (Uzun and Güzel, 2000), zeolites (Biškup and Subotić, 2004; Cincotti et al., 2006), clays (Gier and Johns, 2000; Koppelman and Dillard, 1977), and agricultural residues (O'Connell et al., 2008; Dang et al., 2009; Zewail and El-Garf, 2010) are used to remove heavy metal ions from wastewater. On the other hand, these adsorbents have low adsorption capabilities and relatively weak metallic interactions and hence encounter difficulties in segregation and rejuvenation from water. It is possible to remove metal ions significantly through ion-exchange resins but they exhibit reduced mechanical strength and low selectivity (Nagarale et al., 2006).

To overcome these drawbacks, organic-inorganic hybrid polymers as become an assuring candidate for the removal of toxic chemicals from contaminated water (Wang et al., 2012; Gao and Gao, 2010; Zaitseva et al., 2013; Simsek et al., 2012; Suchithra et al., 2012; Repo et al., 2011; Ge et al., 2010; Pang et al., 2011; Wang et al., 2011).

Several studies in recent years focused on production of new hybrid materials that enhances adsorption capacity or removal capability of pollutants and intents to promote their potency and sturdiness, removes toxic chemicals from nature due to the blending of diverse materials with varying properties. Hybrid materials are classified based on the size of mixture (Makishima, 2004) as composites, hybrids, and nanobiohybrids. Hybrid materials are subdivided into three classes. Organic-inorganic polymer hybrids are derived by the combination of unique type of organic materials with inorganic substrate that are hard and thermally stable. These materials have strong attraction toward particular metal ions that has high adsorption capabilities. Hybrid polymeric materials are considered as an efficient adsorbent, as metal ions are strongly bonded chemically with organic-inorganic polymer hybrids. Hence, these hybrid materials exhibit tremendous physical, chemical, and mechanical properties (Mercier and Pinnavaia, 1998). Diverse forms of organic-inorganic hybrids have been widely studied due to their interesting properties, resulting in plenty of applications as electro-analytical tool (Walcarius, 2001), as membranes for ultra and nanofiltration (Kim et al., 2021; Paun et al., 2011), super hydrophobic surfaces (Wen et al., 2011; Sparks et al., 2013), highly transparent films (Yu and Chen, 2003; Nagappan et al., 2013), pH sensitive composites (Rottman et al., 1999), gas separation (Murray et al., 2009; Rowsell et al., 2004), catalysts (Raj et al., 2013), biosensors (Fu et al., 2011), and adsorbents of toxic compounds (Wang et al., 2012; Gao and Gao, 2010; Zaitseva et al., 2013; Simsek et al., 2012; Suchithra et al., 2012; Repo et al., 2011; Ge et al., 2010; Pang et al., 2011; Wang et al., 2011).

Recent studies on wastewater treatment revealed that separation technique is more efficient, specifically using adsorption technology and membrane filtration. The porous metal organic framework (MOF) are widely used in segregating applications (Kökçam-Demir et al., 2020; Kumar et al., 2018; Candia-Onfray et al., 2021). These MOF comprises of inorganic metal ions or metal clumps and organic linkers enfolding diverse functions (Dong et al., 2019; Xia et al., 2018; Zhang et al. 2018; Wang et al., 2018a; Zou and Li, 2018; Shan et al., 2021). The exclusive porosity, enormous sites available for adsorption, high specific surface area, adaptable pore sizes (Zhang et al., 2015; Li et al., 2014), all together made these MOF'\s a suitable contributor for the production of membranes for filtration and as a good adsorbents (Yuan et al., 2018; Wang et al., 2016, 2017, 2018b; Fan et al., 2018; Li et al., 2020a, b). These organic materials with different functional groups like amino-functionalized ligands and sulphur–functionalized ligands, stimulate several intermolecular interactions of ions or molecules, and gain proficiency for the segregation and removal of contaminants (Liu et al., 2017; Kumar et al., 2017).

Studies reveal that various types of MOFs are currently used for treating wastewater, like MOF-based composites, graded–pore MOF, and defective MOF. For instance, defective amino-modified MOFs (UiO-66-D-NH_2) showed greater affinity 3.0 and 3.8 times to entangle organo-arsenic forms from wastewater compared to defective (UiO-66-D) without amino modification (Xu et al., 2019; He et al., 2020).

In the previous section, we briefly focused on biopolymers-based nanocomposites, CNTs in nanobiohybrids, organic-inorganic hybrid material in biological systems, and its applications in wastewater treatment. Further section of this chapter provides an overview on engineering efforts that primarily focuses on nanobiohybrids, that is, interfacing of organic-inorganic hybrid materials into biological components to instigate unique functionalities which is effective in controlling the water pollution and also focuses on bioaugmentation approach and its transformations, which is beneficial for the ecosystem and mankind.

1.4.3 BIOREMEDIATION

Bioremediation of water pollutant plays a pivotal role in restoring the water reserves. "Bioaugmentation" and "Biostimulation" has become a constant practice employed by the environment scientist to improve the water quality by introducing biotic and abiotic factors at the contamination site (Fig. 1.3).

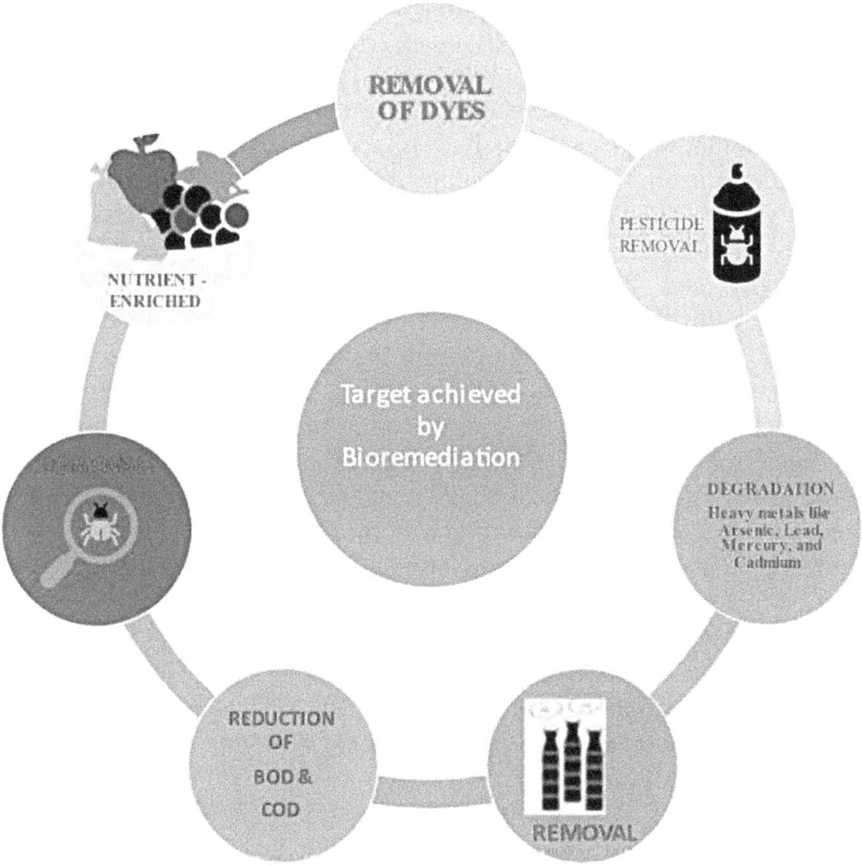

FIGURE 1.3 Schematic representation of various targets achieved through bioremediation.

1.5 IMPORTANCE OF BIOAUGMENTATION AND BIOSTIMULATION IN BIOREMEDIATION

The indigenous microbial species in the polluted site is enriched by the addition of genetically modified or previously selected indigenous flora.[126] In the recent years with the advancement of technology; nanomaterials integrated with the living system—nanohybrid—has emerged as an exponential branch of research in various multidisciplinary fields such as biocatalysis, energy harvesting, bioremediation, medicines, robotics, and biosensing.[127]

For the bioremediation, the engineered synthetic material can be made nanohybrid by adding into the living system (endogenous) or outside the living system (exogenous). For exogenous bioaugmentation various inorganic materials can be used as skeletal for nanohybrid synthesis such as carbon nanotubes (CNTs), silica, hydroxyapatite (HA), calcium carbonate, and semiconductors such as titanium dioxide (TiO_2), cadmium sulfide, and indium phosphide.[128] These material exhibits excellent mechanical strength, optimal surface area, outstanding thermal activity and electrical conductivity, and biocompatibility due to the low cytotoxicity when interfaced with the biological system.[129] CNTs together with the living system has been profusely exploited for the bioremediation by serving as a redox mediator through dye decolorization, pesticide degradation, and heavy metal removal from the contamination site and contributing toward the water management.[130] Similarly certain natural polymers such as HA-modified biochar removed heavy metal such as arsenic and cadmium from aqueous system, in specific and non-specific manner, which is significantly higher as compared to the adsorption rate of heavy metal removal by nonmodified biochar.[131]

Mesoporous silica was coated onto the magnetic multi-walled CNTs with cross linker Glutaraldehyde by enzyme immobilizing laccase into the matrix. The nanohybrid exhibited optimum activity, and storage ability. Moreover, without any mediator, it decolorized dyes (Eriochrome Black T (EBT)), 98% of Acid Red 88 (AR 88), and 66% of Reactive Black 5 (RB5).[132]

In another study, Laccase immobilized into multiwalled carbon nanotubes with the zeolite imidazolate framework via metal affinity adsorption to decolorize dye without any mediator. One of the evident roles of this nanohybrid is that it can be easily separated and laccase enzyme activity remains stable.[133]

In endogenous bioaugmentation, the manipulation in the living system is carried out by the introduction of synthesized particles/nanomaterials example; MOFs loaded with nanoparticle are up taken by living system such as plant cells without being interfered. This technique can be frequently used in bioaugmentation for biosensing and in robotics.[134] Although it is an emerging research area, but still intensive research is carried out to evaluate its practical or doable application.

Generally, whether the created/synthesized nanohybrid is incorporated inside the living cell or immobilized into the material, in either way, nanohybrid should perform both augmentation and biostimulation for achieving bioremediation for water management (Fig. 1.4).

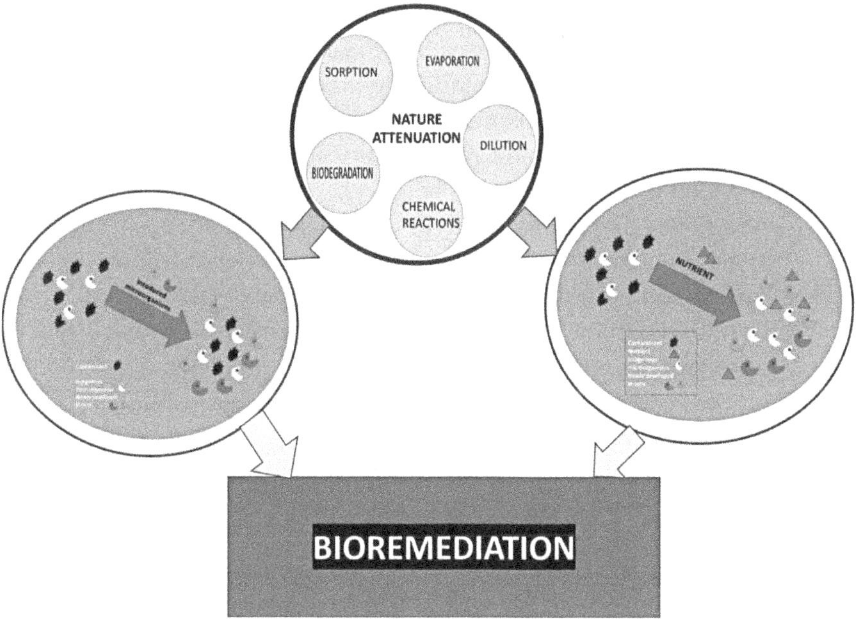

FIGURE 1.4 Bioremediation-mediated growth and reproduction of indigenous microorganism by degradation toxic effluents from wastewater.

Various studies are carried out on a trial-and-error basis, and it is observed and reported that nanohybrids or bioreactors exhibit excellent bioactivity in the laboratory conditions but fail to do so in a large scale or in field. Hence, feasibility of bioaugmentation should be assessed periodically from its preparation to characterization and evaluation in laboratory condition and finally during its field implementation.

Despite admirable applications being shown by metal nanoparticle nanobiohybrids till date, there are some shortcomings which need to be tackled with respect to its design and application are as follows:

i. The broadening of technology with metallic substances like Fe, Co, Ni, etc., which is highly abundant and inexpensive exhibits various oxidation states and hence this issue can be addressed by replacing these metals with other metal species.
ii. The widening of technology to auxiliary proteins leads to achieve highly sturdy nanobiohybrids with thermally stable enzymes having extensive applications even under severe conditions.

iii. Extension of metal nanoparticles biohybrids in synthetic organic chemistry cascade processes by enzymatic activity comprising two metals pave the way to manifold synthesis.
iv. Alternatively, durable metal nanoparticle biohybrids need to be synthesized to avoid low recyclability and stability issues and hence to widen its remediation applications.
v. Apart from these direct catalytic activities, other artificial metalloenzymes, synthesis of metal nanoparticles biohybrids on mesoporous surface can be suitable for heterogeneous catalysis.
vii. In the direction of futuristic applications of highly dispersed nanoparticles in the area of biomedicine, fingerprint for forensic process and designing battery electrodes for solar cell.

KEYWORDS

- **nanotechnology**
- **nanobiohybrids**
- **bio-augmentation**
- **wastewater treatment**
- **biological systems**
- **bio polymers.**

REFERENCES

Ahmed, S. F.; Mofijur, M.; Ahmed, B.; Mehnaz, T.; Mehejabin, F.; Maliat, D.;& Shafiullah, G.M. Nanomaterials as a Sustainable Choice for Treating Waste Water. *Environ. Res.* **2022,** *214*, 113807.

Ahmed, F.; Qayyum, S.; Husain, Q. Benign Nano-Assemblages of Silver Induced by β Galactosidase with Augmented Antimicrobial and Industrial Dye Degeneration Potential. *Mater. Sci. Eng.: C* **2018,** *91*, 570–578.

Aji, M. M.; Narendren, S.; Purkait, M. K.; Katiyar, V. Utilization of Waste Polyvinyl Chloride (PVC) for Ultrafiltration Membrane Fabrication and Its Characterization. *J. Environ. Chem. Eng.* **2020,** *8* (2),103650; Nwaila, G. T.; Ghorbani, Y.; Zhang, S. E.; Frimmel, H. E.; Tolmay, L. C.; Rose, D. H. et al. Valorisation of Mine Waste-Part I: Characteristics of, and Sampling

Methodology for, Consolidated Mineralised Tailings by Using Witwatersrand Gold Mines (South Africa) as an Example. *J. Environ. Manage.* **2021,** *295*, 113013.

Alcântara, A. C.; Darder, M.; Aranda, P.; Ruiz-Hitzky, E. Zein-Layered Hydroxide Biohybrids: Strategies of Synthesis and Characterization. *Materials* **2020,** *13* (4), 825.

Ali, M. E.; Das, R.; Maamor, A.; Hamid, S. B. A. Multifunctional Carbon Nanotubes (CNTs): A New Dimension in Environmental Remediation. *Adv. Mater. Res.* **2014,** *832*, 328–332.

Asuri, P.; Bale, S. S.; Karajanagi, S. S.; Kane, R. S. The Protein–Nanomaterial Interface. *Curr. Opin. Biotechnol.* **2006a,** *17* (6), 562–568.

Asuri, P.; Karajanagi, S. S.; Sellitto, E.; Kim, D. Y.; Kane, R. S.; Dordick, J. S. Water-Soluble Carbon Nanotube-Enzyme Conjugates as Functional Biocatalytic Formulations. *Biotechnol. Bioeng.* **2006b,** *95* (5), 804–811.

Banerjee, U. C.; Mittal, A. K.; Chisti, Y. Research Review Paper: Synthesis of Metallic Nanoparticles Using Plant Extract. *Biotechnol. Adv.* **2013,** *31*, 346–356; (b) Mashwani, Z.-U.-R.; Khan, T.; Khan, M. A.; Nadhman, A. *App. Microb. Biotechnol.* **2015,** *99*, 9923–9934.

Benavente, R.; Lopez-Tejedor, D.; Perez-Rizquez, C.; Palomo, J. M. Ultra-Fast Degradation of p-Aminophenol by a Nanostructured Iron Catalyst. *Molecules* **1970,** *23* (9), 2166.

Bhat, S. A.; Sher, F.; Hameed, M.; Bashir, O.; Kumar, R.; Vo, D. V. N. et al. Sustainable Nanotechnology Based Wastewater Treatment Strategies: Achievements, Challenges and Future Perspectives. *Chemosphere* **2022,** *288*, 132606.

Biškup, B.; Subotić, B. Kinetic Analysis of the Exchange Processes Between Sodium Ions from Zeolite A and Cadmium, Copper and Nickel Ions from Solutions. *Sep. Purif. Technol.* **2004,** *37* (1), 17–31.

Boroum and Moghaddam, A.; Namvar, F.; Moniri, M.; Md. Tahir, P.; Azizi, S.; Mohamad, R. Nanoparticles Biosynthesized by Fungi and Yeast: A Review of Their Preparation, Properties, and Medical Applications. *Molecules* **2015,** *20* (9), 16540–16565.

Brena, B.; González-Pombo, P.; Batista-Viera, F. Immobilization of Enzymes: A Literature Survey. *Immobilization Enzymes Cells* **2013,** 15–31.

Candia-Onfray, C.; Rojas, S.; Zanoni, M. V. B.; Salazar, R. An Updated Review of Metal–Organic Framework Materials in Photo (Electro) Catalytic Applications: From CO_2 Reduction to Wastewater Treatments. *Curr. Opin. Electrochem.* **2021,** *26*, 100669.

Carballares, D.; Morellon-Sterling, R.; Fernandez-Lafuente, R. Design of Artificial Enzymes Bearing Several Active Centers: New Trends, Opportunities and Problems. *Int. J. Mol. Sci.* **2022,** *23* (10), 5304. (b) Baghayeri, M.; Mahdavi, B.; Hosseinpor-Mohsen Abadi, Z.; Farhadi, S. Green Synthesis of Silver Nanoparticles Using Water Extract of *Salvia leriifolia*: Antibacterial Studies and Applications as Catalysts in the Electrochemical Detection of Nitrite. *Appl. Organometall. Chem.* **2018,** *32* (2), e4057; (c) Wang, W.; Zhang, B.; Liu, Q.; Du, P.; Liu, W.; He, Z. Biosynthesis of Palladium Nanoparticles Using *Shewanella loihica* PV-4 for Excellent Catalytic Reduction of Chromium (VI). *Environ. Sci.: Nano* **2018,** *5* (3), 730–739.

(a) Chinnadayyala, S. R.; Santhosh, M.; Singh, N. K.; Goswami, P. *Biosen. Bioelec.* **2015,** *69*, 155–161; (b) Sousa, A. A.; Hassan, S. A.; Knittel, L. L.; Balbo, A.; Aronova, M. A.; Brown, P. H. et al. Biointeractions of Ultrasmall Glutathione-Coated Gold Nanoparticles: Effect of Small Size Variations. *Nanoscale* **2016,** *8* (12), 6577–6588.

Cincotti, A.; Mameli, A.; Locci, A. M.; Orrù, R.; Cao, G. Heavy Metals Uptake by Sardinian Natural Zeolites: Experiment and Modeling. *Ind. Eng. Chem. Res.* **2006,** *45* (3), 1074–1084.

Dang, V. B. H.; Doan, H. D.; Dang-Vu, T.; Lohi, A. Equilibrium and Kinetics of Biosorption of Cadmium (II) and Copper (II) Ions by Wheat Straw. *Bioresour. Technol.* **2009,** *100* (1), 211–219.

Das, R.; Abd Hamid, S. B.; Ali, M. E. Nanobiohybrid: A Favorite Candidate for Future Water Purification Technology. In: *Advanced Materials Research*, Vol. **1131**; Trans Tech Publications Ltd, 2016; , pp193–197.

(a) Dodekatos, G.; Schünemann, S.; Tüysüz, H. Recent Advances in Thermo-, Photo-, and Electrocatalytic Glycerol Oxidation. *ACS Catal* **2018,** *8* (7), 6301–6333; (b) Hanske, C.; Sanz-Ortiz, M. N.; Liz-Marzán, L. M. Silica-Coated Plasmonic Metal Nanoparticles in Action. *Colloidal Synthesis Plasmonic Nanometals* **2020,** 755–820. (c) Li, G.; Tang, Z. Noble Metal Nanoparticle@ Metal Oxide Core/Yolk–Shell Nanostructures as Catalysts: Recent Progress and Perspective. *Nanoscale* **2014,** *6* (8), 3995–4011.

Dong, W.; Wang, D.; Wang, H.; Li, M.; Chen, F.; Jia, F.; Ye, J. Facile Synthesis of In2S3/UiO-66 Composite with Enhanced Adsorption Performance and Photocatalytic Activity for the Removal of Tetracycline Under Visible Light Irradiation. *J. Colloid Interface Sci.* **2019,** *535*, 444–457.

Fan, H.; Mundstock, A.; Feldhoff, A.; Knebel, A.; Gu, J.; Meng, H.; Caro, J. Covalent Organic Framework–Covalent Organic Framework Bilayer Membranes for Highly Selective Gas Separation. *J. Am. Chem. Soc.* **2018,** *140* (32), 10094–10098.

Feng, W.; Ji, P. Enzymes Immobilized on Carbon Nanotubes. *Biotechnol. Adv.* **2011,** *29* (6), 889–895.

Filice, M.; Marciello, M.; del Puerto Morales, M.; Palomo, J. M. Synthesis of Heterogeneous Enzyme–Metal Nanoparticle Biohybrids in Aqueous Media and Their Applications in C–C Bond Formation and Tandem Catalysis. *Chem. Commun.* **2013,** *49* (61), 6876–6878.

Foroutan, R.; Mohammadi, R.; Peighambardoust, S. J.; Jalali, S.; Ramavandi, B. Application of Nano-Silica Particles Generated from Offshore White Sandstone for Cadmium Ions Elimination from Aqueous Media. *Environ. Technol. Innov.* **2020,** *19*, 101031.

Fu, G.; Yue, X.; Dai, Z. Glucose Biosensor Based on Covalent Immobilization of Enzyme in Sol–Gel Composite Film Combined with Prussian Blue/Carbon Nanotubes Hybrid. *Biosens. Bioelectron.* **2011,** *26* (9), 3973–3976.

Gao, B.; Gao, Y.; Li, Y. Preparation and Chelation Adsorption Property of Composite Chelating Material Poly (Amidoxime)/SiO_2 Towards Heavy Metal Ions. *Chem. Eng. J.* **2010,** *158* (3), 542–549.

Gao, Y.; Kyratzis, I. Covalent Immobilization of Proteins on Carbon Nanotubes Using the Cross-Linker 1-Ethyl-3- (3-dimethylaminopropyl) Carbodiimide—A Critical Assessment. *Bioconjugate Chem.* **2008,** *19* (10), 1945–1950.

Ge, P.; Li, F.; Zhang, B. Synthesis of Modified Mesoporous Materials and Comparative Studies of Removal of Heavy Metal from Aqueous Solutions. *Polish J. Environ. Stud.* **2010,** *19* (2).

Ghernaout, D.; Naceur, M. W.; Ghernaout, B. A Review of Electrocoagulation as a Promising Coagulation Process for Improved Organic and Inorganic Matters Removal by Electrophoresis and Electroflotation. *Desalin. Water Treatment* **2011,** *28* (1–3), 287–320.

Gier, S.; Johns, W. D. Heavy Metal-Adsorption on Micas and Clay Minerals Studied by X-ray Photoelectron Spectroscopy. *Appl. Clay Sci.* **2000,** *16* (5–6), 289–299.

Gonzalez-Moragas, L.; Maurer, L. L.; Harms, V. M.; Meyer, J. N.; Laromaine, A.; Roig, A. Materials and Toxicological Approaches to Study Metal and Metal-Oxide Nanoparticles in the Model Organism *Caenorhabditis elegans*. *Mater. Horiz.* **2017,***4* (5) 719–746.

Guiseppi-Elie, A.; Lei, C.; Baughman, R. H. Direct Electron Transfer of Glucose Oxidase on Carbon Nanotubes. *Nanotechnology* **2002,** *13* (5), 559.

Guo, Z.; Richardson, J. J.; Kong, B.; Liang, K. Nanobiohybrids: Materials Approaches for Bioaugmentation. *Sci. Adv.* **2020,** *6* (12), eaaz0330.

He, J.; Xu, Y.; Xiong, Z.; Lai, B.; Sun, Y.; Yang, Y.; Yang, L. The Enhanced Removal of Phosphate by Structural Defects and Competitive Fluoride Adsorption on Cerium-Based Adsorbent. *Chemosphere* **2020,** *256*, 127056.

https://www.watertechnologies.com/handbook/handbook-industrial-water-treatment

Huang, W.; Taylor, S.; Fu, K.; Lin, Y.; Zhang, D.; Hanks, T. W.; Sun, Y. P. Attaching Proteins to Carbon Nanotubes via Diimide-Activated Amidation. *Nano Lett.* **2002,** *2* (4), 311–314.

Hwang, E. T.; Gu, M. B. Enzyme Stabilization by Nano/Microsized Hybrid Materials. *Eng. Life Sci.* **2013,** *13* (1), 49–61.

Jiang, K.; Schadler, L. S.; Siegel, R. W.; Zhang, X.; Zhang, H.; Terrones, M. Protein Immobilization on Carbon Nanotubes via a Two-Step Process of Diimide-Activated Amidation. *J. Mater. Chem.* **2004,** *14* (1), 37–39.

Kim, D. G.; Kang, H.; Han, S.; Lee, J. C. Dual Effective Organic/Inorganic Hybrid Star-Shaped Polymer Coatings on Ultrafiltration Membrane for Bio-and Oil-Fouling Resistance. *ACS Appl. Mater. Interfaces* **2012,** *4* (11), 5898–5906.

Kökçam-Demir, Ü.; Goldman, A.; Esrafili, L.; Gharib, M.; Morsali, A.; Weingart, O.; Janiak, C. Coordinatively Unsaturated Metal Sites (Open Metal Sites) in Metal–Organic Frameworks: Design and Applications. *Chem. Soc. Rev.* **2020,** *49* (9), 2751–2798.

Koppelman, M. H.; Dillard, J. G. A Study of the Adsorption of Ni (II) and Cu (II) by Clay Minerals. *Clays Clay Minerals* **1977,** *25* (6), 457–462.

Kumar, P.; Bansal, V.; Kim, K. H.; Kwon, E. E. Metal-Organic Frameworks (MOFs) as Futuristic Options for Wastewater Treatment. *J. Ind. Eng. Chem.* **2018,** *62*, 130–145.

Kumar, P.; Pournara, A.; Kim, K. H.; Bansal, V.; Rapti, S.; Manos, M. J. Metal-Organic Frameworks: Challenges and Opportunities for Ion-Exchange/Sorption Applications. *Progr. Mater. Sci.* **2017,** *86*, 25–74.

Lauth, V.; Maas, M.; Rezwan, K. An Evaluation of Colloidal and Crystalline Properties of $CaCO_3$ Nanoparticles for Biological Applications. *Mater. Sci. Eng. C* **2017,** *78*, 305–314.

Lawrence, N. S.; Deo, R. P.; Wang, J. Comparison of the Electrochemical Reactivity of Electrodes Modified with Carbon Nanotubes from Different Sources. *Electroanalysis: Int. J. Devoted Fundamental Pract. Aspects Electroanal.* **2005,** *17* (1), 65–72.

Lee, Y. M.; Kwon, O. Y.; Yoon, Y. J.; Ryu, K. Immobilization of Horseradish Peroxidase on Multi-Wall Carbon Nanotubes and Its Electrochemical Properties. *Biotechnol. Lett.* **2006,** *28* (1), 39–43.

Li, M.; Li, D.; O'Keeffe, M.; Yaghi, O. M. Topological Analysis of Metal–Organic Frameworks with Polytopic Linkers and/or Multiple Building Units and the Minimal Transitivity Principle. *Chem. Rev.* **2014,** *114* (2), 1343–1370.

Li, T.; Liu, L.; Zhang, Z.; Han, Z. Preparation of Nano Fibrous Metal-Organic Framework Filter for Rapid Adsorption and Selective Separation of Cationic Dye from Aqueous Solution. *Sep. Purif. Technol.* **2020a,** *237*, 116360.

Li, Y.; Li, W.; Jarvis, P.; Zhou, W.; Zhang, J.; Chen, J. et al. Occurrence, Removal and Potential Threats Associated with Microplastics in Drinking Water Sources. *J. Environ. Chem. Eng.* **2020b,** *8* (6), 104527.

Liang, K.; Richardson, J. J.; Cui, J.; Caruso, F.; Doonan, C. J.; Falcaro, P. Metal–Organic Framework Coatings as Cytoprotective Exoskeletons for Living Cells. *Adv. Mater.* **2016,** *28* (36), 7910–7914.

Liu, C. S.; Zhang, Z. H.; Chen, M.; Zhao, H.; Duan, F. H.; Chen, D. M.; Du, M. Pore Modulation of Zirconium–Organic Frameworks for High-Efficiency Detection of Trace Proteins. *Chem. Commun.* **2017,** *53* (28), 3941–3944.

Liu, Y.; Qu, X.; Guo, H.; Chen, H.; Liu, B.; Dong, S. Facile Preparation of Amperometric Laccase Biosensor with Multifunction Based on the Matrix of Carbon Nanotubes–Chitosan Composite. *Biosens. Bioelectron.* **2006,** *21* (12), 2195–2201.

Lopez-Tejedor, D.; De las Rivas, B.; Palomo, J. M. Ultra-Small Pd (0) Nanoparticles into a Designed Semisynthetic Lipase: An Efficient and Recyclable Heterogeneous Biohybrid Catalyst for the Heck Reaction Under Mild Conditions. *Molecules* **2018,** *23* (9), 2358.

Lykourinou, V.; Chen, Y.; Wang, X. S.; Meng, L.; Hoang, T.; Ming, L. J.; Ma, S. Immobilization of MP-11 into a Mesoporous Metal–Organic Framework, MP-11@ mesoMOF: A New Platform for Enzymatic Catalysis. *J. Am. Chem. Soc.* **2011,** *133* (27), 10382–10385.

Lynge, M. E.; van der Westen, R.; Postma, A.; Städler, B. Polydopamine—A Nature-Inspired Polymer Coating for Biomedical Science. *Nanoscale* **2011,** *3* (12), 4916–4928.

Makishima, A. Possibility of Hybrid Materials. *Ceram. Jap.* **2004,** *39* (2), 90–91.

Massoud, M. A.; Tarhini, A.; Nasr, J. A. Decentralized Approaches to Wastewater Treatment and Management: Applicability in Developing Countries. *J. Environ. Manage.* **2009,** *90* (1), 652–659.

Mercier, L.; Pinnavaia, T. J.Heavy Metal Ion Adsorbents Formed by the Grafting of a Thiol Functionality to Mesoporous Silica Molecular Sieves: Factors Affecting Hg (II) Uptake. *Environ. Sci. Technol.* **1998,** *32* (18), 2749–2754.

Mpungose, P. P.; Vundla, Z. P.; Maguire, G. E.; Friedrich, H. B. The Current Status of Heterogeneous Palladium Catalysed Heck and Suzuki Cross-Coupling Reactions. *Molecules* **2018,** *23* (7), 1676.

Murray, L.J.; Dincă, M.; Long, J. R. Hydrogen Storage in Metal–Organic Frameworks. *Chem. Soc. Rev.* **2009,** *38* (5), 1294–1314.

Nagappan, S.; Choi, M. C.; Sung, G.; Park, S. S.; Moorthy, M. S.; Chu, S. W. et al. Highly Transparent, Hydrophobic Fluorinated Polymethylsiloxane/Silica Organic-Inorganic Hybrids for Anti-Stain Coating. *Macromol. Res.* **2013,** *21* (6), 669–680.

Nagarale, R. K.; Gohil, G. S.; Shahi, V. K. Recent Developments on Ion-Exchange Membranes and Electro-Membrane Processes. *Advances Colloid Interface Sci.* **2006,** *119* (2–3), 97–130.

Nelson, D. L.; Lehninger, A. L.; Cox, M. M. *Lehninger Principles of Biochemistry*; Macmillan, 2008.

Nepal, D.; Geckeler, K. E. pH-Sensitive Dispersion and Debundling of Single-Walled Carbon Nanotubes: Lysozyme as a Tool. *Small* **2006,** *2* (3), 406–412.

Niu, J.; Lunn, D. J.; Pusuluri, A.; Yoo, J. I.; O'Malley, M. A.; Mitragotri, S.; Hawker, C. J. Engineering Live Cell Surfaces with Functional Polymers via Cytocompatible Controlled Radical Polymerization. *Nat. Chem.* **2017,** *9* (6), 537–545.

O'Brien, P.; Lopez-Tejedor, D.; Benavente, R.; Palomo, J. M. Pd Nanoparticles-Polyethylenemine-Lipase Bionanohybrids as Heterogeneous Catalysts for Selective Oxidation of Aromatic Alcohols. *ChemCatChem* **2018,** *10* (21), 4992–4999.

O'Connell, D. W.; Birkinshaw, C.; O'Dwyer, T. F. Heavy Metal Adsorbents Prepared from the Modification of Cellulose: A Review. *Bioresour. Technol.* **2008,** *99* (15), 6709–6724.

Palani, G.; Arputhalatha, A.; Kannan, K.; Lakkaboyana, S. K.; Hanafiah, M. M.; Kumar, V.; Marella, R. K. Current Trends in the Application of Nanomaterials for the Removal of Pollutants from Industrial Wastewater Treatment—A Review. *Molecules* **2021,** *26* (9), 2799.

Pang, Y.; Zeng, G.; Tang, L.; Zhang, Y.; Liu, Y.; Lei, X. et al. PEI-Grafted Magnetic Porous Powder for Highly Effective Adsorption of Heavy Metal Ions. *Desalination* **2011,** *281*, 278–284.

Patil, M. P.; Kim, G. D. Marine Microorganisms for Synthesis of Metallic Nanoparticles and Their Biomedical Applications. *Colloids Surfaces B: Biointerfaces* **2018,** *172*, 487–495. (b) Ghosh, S. *Appl. Microb. Biotechnol.* **2018,** *102*, 7693–7701; (c) Makarovsky, D.; Fadeev, L.; Salam, B. B.; Zelinger, E.; Matan, O.; Inbar, J.; Jurkevitch, E.; Gozin, M.; Burdman, S. *Appl. Environ. Microbiol.* **2018,** *84*, Art. No. e02212-17.

Paun, G.; Neagu, E.; Tache, A.; Radu, G. L.; Parvulescu, V. Application of the Nanofiltration Process for Concentration of Polyphenolic Compounds from *Geranium robertianum* and *Salvia officinalis* Extracts. *Chem. Biochem. Eng. Quart.* **2011,** *25* (4), 453–460.

Raj, G.; Swalus, C.; Guillet, A.; Devillers, M.; Nysten, B.; Gaigneaux, E. M. Supramolecular Organization in Organic–Inorganic Heterogeneous Hybrid Catalysts Formed from Polyoxometalate and Poly (ampholyte) Polymer. *Langmuir* **2013,** *29* (13), 4388–4395.

Repo, E.; Warchoł, J. K.; Bhatnagar, A.; Sillanpää, M. Heavy Metals Adsorption by Novel EDTA-Modified Chitosan–Silica Hybrid Materials. *J. Colloid Interface Sci.* **2011,** *358* (1), 261–267.

Richardson, J. J.; Liang, K. Nano-Biohybrids: In Vivo Synthesis of Metal–Organic Frameworks Inside Living Plants. *Small* **2018,** *14* (3), 1702958.

Rottman, C.; Grader, G.; De Hazan, Y.; Melchior, S.; Avnir, D. Surfactant-Induced Modification of Dopants Reactivity in Sol−Gel Matrixes. *J. Am. Chem. Soc.* **1999,** *121* (37), 8533–8543.

Rowsell, J. L.; Millward, A. R.; Park, K. S.; Yaghi, O. M. Hydrogen Sorption in Functionalized Metal− Organic Frameworks. *J. Am. Chem. Soc.* **2004,** 126 (18), 5666–5667.

Russo, T.; Fucile, P.; Giacometti, R.; Sannino, F. Sustainable Removal of Contaminants by Biopolymers: A Novel Approach for Wastewater Treatment. *Curr. State Future Perspect. Processes* **2021,** *9* (4), 719; (b) Liu, R.; Tan, K. T.; Gong, Y.; Chen, Y.; Li, Z.; Xie, S.; Jiang, D. Covalent Organic Frameworks: An Ideal Platform for Designing Ordered Materials and Advanced Applications. *Chem. Soc. Rev.* **2021,** *50* (1), 120–242.

San, B. H.; Ravichandran, S.; Park, K. S.; Subramani, V. K.; Kim, K. K. Bioinorganic Nanohybrid Catalyst for Multistep Synthesis of Acetaminophen, an Analgesic. *ACS Appl. Mater. Interfaces* **2016,** *8* (44), 30058–30065.

Setyawati, M. I.; Tay, C. Y.; Leong, D. T. Mechanistic Investigation of the Biological Effects of SiO2,TiO2, and ZnO Nanoparticles on Intestinal Cells. *Small* **2015,** *11* (28), 3458–3468.

Shan, Y.; Chen, L.; Pang, H.; Xu, Q. Metal–Organic Framework-Based Hybrid Frameworks. *Small Struct.* **2021,** *2* (2), 2000078.

Siddique, M. H.; St Pierre, C. C.; Biswas, N.; Bewtra, J. K.; Taylor, K. E. Immobilized Enzyme Catalyzed Removal of 4-Chlorophenol from Aqueous Solution. *Water Research* **1993,** *27* (5), 883–890.

Simsek, E. B.; Duranoglu, D.; Beker, U. Heavy Metal Adsorption by Magnetic Hybrid-Sorbent: An Experimental and Theoretical Approach. *Sep. Sci. Technol.* **2012,** *47* (9), 1334–1340.

Sousa, J. C.; Ribeiro, A. R.; Barbosa, M. O.; Pereira, M. F. R.; Silva, A. M. A Review on Environmental Monitoring of Water Organic Pollutants Identified by EU Guidelines. *J. Hazard. Mater.* **2018,** *344*, 146–162.

Sparks, B. J.; Hoff, E. F.; Xiong, L.; Goetz, J. T.; Patton, D. L. Superhydrophobic Hybrid Inorganic–Organic Thiol-ene Surfaces Fabricated via Spray-Deposition and Photopolymerization. *ACS Appl. Mater. Interfaces* **2013,** *5* (5), 1811–1817.

Su, D.; Liu, X.; Wang, L.; Ma, C.; Xie, H.; Zhang, H.; Huang, X. Bio-Inspired Engineering Proteinosomes with a Cell-Wall-Like Protective Shell by Self-Assembly of a Metal-Chelated Complex. *Chem. Commun.* **2016,** *52* (95), 13803–13806.

Subrizi, F.; Crucianelli, M.; Grossi, V.; Passacantando, M.; Pesci, L.; Saladino, R. Carbon Nanotubes as Activating Tyrosinase Supports for the Selective Synthesis of Catechols. *ACS Catal.* **2014,** *4* (3), 810–822.

Suchithra, P. S.; Vazhayal, L.; Mohamed, A. P.; Ananthakumar, S. Mesoporous Organic–Inorganic Hybrid Aerogels Through Ultrasonic Assisted Sol–Gel Intercalation of Silica–PEG in Bentonite for Effective Removal of Dyes, Volatile Organic Pollutants and Petroleum Products from Aqueous Solution. *Chem. Eng. J.* **2012,** *200*, 589–600.

Tao, L. Y.; Gong, J. S.; Su, C.; Jiang, M.; Li, H.; Li, H.; Shi, J. S. Mining and Expression of a Metagenome- Derived Keratinase Responsible for Biosynthesis of Silver Nanoparticles. *ACS Biomater. Sci. Eng.* **2018,** *4* (4), 1307–1315.

Udayakumar, G. P.; Muthusamy, S.; Selvaganesh, B.; Sivarajasekar, N.; Rambabu, K.; Sivamani, S.; Hosseini-Bandegharaei, A. Ecofriendly Biopolymers and Composites: Preparation and Their Applications in Water-Treatment. *Biotechnol. Adv.* **2021,** *52*, 107815; (b) Biswas, S.; Pal, A. Application of Biopolymers as a New Age Sustainable Material for Surfactant Adsorption: A Brief Review. *Carbohydr. Polym. Technol. App.* **2021,** *2*, 100145.

Uzun, I.; Güzel, F. Adsorption of Some Heavy Metal Ions from Aqueous Solution by Activated Carbon and Comparison of Percent Adsorption Results of Activated Carbon with Those of Some Other Adsorbents. *Turk. J. Chem.* **2000,** *24* (3), 291–298.

Vetchinkina, E. P.; Loshchinina, E. A.; Vodolazov, I. R.; Kursky, V. F.; Dykman, L. A.; Nikitina, V. E. Biosynthesis of Nanoparticles of Metals and Metalloids by Basidiomycetes: Preparation of Gold Nanoparticles by Using Purified Fungal Phenol Oxidases. *Appl. Microbiol. Biotechnol.* **2017,** *101* (3), 1047–1062.

Walcarius, A. Electrochemical Applications of Silica-Based Organic−Inorganic Hybrid Materials. *Chem. Mater.* **2001,** *13* (10), 3351–3372.

Wang, C.; Kaneti, Y. V.; Bando, Y.; Lin, J.; Liu, C.; Li, J.; Yamauchi, Y. Metal–Organic Framework-Derived One-Dimensional Porous or Hollow Carbon-Based Nanofibers for Energy Storage and Conversion. *Mater. Horiz.* **2018a,** *5* (3), 394–407.

Wang, D.; Jia, F.; Wang, H.; Chen, F. Fang, Y.; Dong, W.; Yuan, X. Simultaneously Efficient Adsorption and Photocatalytic Degradation of Tetracycline by Fe-Based MOFs. *J. Colloid Interface Sci.* **2018b,** *519*, 273–284.

Wang, H.; Yuan, X.; Wu, Y.; Zeng, G.; Dong, H.; Chen, X.; Peng, L. In Situ Synthesis of In2S3@ MIL-125 (Ti) Core–Shell Microparticle for the Removal of Tetracycline from Wastewater by Integrated Adsorption and Visible-Light-Driven Photocatalysis. *Appl. Catal. B: Environ.* **2016,** *186*, 19–29.

Wang, L.; Wu, X. L.; Xu, W. H.; Huang, X. J.; Liu, J. H.; Xu, A. W. Stable Organic–Inorganic Hybrid of Polyaniline/α-Zirconium Phosphate for Efficient Removal of Organic Pollutants in Water Environment. *ACS Appl. Mater. Interfaces* **2012,** *4* (5), 2686–2692.

Wang, L.; Zhang, J.; Wang, A. Fast Removal of Methylene Blue from Aqueous Solution by Adsorption onto Chitosan-g-Poly (Acrylic Acid)/Attapulgite Composite. *Desalination* **2011,** *266* (1–3), 33–39.

Wang, X.; Chi, C.; Zhang, K.; Qian, Y.; Gupta, K. M.; Kang, Z.; Zhao, D. Reversed Thermo-Switchable Molecular Sieving Membranes Composed of Two-Dimensional Metal-Organic Nanosheets for Gas Separation. *Nat. Commun.* **2017,** *8* (1), 1–10.

Wen, X. F.; Wang, K.; Pi, P. H.; Yang, J. X.; Cai, Z. Q.; Zhang, L. J. et al. Organic–Inorganic Hybrid Superhydrophobic Surfaces Using Methyltriethoxysilane and Tetraethoxysilane Sol–Gel Derived Materials in Emulsion. *Appl. Surface Sci.* **2011,** *258* (3), 991–998.

Xia, Q.; Huang, B.; Yuan, X.; Wang, H.; Wu, Z.; Jiang, L.; Wang, H. Modified Stannous Sulfide Nanoparticles with Metal-Organic Framework: Toward Efficient and Enhanced Photocatalytic Reduction of Chromium (VI) Under Visible Light. *J. Colloid Interface Sci.* **2018,** *530*, 481–492.

Xu, Y.; Lv, J.; Song, Y.; Zhou, X.; Tian, C.; Hong, X.; Lin, Z. Efficient Removal of Low-Concentration Organo Arsenic by Zr-Based Metal–Organic Frameworks: Cooperation of Defects and Hydrogen Bonds. *Environ. Sci.: Nano* **2019,** *6* (12), 3590–3600.

(a) Yaashikaa, P. R.; Kumar, S.; Karishma, S. Review on Biopolymers and Composites—Evolving Material as Adsorbents in Removal of Environmental Pollutants. *Environ. Res.* **2022,** *212* (Part A), 113114; (b) Foroutan, R.; Peighambardoust, S. J.; Latifi, P.; Ahmadi, A.; Alizadeh, M.; Ramavandi, B. Carbon Nanotubes/β-Cyclodextrin/MnFe2O4 as a Magnetic Nanocomposite Powder for Tetracycline Antibiotic Decontamination from Different Aqueous Environments. *J. Environ. Chem. Eng.* **2021,** *9* (6), 106344.

Yu, Y. Y.; Chen, W. C. Transparent Organic–Inorganic Hybrid Thin Films Prepared from Acrylic Polymer and Aqueous Monodispersed Colloidal Silica. *Mater. Chem. Phys.* **2003,** *82* (2), 388–395.

Yuan, S.; Feng, L.; Wang, K.; Pang, J.; Bosch, M.; Lollar, C.; Zhou, H. C. Stable Metal–Organic Frameworks: Design, Synthesis, and Applications. *Adv. Mater.* **2018,** *30* (37), 1704303.

Zaitseva, N.; Zaitsev, V.; Walcarius, A. Chromium (VI) Removal via Reduction–Sorption on Bi-Functional Silica Adsorbents. *J. Hazard. Mater.* **2013,** *250*, 454–461.

Zewail, T. M.; El-Garf, S. A. M. Preparation of Agriculture Residue Based Adsorbents for Heavy Metal Removal. *Desalination Water Treat.* **2010,** *22* (1–3), 363–370.

Zhang, M.; Wang, C.; Liu, C.; Luo, R.; Li, J.; Sun, X.; Wang, L. Metal–Organic Framework Derived Co_3O_4/C@ SiO_2 Yolk–Shell Nanoreactors with Enhanced Catalytic Performance. *J. Mater. Chem. A* **2018,** *6* (24), 11226–11235.

Zhang, X.; Yan, S.; Tyagi, R. D.; Surampalli, R. Y. *Chemosphere* **2011,** *82*, 489–494.

Zhang, Y. B.; Furukawa, H.; Ko, N.; Nie, W.; Park, H. J.; Okajima, S.; Yaghi, O. M. Introduction of Functionality, Selection of Topology, and Enhancement of Gas Adsorption in Multivariate Metal–Organic Framework-177. *J. Am. Chem. Soc.* **2015,** *137* (7), 2641–2650.

Zou, K. Y.; Li, Z. X. Controllable Syntheses of MOF-Derived Materials. *Chem.—Eur. J.* **2018,** *24* (25), 6506–6518.

CHAPTER 2

Biocatalysts in Remediation of Wastewater

V. SWARUPA, RUBY VARGHESE, BHASKAR GAONKAR, R. ROOPASHREE, and G. SUBBULAKSHMI

Department of Chemistry and Biochemistry, Jain Deemed to-be University, JC Road, Bengaluru, Karnataka, India

ABSTRACT

A profuse number of recalcitrant compounds in wastewater is dispensed from domestic and several industrial processes which pose an alarming threat to environmental sustainability. Additionally, the emerging pollutants as a result of increasing population and urbanization are a great concern globally. Though various physical and chemical methods are available to treat wastewater, the advantages of the application of biocatalytic tools for the remediation of pollutants are that they can function in milder conditions, are biodegradable, and can transform toxicological affluents into harmless end products. Hence, the enzyme-based biotechnological approach is a promising strategy to treat wastewater bodies with efficient and economical affordability. This chapter highlights the different classes of enzymes, focusing on the immobilized enzymes, enzymatic procedures in pollutants remediation, and enzyme reactors to degrade diverse water pollutants. Furthermore, considerable challenges and future aspects of the enzyme-based treatment of water pollutants are also conferred.

2.1 INTRODUCTION

Water is an indispensable source of life for all living beings and human body contains 65–70% water. Human dominance and the evolvement of powerful

Application of Engineering Principles and Practices in Biotechnology.
Ann Rose Abraham, Leonardo Sepúlveda Torre, Tamara Tatrishvili, and A. K. Haghi (Eds.)

technology has resulted in the alteration of various earth's ecosystem like terrestrial, air, and marine ecosystems. About 71% of earth's surface is covered by water (https://www.usbr.gov/mp/arwec/water-facts-ww-water-sup.html). However, the quality of water is adversely affected by diverse human activities, and the affected water is called wastewater. Novel pollution risk factors because of industrialization and urbanization have increased by 66% from 2000. In 2019, globally water pollution was the cause of 1.4 million premature deaths (Richard Fuller et al., 2022). The sources that generate wastewater includes industrial, agricultural, and domestic practices and the contaminants or the compounds present also are many and varied. More frequently detected organic pollutants in wastewater includes pesticides, phenols, dyes, pharmaceuticals, and estrogens (Aleya and Uddin, 2020). The uncontrolled dose and the unknown chemicals present disturbs the water quality and when it is mixed with other water bodies as well other ecosystems, it is dangerous to human beings and other living organisms. Some of their detrimental effects include physiological disorders majorly reproductive and neurological impairment, increased risk of cancer in aquatic and terrestrial organisms, and evolvement of new antibiotic resistant microorganisms.

Apart from the unknown chemicals in wastewater, properties of many existing chemicals itself, like structure, class, its toxicity mechanism, dose, biodegradability, and its impact on humans and environment are still unknown. Hence, proper treatment of wastewater is important before discharging into the environment to protect human health and the environment. Tragically, some chemicals are stubborn to currently applied conventional approaches and some chemicals leave undesirable by-products resulting in inefficient wastewater treatment (Ho et al., 2022). Additionally, some purification strategies used in wastewater treatment, namely, photocatalysis and ozonation uses toxic solvents which upon degradation leaves toxic products and these methods are energy-intensive and expensive. Therefore, it is worthwhile to develop or modify the methods that are sustainable and environment friendly. In the context of this as a modern technology, biotechnological processes using microorganisms and/or enzymes are more satisfactory. Specifically, enzymes like tyrosinases, laccases, and peroxidases play a vital role in diminishing any kind of contaminants including phenol-based compounds, which are widely found in wastewater (Stadlmair et al., 2018). The benefits of enzyme-based approaches are low cost, require low energy, operate at mild conditions, are less toxicity, and produce reduced amount of by-products (Jager and Croft et al., 2018). Hence, this review will underline the research achievements pertaining to the enzymatic approaches for the bioremediation of wastewater, its advantages and disadvantages, and various enzyme reactors used for the removal of toxic contaminants in wastewater.

2.2 METHODS OF WASTEWATER TREATMENT

Elimination of organic pollutants in surface water is essential to provide pure drinking water and to protect aquatic ecosystem. Various treatment methods that have been applied till date are classified as chemical, physical, and biological methods. The chemical methods comprise treatments like ozonation, oxidative processes, electrochemical, and photochemical destruction. The chemicals most commonly used are hydrochloric acid, sodium hypochlorite, and magnesium hydroxide (Fig. 2.1) These processes help in the eradication of both organic and inorganic compounds. Physical methods employed are filtration, reverse osmosis, foam separation, electrodialysis, and porous bed filtration. These physical procedures help in the removal of liquid and solid waste and ensure the better quality of water to be discharged or reused. However, the main disadvantages are the production of more sludge and toxic by-products, sophisticated equipment, and high cost (Eggen et al., 2014).

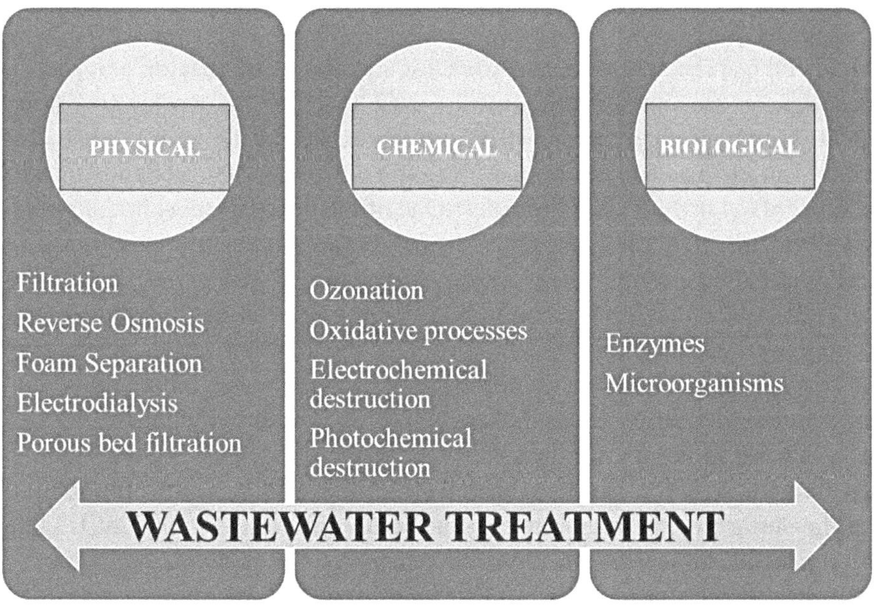

FIGURE 2.1 Wastewater treatment methods.

Currently, wastewater treatment by biological methods have attained greater attention because of its simplicity, cost-effectiveness, and lesser toxic residues. Removal of pollutants by biological methods are of two types—(i) treatment using free or immobilized form of enzymes and (ii) by microorganisms. The whole microorganisms like bacteria (e.g., *Streptomyces* and *Pseudomonas*) and fungi (e.g., *Trametes versicolor* and *Pleurotus ostreatus*) remove pollutants from wastewater by converting them into low toxic or by direct adsorption of the pollutants (Zhu et al., 2020). Although microbiological strategies are efficient in the elimination of major pollutants, they are less useful in the removal of dyes, pharmaceutical compounds, and phenols. Enzymes belonging to oxidoreductase class particularly which comprises peroxidases, laccases, and tyrosinases act as an alternative for biological treatment of wastewater. These enzymes catalyzes the oxidation reactions of several phenolic molecules and its derivatives. Biocatalysts has attained greater attention because it converts harmful substrates to lesser toxic products. The disadvantage of using free enzymes is its lower stability; however; replacing it with immobilized enzymes lead to increased stability and reusability (Thwaites et al., 2018).

2.3 ENZYMATIC BIOREACTORS

Fluidized bed reactor, stirred tank reactor, membrane bioreactor, and packed bed reactor are the most frequently used reactors for wastewater treatment. Membrane bioreactor (MBR) plants are fabricated with the blend of biological process and membrane filtration which confers more advantages compared to conventional strategies. One of the developments in the wastewater treatment is the generation of membrane bioreactors by employing enzymes called enzymatic membrane bioreactors (EMBRs) (Fig. 2.2).

EMBRs are designed by immobilizing enzymes on the membrane used for the separation. Common methods of enzyme immobilization are physical adsorption, cross linking, immobilization through ionic interactions, and entrapment in a polymeric gel. Across the membrane by applying pressure as a driving force, the products formed by the enzymatic catalysis can be discharged from the reaction chamber. As the enzymes are immobilized on the surface of the membrane, it facilitates substrate enrichment leading to enhanced enzymatic reaction efficiency. As the products are removed regularly in time, it reduces product inhibition, and membranes aid in the enhanced enzyme stability and continuous operation, and facilitates reuse

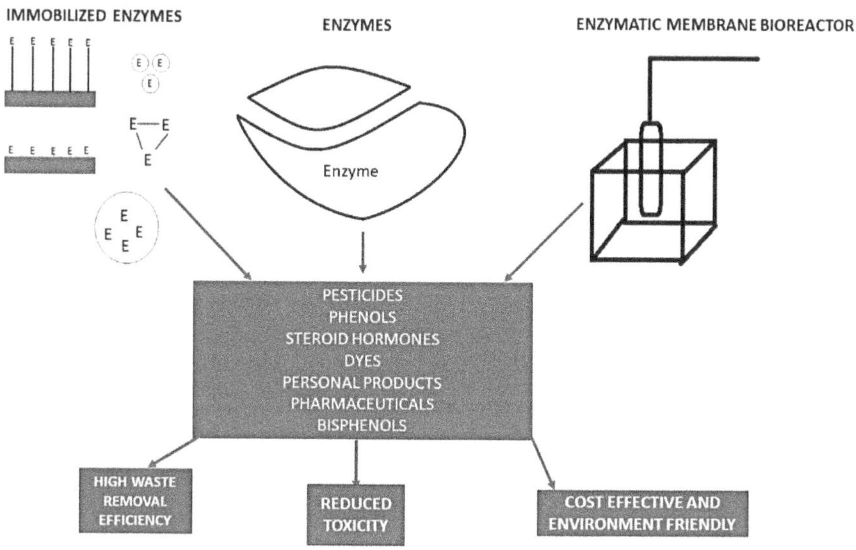

FIGURE 2.2 Multifaceted role of enzyme (immobilized enzyme/enzyme/enzymatic membrane reactor) in the wastewater treatment.

of the enzyme (Luo et al., 2020). Widely used immobilized enzymes in the wastewater treatment are oxidoreductases, laccases, tyrosinases, esterases, hydrolases, etc.

Membrane surface holds limited area for enzyme loading leading to weak catalytic efficiency. Currently, in order to enhance the enzyme loading and stability, nanomaterials have been incorporated into the membrane system. Frequently used nanomaterials are graphene oxides, magnetic nanoparticles, metal organic frameworks, and carbon nanotubes. The application of immobilized enzymes and nanomaterials-based immobilized enzymes in the elimination of toxic chemicals like antibiotics, dyes, phenols, and pesticides in wastewater will be discussed below.

2.3.1 *ANTIBIOTICS*

Antibiotics which are one of the modern medicines has revolutionized the medical fields which are used to treat various diseases of animals and humans. The major user of antibiotics is agriculture industries which are used to enhance the production followed by aquaculture, which are used to treat infected marine animals (Meek et al., 2015). However, identification of antibiotics in different water sources including drinking water has become an emerging pollutant due to its toxicity potential, development of antibiotic resistance, and genotoxicity on aquatic organisms especially (Bilal et al., 2020). Zumstein and Helbling (2019) have assessed the biotransformation of various antibiotics using enzymes extracted from the wastewater microbial community and reported that extracellular enzymes lead to loss of antibiotic activity by removing the functional groups involved in antibiotic activity. Nanoparticles-based immobilization of β-lactamase and its efficiency in penicillin degradation was evaluated by Gao et al. (2017) (Fig. 2.3). The study revealed that the efficiency of enzyme retained 95% even after 35 times of continuous use. Various studies have reported the successful application of immobilized to laccase to degrade different antibiotics like ampicillin, tetracyclin, and carbamazepine (Zhang et al., 2020; Simon-Herrero et al., 2019; Zdarta et al., 2019). Combination of immobilized eugenol and laccase were used in enzyme membrane reactor and described the effect of combined enzymes for the transformation of 32 antibiotics out of 38 antibiotics.

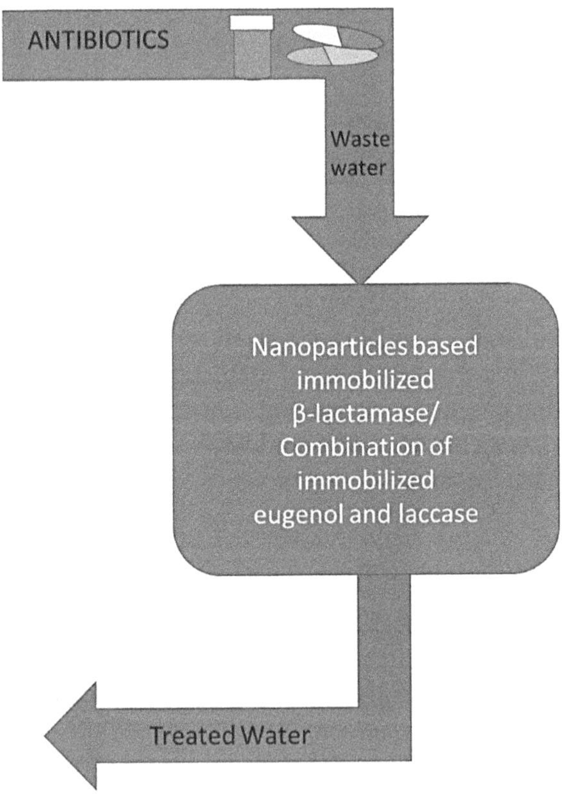

FIGURE 2.3 Nanoparticle-based immobilized enzyme for treatment of wastewater plant.

2.3.2 PESTICIDES

The agricultural sector is the major user of pesticides and pesticide application has increased the production of vegetables and fruits to more than 50% and cereals to more than 30% (Pimentel, 2007). Though pesticides aid in limiting the pest growth, their unsystematic and unregulated usage for the application of pest control and its seepage into water bodies cause detrimental effects to different living beings including human health and to the ecosystem. Organophosphate chemicals are the most frequently used pesticide in agricultural field which has resulted in contamination of water and soil across the globe.

Three majorly used enzyme tools to degrade pesticides are esterases, hydrolases, the mixed function oxidases (MFO), cytochrome p450, and glutathione S-transferases (GSTs) (Diez, 2010). The impact of various organophosphorus insecticides on freshwater planarians was evaluated by Poirier et al. (2017) and revealed that enzyme SsoPox degraded organophosphates efficiently and decreased the detrimental effect in planarians drastically. Recently application of microbial-enzyme systems including immobilized and biosensor approaches for the degradation of organophosphates was reported by various studies (Himanshu et al., 2023, Thakur et al., 2019) (Fig. 2.4). Examples of other pesticides that were bioremediated using enzymes derived from microbial sources were endosulphan (monooxygenases), glyphosate (oxidoreductase), hexachlorocyclohexane, and dicamba (dehalogenases), etc.

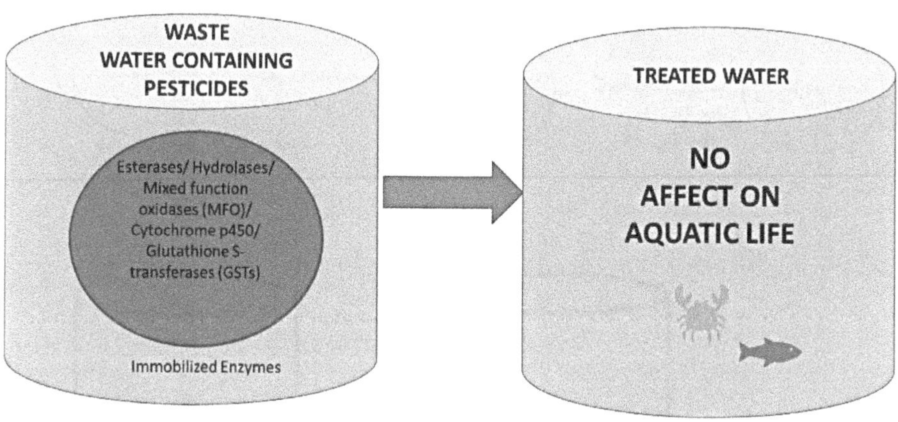

FIGURE 2.4 Pesticide-contained water treatment using immobilized enzymes.

2.3.3 DYES

Synthetic dyes are broadly utilized in food, textile, paper, leather, cosmetics, and pharmaceutical industries. Commonly used dyes include azo and anthraquinone dyes which contains azo group (-N=N-) as the functional group linked to aromatic rings and are difficult to destroy (Popli and Patel., 2015). They are toxic and carcinogenic and hence they are harmful to living beings when released to waterbodies. Enzymatic tools were identified as one of the efficient strategies to remove dyes in wastewater (Fig. 2.5). Liu et al. (2020) has represented the potential role of lignolytic enzymes namely laccase, lignin peroxidase, and manganese peroxidase in the degradation azo dyes including anthracene and triphenyl methane dyes. Recently, many research articles have described the application of laccase enzymes in the elimination of color from textile dye effluents (Iracheta-Cardenas et al., 2016; Collivignarelli et al., 2019). Efficacy of commercial laccase enzyme for decolorization of various dyes, which includes RB220, RB19, and AR42, was found to be more than 90% (Cifci et al., 2019). Soyabean peroxidase influenced 85% efficiency in decolorization of methyl orange (azo dye) present in liquid effluents (Chiong et al., 2016). Potential role of oxidoreductase enzymes like laccases, tyrosinases, and peroxidases produced by bacterial consortium in decolorization of anthraquinone dyes present in textile wastewater (Indanthrene Blue RS dye) was reported by Mohanty et al. (2021). Multicopper oxidase enzyme derived

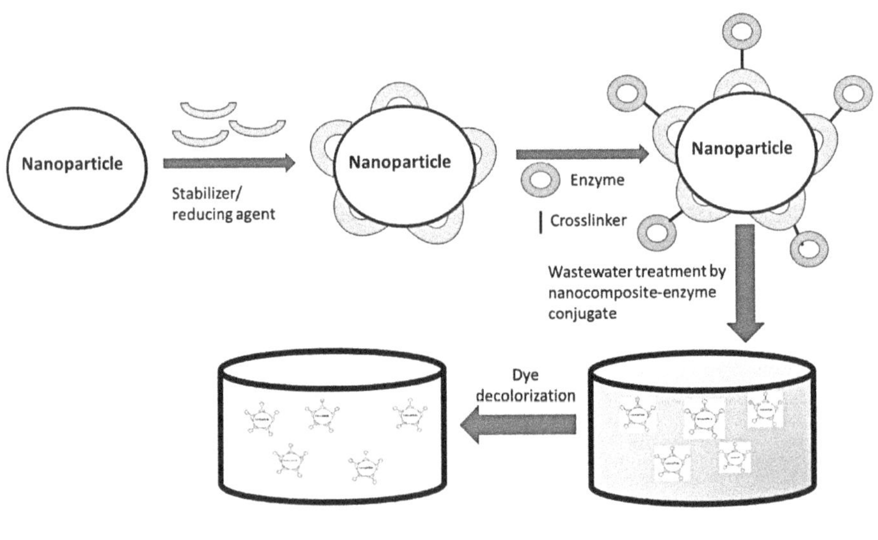

FIGURE 2.5 Nanobiocatalyst for removing dye from fresh water.

from *E.Coli* was immobilized on polyhydroxy butyrate and its efficiency of 80% on decolorization of Cibacron Blue 3GA and reactive blue 19 dye solutions used in textile industry was proclaimed (Bello-Gil et al., 2018). Similarly, nanoparticle-based immobilized peroxidase showing 100% elimination of Direct Brown 27 dye from wastewater was reported by Klanovicz et al. (2022). The literature survey suggests that enzyme-based strategies are the promising technology for the removal of dyes from wastewater.

2.3.4 PHENOLS

Phenolic compounds are the major component present in the effluents of range of industries like pharmaceuticals, paper, oil refining, paint, petrochemicals, plastic, wood products, phenolic resin, and textile (Villegas et al., 2016; Saputera et al., 2021). Most studied enzymes for the removal of phenols are tyrosinases, laccases, and especially peroxidase in both free and immobilized form. Peroxidases catalyze the conversion of different inorganic and organic chemicals in the presence of H_2O_2 by oxidative transformation. Peroxidases from various plant resources that includes soyabean peroxidase, potato peroxidase, and horseradish peroxidase have proved potential bioremediation properties on different toxic products, especially phenols. Kurnik et al. (2015) group has determined 90% efficiency in removal of phenols using peroxidases extracted from potato pulp. Several other studies were published on the peroxidase-based bioremediation of phenols (Ai et al., 2016; Chang et al., 2016; Zheng et al., 2019). Recent study observed by Ely et al. (2021) presents maximum bioconversion of the phenols that are present in biorefinery, using the combination of horseradish peroxidase enzyme with Fenton process. About 99% efficiency of phenol degradation using polyphenol oxidase enzyme extracted from potato in combination with amine-functionalized graphene oxide was reported by Pravin et al. (2018).

Laccases catalyzes the cleavage of spectrum of substrates including phenols by oxidation mechanism. A study conducted by Asadgol et al. (2014) observed that treatment of phenolic pollutants with laccase enzyme resulted in the removal of 80% of phenols. Increase in bisphenol degradation rate by using membrane reactor developed with immobilized laccase enzyme was reported by Barrios-Estrada et al. (2018). Laccase enzyme immobilized on the polyethylenimine (PEI)-based nanoparticles under magnetic field showed phenol industrial wastewater degradation rate of 70.30% (Xia et al., 2021). Immobilized tyrosinase on the polyacrylonitrile (PAN)-based beads with glutaraldehyde was investigated for the removal of phenols in wastewater based on toxicity studies. Substantial decrease in the toxicity posttreatment with the tyrosinase-immobilized beads was identified by Wu et al. (2017). Nano-biocatalyst strategy where tyrosinase was immobilized on magnetic iron oxide and the potential removal of phenolics in wastewater was analyzed. The study displayed 100% removal of phenols including high efficiency and reuse of nano-biocatalyst (Abdollahi et al., 2018). Complete removal of phenolic compounds in wastewater like *p*-chlorophenol, phenol, and, *p*-cresol by employing tyrosinase enzyme, which was immobilized on zeolitic imidazolate frameworks (ZIFs) was reported (Wei et al., 2021). These studies imply that immobilized laccases, tyrosinases, and especially peroxidases in combination with nanomaterials can be used efficiently in wastewater treatment in the future.

2.4 CONCLUSION AND FUTURE PROSPECTS

The comprehensive review on biocatalysts, the application of free, and especially biocatalysts immobilization shows great potential in the treatment of wastewater treatment. Recent advancements in the field of biotechnology proved various other strategies that are more efficient in the removal of toxics in wastewater. It comprises the novel designing of bioreactors containing membranes immobilized with the enzymes, microbial consortium-based immobilization, and nanomaterials-based immobilization of enzymes, which enhances substrate binding efficiency, storage facility, catalytic activity, stability, and reusability. However, the undetermined question is whether this successful laboratory or small-scale improvements can be transferred into large scale? Several impediments need to be resolved to transfer the lab achievements into industry scale, which are summarized as follows: (a) identifying new or optimizing the existing procedures to develop long-term stable enzymes, (b) scaling down the cost of enzyme production, (c) fabrication of the specialized enzyme bioreactors that help in the removal broad range of chemicals and emerging pollutants in the wastewater, (d) standardization of the biotransformation procedure to elevate the removal rate, (e) need to design strategies to overcome the effect of inhibitors on enzyme activity during the biodegradation process, and (f) development of improved support/matrix and cross-linkers.

KEYWORDS

- **antimicrobial**
- **biodegradable**
- **bioreactors**
- **enzyme immobilization**
- **pollutants**
- **remediation**

REFERENCES

Abdollahi, K.; Yazdani, F.; Panahi, R.; Mokhtarani, B. Biotransformation of Phenol in Synthetic Wastewater Using the Functionalized Magnetic Nano-Biocatalyst Particles Carrying Tyrosinase. *3 Biotech* **2018,** *8* (10), 419.

Ai, J.; Zhang, W.; Liao, G.; Xia, H.; Wang, D. *RSC Adv.* **2016,** *6*, 38117–38123.

Aleya, L.; Uddin, M. S. Environmental Pollutants and the Risk of Neurological Disorders. *Environ. Sci. Pollut. Res.* **2020,** *27*, 44657–44658. https://doi.org/10.1007/s11356-020-11272-3

Asadgol, Z.; Forootanfar, H.; Rezaei, S. et al. Removal of Phenol and Bisphenol—A Catalyzed by Laccase in Aqueous Solution. *J. Environ. Health Sci. Eng.* **2014,** *12*, 93.

Barrios-Estrada, C.; de Jesús Rostro-Alanis, M.; Parra, A. L.; Belleville, M.-P.; Sanchez-Marcano, J.; Iqbal, H. M. N.; Parra-Saldívar, R. Potentialities of Active Membranes with Immobilized Laccase for Bisphenol A Degradation. *Int. J. Biol. Macromol.* **2018,** *108*, 837–844.

Bello-Gil, D.; Roig-Molina, E.; Fonseca, J.; Sarmiento-Ferrandez, M. D.; Ferrándiz, M.; Franco, E.; Mira, E.; Maestro, B.; Sanz, J. M. An Enzymatic System for Decolorization of Wastewater Dyes Using Immobilized CueO Laccase-Like Multicopper Oxidase on Poly-3-Hydroxybutyrate. *Microb. Biotechnol.* **2018,** *11* (5), 881–892.

Bilal, M.; Mehmood, S.; Rasheed, T.; Iqbal, H. M. Antibiotics Traces in the Aquatic Environment: Persistence and Adverse Environmental Impact. *Curr. Opin. Environ. Sci. Health.* **2020,** *13*, 68–74. https:// doi.org/10.1016/j.coesh.2019.11.005.

Chang, Q.; Huang, J.; Ding, Y.; Tang, H. Catalytic Oxidation of Phenol and 2,4-Dichlorophenol by Using Horseradish Peroxidase Immobilized on Graphene Oxide/Fe_3O_4. *Molecules* **2016,** *21*, 1044.

Chiong, T.; Lau, S. Y.; Lek, Z. H.; Koh, B. Y.; Danquah, M. K. Enzymatic Treatment of Methyl Orange Dye in Synthetic Wastewater by Plant-Based Peroxidase Enzymes. *J. Environ. Chem. Eng.* **2016,** *4* (2), 2500–2509.

Çifçi, D. İ.; Atav, R.; Güneş, Y.; Güneş, E. Determination of the Color Removal Efficiency of Laccase Enzyme Depending on Dye Class and Chromophore. *Water Sci. Technol.* **2019,** *80* (1), 134–143.

Collivignarelli, M. C.; Abba, A.; Carnevale Miino, M.; Damiani, S. Treatments for Color Removal from Wastewater: State of the Art. *J. Environ. Manage.* **2019,** *236*, 727–745.

Diez, M. C. Biological Aspects Involved in the Degradation of Organic Pollutants. *J. Soil. Sci. Plant. Nutr.* **2010,** *10* (3), 244–267.

Eggen, R.I.L.; Hollender, J.; Joss, A.; Schärer, M.; Stamm, C. Reducing the Discharge of Micropollutants in the Aquatic Environment: The Benefits of Upgrading Wastewater Treatment Plants. *Environ. Sci. Technol.* **2014,** *48*, 7683–7689.

Ely, C.; Souza, D. H.; Fernandes, M.; Trevisan, V.; Skoronski, E. Enhanced Removal of Phenol from Biorefinery Wastewater Treatment Using Enzymatic and Fenton Process. *Environ. Technol.* **2021,** *42* (17), 2733–2739.

Fuller, R.; Landrigan, P. J.; Balakrishnan, K. et al. Pollution and Health: A Progress Update. *Lancet Planetary Health* **2022,** *6* (6), e535–e547.

Gao, X. J.; Fan, X. J.; Chen, X. P.; Ge, Z. Q. Immobilized β-Lactamase on Fe3O4 Magnetic Nanoparticles for Degradation of β-lactam Antibiotics in Wastewater. *Int. J. Environ. Sci. Technol.* **2017,** *15*, 2203–2212. DOI: 10.1007/s13762- 017-1596-4

Ho, K. C.; Teow, Y. H.; Sum, J. Y.; Ng, Z. J.; Mohammad, A. W. Water Pathways Through the Ages: Integrated Laundry Wastewater Treatment for Pollution Prevention. *Sci. Total Environ.* **2021,** *760*, 143966. https:// doi.org/10.1016/j.scitotenv.2020.143966.

Iracheta-Cárdenas, M. M.; Rocha-Pena, M. A.; Galan-Wong, L. J.; Arevalo-Nino, K.; Tovar-Herrera, O. E. A Pycnoporus Sanguineus Laccase for Denim Bleaching and Its Comparison with an Enzymatic Commercial Formulation. *J. Environ. Manage.* **2016,** *177*, 93–100.

Jager, C. M.; Croft, A. K. Anaerobic Radical Enzymes for Biotechnology. *Chem. Bio. Eng. Rev.* **2018,** *5*, 143–162. https://doi.org/10.1002/ cben.201800003

Klanovicz, N.; Stefanski, F. S.; Camargo, A. F.; Treichel, W. M. H.; Silva, A. C.; Teixeira, C. Complete Wastewater Discoloration by a Novel Peroxidase Source with Promising Bioxidative Properties. *J. Chem. Technol. Biotechnol.* **2022,** *97* (9), 2613–2625.

Kurnik, K.; Treder, K.; Skorupa-Kłaput, M.; Tretyn, A.; Tyburski, J. Removal of Phenol from Synthetic and Industrial Wastewater by Potato Pulp Peroxidases. *Water Air Soil Pollut.* **2015,** *226* (8), 254. DOI: 10.1007/s11270-015-2517-0.

Liu, S.; Xu, X.; Kang, Y.; Xiao, Y.; Liu, H. Degradation and Detoxification of Azo Dyes with Recombinant Ligninolytic Enzymes from Aspergillus sp. with Secretory Overexpression in *Pichia pastoris*. *R. Soc. Open Sci.* **2020,** *7*, 200688.

Luo, J.; Song, S.; Zhang, H.; Zhang, H.; Zhang, J.; Wan, Y. Biocatalytic Membrane: Go Far Beyond Enzyme Immobilization. *Eng. Life Sci.* **2020,** *20* (11), 441–450.

Mali, H.; Shah, C.; Raghunandan, B. H.; Prajapati, A. S.; Patel, D. H.; Trivedi, U.; Subramanian, R. B. Organophosphate Pesticides an Emerging Environmental Contaminant: Pollution, Toxicity, Bioremediation Progress, and Remaining Challenges. *J. Environ. Sci.* **2023,** 127, 234–250.

Meek, R. W.; Vyas, H.; Piddock, L. J. V. Nonmedical Uses of Antibiotics: Time to Restrict Their Use? *PLoS Biol.* **2015,** *13* (10). DOI: 10.1371/journal.pbio.1002266.

Mohanty, S. S.; Kumar, A. Enhanced Degradation of Anthraquinone Dyes by Microbial Monoculture and Developed Consortium Through the Production of Specific Enzymes. *Sci. Rep.* **2021,** *11*, 7678.

Pimentel, D. Environmental and Economic Costs of the Application of Pesticides Primarily in the United States. In: *Food, Energy, and Society*; Pimentel, M.; Pimentel, D., Eds., 3rd ed.; CRC Press, 2007.

Poirier, L.; Brun, L.; Jacquet, P.; Lepolard, C.; Armstrong, N.; Torre, C.; Daudé, D.; Ghigo, E.; Chabrière, E. Enzymatic Degradation of Organophosphorus Insecticides Decreases Toxicity in Planarians and Enhances Survival. *Sci. Rep.* **2017,** *7* (1), 15194. DOI: 10.1038/s41598-017-15209-8. PMID: 29123147; PMCID: PMC5680213.

Popli, S.; Patel, U. D. Destruction of Azo Dyes by Anaerobic–Aerobic Sequential Biological Treatment: A Review. *Int. J. Environ. Sci. Technol.* **2015,** *12* (1), 405–420.

Pravin, M. D.; Chris Felshia, S.; Gnanamani, A. *RSC Adv.* **2018, 8**, 38416–38424.

Saputera, W. H.; Putrie, A. S.; Esmailpour, A. A.; Sasongko, D.; Suendo, V.; Mukti, R. R. Technology Advances in Phenol Removals: Current Progress and Future Perspectives. *Catalysts* **2021,** *11*, 998.

Simon-Herrero, C.; Naghdi, M.; Taheran, M.; Kaur Brar, S.; Romero, A.; Valverde, J. L. et al. Immobilized Laccase on Polyimide Aerogels for Removal of Carbamazepine. *J. Hazard. Mater.* **2019,** *376*, 83–90.

Stadlmair, L. F.; Letzel, T.; Drewes, J. E.; Grassmann, J. Enzymes in Removal of Pharmaceuticals from Wastewater: A Critical Review of Challenges, Applications and Screening Methods for Their Selection. *Chemosphere* **2018,** *205*, 649–661. https://doi.org/10.1016/j.chemosphere.2018.04.142.

Thakur, M.; Medintz, I. L.; Walper, S. A. Enzymatic Bioremediation of Organophosphate Compounds-Progress and Remaining Challenges. *Front. Bioeng. Biotechnol.* **2019,** *7*, 289. DOI: 10.3389/fbioe.2019.00289. PMID: 31781549; PMCID: PMC6856225.

Thwaites, B. J.; Short, M. D.; Stuetz, R. M.; Reeve, P. J.; Alvarez Gaitan, J.-P.; Dinesh, N. et al. Comparing the Performance of Aerobic Granular Sludge Versus Conventional Activated Sludge for Microbial Log Removal and Effluent Quality: Implications for Water Reuse. *Water Res.* **2018,** *145*, 442–453.

Villegas, L. G. C.; Mashhadi, N.; Chen, M. et al. A Short Review of Techniques for Phenol Removal from Wastewater. *Curr. Pollut. Rep.* **2016,** *2*, 157–167.

Wei, C. M.; Feng, C. Y.; Li, S.; Zou, Y.; Yang, Z. Mushroom Tyrosinase Immobilized in Metal-Organic Frameworks as an Excellent Catalyst for Both Catecholic Product Synthesis and Phenolic Wastewater Treatment. *J. Chem. Technol. Biotechnol.* **2021,** *97* (4), 962–972.

Wu, Q.; Xu, Z.; Duan, Y.; Zhu, Y.; Oua, M.; Xu, X. *RSC Adv.* **2017,** 7, 28114–28123.

Xia, T. T.; Feng, M.; Liu, C. L.; Liu, C. Z.; Guo, C. Efficient Phenol Degradation by Laccase Immobilized on Functional Magnetic Nanoparticles in Fixed Bed Reactor Under High-Gradient Magnetic Field. *Eng. Life Sci.* **2021,** *21* (6), 374–381.

Zdarta, J.; Jankowska, K.; Bachosz, K.; Kijenska-Gawronska, E.; Zgo´łaGrze´skowiak, A.; Kaczorek, E. et al. A Promising Laccase Immobilization Using Electrospun Materials for Biocatalytic Degradation of Tetracycline: Effect of Process Conditions and Catalytic Pathways. *Catal. Today* **2020,** *348*, 127–136.

Zhang, C.; You, S.; Zhang, J.; Qi, W.; Su, R.; He, Z. An Effective In-Situ Method for Laccase Immobilization: Excellent Activity, Effective Antibiotic Removal Rate and Low Potential Ecological Risk for Degradation Products. *Bioresour. Technol.* **2020,** *308*, 123271.

Zheng, G.; Liu, S.; Zha, J.; Zhang, P.; Xu, X.; Chen, Y.; Jiang, S. Protecting Enzymatic Activity via Zwitterionic Nanocapsulation for the Removal of Phenol Compound from Wastewater. *Langmuir* **2019,** *35*, 1858–1863.

Zhu, Y.; Wang, W.; Ni, J.; Hu, B. Cultivation of Granules Containing Anaerobic Decolorization and Aerobic Degradation Cultures for the Complete Mineralization of Azo Dyes in Wastewater. *Chemosphere* **2020,** *246*, 125753. https://doi.org/10.1016/j.chemosphere.2019.125753

Zumstein, M. T.; Helbling, D. E. Biotransformation of Antibiotics: Exploring the Activity of Extracellular and Intracellular Enzymes Derived from Wastewater Microbial Communities. *Water Res.* **2019,** *155*, 115–123.

PART 2

FRONTIERS IN BIOENGINEERING AND BIOTECHNOLOGY

CHAPTER 3

Biomaterials from Sustainable Natural Sources for Tissue Engineering

NEBU GEORGE THOMAS[1], SHILPA JOY[2], P. K. BINCI[3], V. P. JAYACHANDRAN[4], PREETHA G. PRASAD[5], SHERIN JACOB[6], SHERIN SARA GEORGE[7], and ANIL SUKUMARAN[8]

[1]Pushpagiri Research Centre, Tiruvalla, Kerala, India

[2]Biotechnology, Sri Shakthi Institute of Engineering and Technology, Coimbatore, Tamil Nadu, India

[3]ICAR-Central Institute OF Fisheries Technology, Cochin, Kerala, India

[4]Applied Biology Section, Department of Applied Sciences, University of Technology and Applied Sciences, Muscat, Sultanate of Oman

[5]Department of Chemistry, Kumbalathu Sankupillai Memorial Devaswom Board College, Sasthamcotta, Kerala, India

[6]Faculty, School of Biosciences, MG University, Kottayam, Kerala, India

[7]Department of Pediatric and Preventive Dentistry, Pushpagiri College of Dental Sciences, Thiruvalla, Kerala, India

[8]Department of Dentistry, Oral Health Institute, Hamad Medical Corporation, Doha, Qatar

ABSTRACT

A wide range of tissue engineering scaffolds is developed from different biomaterials by various manufacturing methods that have been applied to regenerate different tissues and body organs. Many factors such as biodegradability, biocompatibility, mechanical properties, scaffold structures,

Application of Engineering Principles and Practices in Biotechnology.
Ann Rose Abraham, Leonardo Sepúlveda Torre, Tamara Tatrishvili, and A. K. Haghi (Eds.)

and manufacturing techniques are important in designing scaffolds used in regenerative medicine, regardless of tissue type. Natural polymers derived from environmentally friendly and sustainable resources like plants and marine sources meet the need for such novel biomaterials with desirable properties for tissue engineering which promise minimal chemical treatment for industrial applications. This chapter describes the development of biomaterials from sustainable natural plant and marine sources. The chapter also has pointed out the current limitations and challenges that must be addressed for the imperturbable application of these biomaterials in green chemistry and clinical application in tissue engineering.

3.1 INTRODUCTION

Tissue engineering requires the use of biomaterials throughout every step. In order to promote cell development and ultimate tissue repair, they are designed to construct an architectural framework that seems to be similar to natural extracellular matrix. Tissue engineering is devoted to the rebuilding of functional human tissues. Despite the fact that the body has inherent self-healing capacities, the degree of regeneration differs between tissues and can also be hampered by the intensity of an ailment or injury (Sell et al., 2020). The traditional paradigm orchestrates tissue creation and incorporation inside the host environment by utilizing a mix of biomaterial scaffolds, cells, and bioactive compounds. The creation of biomaterials that can facilitate regeneration processes by efficiently conveying cellular components and therapeutic substances as well as providing structural scaffolding that provides tissues appropriate mechanical characteristics is a key area of tissue engineering. Additionally, the biomaterial must preferably disintegrate at a pace that is equivalent to the formation of new tissue at the implantation site. Natural biomaterials are designed to imitate the biological and physical characteristics of the extracellular matrix that naturally occurs in all bodily tissues. Protein-based biomaterials, polysaccharide-based biomaterials, glycosaminoglycan-derived biomaterials, and tissue/organ-derived biomaterials are the four subtypes that make up natural biomaterials (Chen and Liu, 2016).

Many people worldwide suffer from end-stage organ disorders, and the only permanent treatment for such patients is organ transplantation. However, due to the ongoing organ scarcity, there is a sizable disparity seen between number of patients on the transplant waiting list, total quantity of donors, as well as the number of individuals who pass away while awaiting a transplant each year. In recent decades, several approaches and remedies have been attempted to address this issue; at the present, whole-organ bioengineering appears promising and has the potential to shift the current paradigm of organ scarcity in the near future. The perfect transplantable natural bioscaffold that contains all the required microarchitecture and extracellular signals for cell adhesion, differentiation, vascularization, and function is provided by the creation of decellularization procedures for the formation of whole-organ engineering. There have been various initiatives to produce whole organs. The liver, heart, kidney, and lung are a few of the key organs that are most widely used. Although there has been a lot of development so far, there are still considerable obstacles in whole-organ bioengineering that need to be addressed before this new technology may be used in clinical settings. These include choosing the best cell sources, locating signals for differentiation, accomplishing strong vascularization, optimizing bioreactor perfusion technology together with scalability, and avoiding graft immunological rejection. Suitable species that supply resorbable tissues are also identified (Charbe et al., 2022).

3.2 BIOMATERIALS BASED ON PLANT CELLULOSE AND PLANT-BASED POLYMERS

Recent years have witnessed substantial attention on regenerative medicine from scientific communities. There exists an imbalance between the number of availability of organs/graft materials and the population that needs them. Development of artificial organ substitutes as well as tissue regeneration would be an essential approach to fill in the void. The real-time solution for this issue is innovative approaches in the development and fabrication of economical, biodegradable, and biocompatible scaffolds bearing desirable geometrical structures and mechanical properties. This can be a great leap in the field of green medicine that utilizes ecofriendly materials in medicine. Biomaterials are transformed into scaffolds in various forms as hydrogels, sponges, decellularized ghost organs, pastes, micro- and nano-fibers, solid inert scaffolds, powders microsphere scaffolds, etc. Natural polymers may have undesirable effects possessing poor mechanical strength and this can be enhanced by combining them with synthetic polymers (Jahangirian et al., 2019).

In the recent past research communities got massively attracted to the creation and improvement of economically feasible as well as safer alternatives to, mammalian-based biomaterials. Scaffold proteins irrespective of being natural or synthetic by origin proffer enterprising and groundbreaking way out to the field of regenerative medicine. By rule, both natural and synthetic may have their own share of drawbacks and benefits. Even though naturally occurring materials are biodegradable and biocompatible many times they bear issues related to mechanical properties and contribute to concerns in easy handling during the ongoing process. In reality, collagen, keratin, and other proteins of animal origin may be risky from the perspective of the potential for transmitting animal viruses or prions. Certain proteins like silk fibroin bear longer rates of degradation that makes it practically difficult to sandwich into short-term applicability. Also silk fibroin can be associated with undesirable consequences like chronic inflammatory reaction as amylioidosis.

The extracellular matrix (ECM) can be defined as the noncellular component seen within all tissues and organs. ECM gives essential physical scaffolding for the cellular constituents as well as opens up significant biomechanical and biochemical signals that necessitate homeostasis tissue morphogenesis and differentiation. This noncellular component forms complex chemical and physical environment to aid in the cell functions. Proteins are regarded as beneficial factors owing to their bioactivity as well as likeness with the constituents of the native ECM. Residual degradation products from synthetic polymers like polyesters used in the preparation of scaffolds can bring down the pH in the immediate vicinity and lead to inflammatory reactions, cellular/tissue necrosis, as well as undesirable immune reactions. Also to shed off the clings of the noxious polymers and solvents utilized in the preparation of tissue engineering scaffolds, explorative studies are being conducted in the development of scaffolds from renewable resources and environment friendly materials, particularly from the photosynthetic beings viz., plants have gained growing noticeability in the arena of medical innovation. The traits of diversity, adaptability, availability, and cultivability make them attractive sources of biomaterials.

3.2.1 PLANT-DERIVED PROTEINS USED IN THE PREPARATION OF SCAFFOLDS

Reports highlight the possibility of developing scaffolds from plant proteins like soy protein, zein, wheat gluten, etc. underscoring the desirable properties such as biocompatibility, mechanical as well as aqueous stability. Zein and gliadin are considered to be favorable choices over animal components owing to their wide availability, structural diversity, as well as consistent quality. These plant proteins are also easy to blend with other synthetic biopolymers because of their specific solubility and film-forming properties. Zein and gliadin are favorable choices due to their wide availability, consistent quality, and structural diversity (Pascoli et al., 2018).

Even though plant proteins are highlighted for their advantageous traits, plant-based biomaterials generally are dimmed by their irrelevant physiochemical properties. Plant proteins (particularly soy proteins and gluten) have limited organic solvents (although less toxic compared to the conventional solvents such as chloroform used in tissue engineering); therefore, it becomes a difficult task to yield biomaterials from such proteins. Hence opportunities for developing composites are an attractive and efficient approach. Blending plant proteins with synthetic polymers as well as crosslinking are smart modes to be adopted to augment their biological responsiveness, water resistance, and mechanical properties to enable them to be suitable for medical functionalities applications. The possibility is that the cross-linking or blending process can interfere with the surface properties /biodegradability/biocompatibility of proteins (Jahangirian et al., 2019).

3.2.1.1 SOY PROTEIN

This is a globular protein; its source is soy beans scientifically known as Glycine max belonging to the family Fabaceae. This protein has a comparatively longer shelf life because of being relatively stable. Approximately 38% of soy bean is proteins. According to the sedimentation, this protein comprises four fractions viz., 2S, 7S, 11S, and 15S. Conglycinin 7S and glycinin 11S are the two important subunits in soy protein, Glycinin and β-conglycinin along with α- and γ-conglycinin lead to the formation of storage proteins that become the source of proteins for the seedlings. The globular structure of soy protein makes it hydrolysis resistant compared to that of the helical or coiled structures. Therefore, while being immersed in different pH buffer solutions, it can behave as polycation or polyanion. Soy protein has an isoelectric point of approximately 4.8 and at this pH the solubility and swelling of soy protein is low, but the swelling ratio can be enhanced either by increasing or decreasing the pH of the buffer solution. Enhanced solubility by pH increment could aid in the electrospinning-mediated fabrication of soy protein fibers.

The dissolution and solution viscosity of soy protein isolate in aqueous medium can be altered based on the heating time and temperature. In the electrospinning method electric field resulted in the drifting of soy protein hydrogel films to the negative or positive electrodes based on the pH of the solution. In general, soy protein possesses controllable degradability as well as substantial water stability and mechanical properties.

Soy protein isolate hydrogel hydrogels bear notable potential for utilizing in electroactive micro sensors and actuators as well as for biomedical applications. On heating, the 7S and 11S globulins possess the ability to interact and form a strong network. The functional groups like OH, SH, and NH2 enable the protein to be chemically or physically modified or to be composited with other biopolymers (Pascoli et al., 2018).

3.2.1.2 ZEIN

Zein belonging to the prolamin class is considered the major protein seen in maize and it contributes approximately 50% of the total protein content in maize. The composition of zein shows lipophilic amino acid residues. This alcohol-soluble protein comprises various subunits including α, β, γ-zein, and δ-zein, among which α-zein form accounts for approximately above 70% of the total zein protein and is available in commercial form. Low water solubility and negative nitrogen balance make it away from the thought of direct human consumption.

Various properties like cytoaffinity, hydrophobicity, biocompatibility, convertibility to colloidal well as high coating capacity and ability to resist microbial interference, zein finds applications as thin films, porous scaffolds as well as in modified delivery systems for drugs, enzymes etc. Certain studies proved that potential of zein-based porous scaffold to impact the growth and differentiation of mesenchymal cells. Zein is found to possess insufficient mechanical properties as well as poor water stability and therefore can be used in aqueous environment only on further crosslinking or blending with other polymers. This protein has been electrospun to form 2D ultra-fine fibers for biomedical functions. Zein has been electrospun into 2D ultra-fine fibers for biomedical applications (Jahangirian et al., 2019; Reddy and Yang, 2011).

3.2.1.3 GLIADIN

Gliadin is one of the major gluten storage proteins found in wheat and several other cereals classified under the genus Triticum and is composed of single-chain polypeptides with an average molecular weight of 25–100 kDa connected by intramolecular disulfide (S–S) bonds. The presence of S-S bonds and co-operative hydrophobic interactions lead the protein chains to take up a folded shape. It contributes to 30% protein in wheat and it contributes to the flow properties of bread dough. By definition, this is protein group extracted from gluten by 70% ethanol and is insoluble in aqueous and neutral salt solutions. In the presence of extreme pH they show solubility in aqueous solutions. Based on the electrophoretic mobility gliadins are categorized as α-, β-, γ-, and ω-gliadins. This protein possesses significantly low solubility in aqueous solution. It has carrier role for controlled release of cationic and lipophilic drugs owing to its unique physicochemical properties. This protein can deliver sensitive enzymes and protect these enzymes from break down by stomach acids. Gliadin is noted to have drawbacks like low water stability as well as immunogenic toxicity in individuals with celiac disease. Certain study proved that blending a small amount of gliadin with PCL into composite biomaterial inks for scaffold fabrication enhanced cell affinity and suppressed gliadin's side effect. These proteins do not show the common drawbacks of synthetic materials pertaining to the presence of monomer/ initiator residues (Reddy and Yang, 2011). Also certain study highlighted the Electrohydrodynamic printing (EHDP) of polycaprolactone (PCL)-gliadin biomaterial ink resulted in composite scaffold with notable improvement in tensile strength as well as improved cell adhesion and proliferation of mouse embryonic fibroblasts (NIH/3T3). A similar effect was also noticed in case of PCL/zein composite ink derived scaffold (Ramji and Shah, 2014).

3.2.1.4 GLUTENIN

Wheat glutenin is the highly cross-linked protein from wheat and it contributes approximately to 50%, of the total protein in wheat grain. Glutenin contributes to its elasticity and strength of bread dough. This protein is made up of macropolymers of high- and low-molecular weight subunits crosslinked with S-S bonds. The random fusing of these macropolymers with individual gliadins results in aggregates that are held together by noncovalent interactions. It is intrinsically soluble in water due to the presence of 2% cysteine contributing to the amino acid composition (Reddy and Yang, 2011; Jing et al., 2020). Urade et al (2018) reported that disulfide cross links cleaved wheat glutenin after dissolving in aqueous solvent with an anionic surfactant later electro spun to make bulky scaffolds with ultrafine fibers in 3D form.

On incubation in phosphate-buffered saline for 35 days, these 3D scaffolds could retain their fibrous structures and they maintained uniform distribution as well as adipogenic differentiation of adipose-derived mesenchymal stem cells (Xu et al., 2014; Urade et al., 2017).

3.2.1.5 PLANT-DERIVED BIOSYNTHETIC PROTEINS—A RECOMBINANT APPROACH

The turn of the new millennium has led to a gigantic face lift in the field of Biotechnology. Genetic engineering has ship shaped many new tools and techniques and recombinant proteins are one of the essential outcomes of the recent developments. Recombinant proteins can be defined as exogenous proteins that are expressed in a host called production organism and the expressed protein can be used for purposes like in the prevention of therapy of diseases in humans or animals. This approach has become a potent device for fighting various ailments which have previously been considered hard to treat.

Even though the most exploited expression systems include bacteria like *Escherichia coli*, yeast like Pichiapastoris and mammalian system as the Chinese Hamster Ovary cells, they bear pros and cons pertaining to expense, protein size, time of development, yield, growth conditions, posttranslational modifications, size of the proteins, and regulatory approval. Plant Science has developed to a greater extent to device advanced technologies to grow and harvest crops in an economically feasible and efficient manner. To grow plants comparatively simple conditions like water, environment, sunlight, and fertilizers are only needed (Burnett and Burnett, 2020).

Silk worm originated silk and spider silk are considered to be superior materials for tissue regeneration. Spider silk is made up of the spidron protein and it is successfully expressed in tobacco plant (Peng et al., 2020). Table1.1 highlights the advantages and disadvantages associated with plants as expression systems for proteins.

3.3.3 PLANT POLYSACCHARIDES

Plant polysaccharides, also known as glycans, are natural polycarbohydrates with a back bone of many identical or different monosaccharide subunits linked by ether bonds, viz., α- or β-glycosidic linkages. Plants can synthesize diverse polysaccharides with the type of monosaccharide, the nature of their interconnections, and the complexity of the structure. These are structural constituents of the cell wall.

3.3.3.1 APPLICATIONS OF PLANT POLYSACCHARIDES

Plant polysaccharides are attractive biomaterials for the following applications:

Tissue engineering: In bone tissue engineering, scaffolds based on Polysaccharides are preferred due to low cost, biocompatibility, biodegradability, and mechanical properties. Moreover, these scaffolds can enhance the rate of cell proliferation and adhesion. The cell adhesion and proliferation properties can be further enhanced by increase of surface area via reinforcement of native polysaccharide by nanomaterials. The nontoxicity and gel-forming ability of the polysaccharides are explored for the fabrication of easily removable antimicrobial and anti-inflammatory wound dressings for skin tissue engineering applications. The healing can be improved by the encapsulation of antimicrobial and anti-inflammatory drugs into wound dressing (Buck et al., 2018). Recent studies explore the efficacies by incorporation of other antimicrobial agents such as essential oils in the wound dressing (Wang et al., 2021).

Drug delivery: Recent studies showed the plant polysaccharides as potent drug delivery system because they can act as low surface energy neutral coating excluding the binding of nonspecific proteins encountering low immunogenicity. They also show the ability to encapsulate and protect the drug (Raeisi and Raeisi, 2020)

Bioactive Plant Polysaccharides for biomedical applications

The recent trends of research confronting biomedical applications stimulated the development of plant polysaccharides for potential biomedical applications. The compounds that are widely in use are: starch, cellulose, hemicellulose, pectins, inulin, and gums.

3.3.3.2 STARCH

Starch is formed from two structurally different polysaccharides, amylose and amylopectin. Both these residues contain only D-glucose molecules connected by α-(1,4) linkages in amylose and α-(1,4) linkages and α-(1,6) linkages at branching points. The structure is given in Fig. 1. The size, shape, and morphology of the starch depend on the biological source. It is a suitable biomaterial for the formation of films and gels which could be further employed for the incorporation of bioactive components for controlled release for wound healing (Aliabadi et al., 2020), drug delivery (Koev et al., 2020), and bone tissue engineering (Mohammadinejad et al., 2019). Recently, the limitations of poor mechanical properties and water sensitivity afforded by starch are improved by the chemical modification of native starch which broadened their scope in bioengineering applications (Jelkmann et al., 2019).

3.3.3.3 CELLULOSE

Cellulose is the most abundant polymeric material on our planet, made up of β- (1→4) glucose units. It is a linear homopolymer with extensive hydrogen-bonding forces acting to promote its crystalline properties. The glucose units in cellulose are linked by β glycosidic bonds. The interconnectivity and porosity offer it for biomedical drug delivery and food packaging applications (Gopinath et al., 2022).

3.3.3.4 HEMICELLULOSE

Hemicelluloses (pylose) have shorter polymeric chains than cellulose. This branched copolymer formed from both pentoses and hexoses and is the second most abundant chemical constituent present along with cellulose in plant cell walls. The possibility of chemical modification of the hydroxyl and carboxylic groups makes it highly suitable for a variety of biomedical applications (Liu et al., 2020). It is versatile for food packaging functional material (Nechita et al., 2021)

3.3.3.5 PECTIN

Pectin is essential for the initial growth and ripening process of fruit and waste material from the food and fruit processing industry. The main component of pectin is α-1,4-linked D-galacturonic acid units. It has got immense biomedical applications due to the health effects including hypoglycemic and hypocholesterolemic properties. Usually, pectin is modified with selected organic, inorganic, or polymeric molecules and synthesized in the form of capsules, hydrogels etc. to improve the inherently low mechanical strength and fast degradation. Such blends of pectin are widely in use for the preparation of hydrogels for tissue regeneration applications (Bostancı et al., 2022).

3.3.3.6 INULIN

Structure of inulin consists of a mixture of oligomers and polymers that belong to the group of gluco-fructanslinked by β-2,1-bonds. Gels made from Inulin are ideal drug delivery biomaterial despite its swelling in physiological fluids (Afinjuomo et al., 2021).

Guar Gum: Guar gum is a water-soluble plant polysaccharide composed of linear chain of (1 → 4)-linked β-D-mannopyranosyl units with (1 → 6)-linked α-D-galactopyranosyl residues as side chains. This polymer is very used in the development of hydrogels with potent applications as biomaterial because of its easy dispersion in water (Das et al., 2011).

3.3.3.7 LIGNIN

Lignin being one of the components of plant cell wall is highly abundant in nature. It is a complex and irregular amorphous biopolymer containing randomly crosslinked phenylpropanoid units. They play a significant role in plant cell formation particularly in wood and bark of trees as they provide rigidity. A plant cell wall comprises three layers viz., the primary cell wall, the middle lamella, and the secondary cell wall. The cell wall constituents are cellulose microfibrils, hemicellulose, lignin, pectin, and soluble protein. Due to the versatility and chemical diversity of the polyphenolic chemical structure, the chemical industry has focused on its use as a viable alternative of renewable raw material.

Drug delivery System: Lignin-based scaffolds find immense applications as a renewable material for drug encapsulation. The lignin-derived nanoparticles with lower concentration of silver showed significant broad spectral biocidal activity against both gram-negative and gram-positive human pathogens as well as quaternary amine-resistant bacteria (Richter et al., 2015) gradable particle after the release, thus having a smaller impact on the environment.

Tissue engineering: An alginate–lignin composite prepared as aerogels of nano-sized interconnecting pores showed low stiffness in the range of fibrous tissue without cytotoxic effects on mouse fibroblast-like L929 cells in vitro (Barros et al., 2016).

The higher antioxidant activity reported for lignin is being explored for delivery of selected active ingredients for repairing aged wounded or burned skin in combination with the antiaging efficacies of carbon nanotubes (Morganti et al., 2017).

3.3.4 PLANT SECONDARY METABOLITES: POTENT LEAD FOR BIOLOGICALLY ACTIVE COMPOUNDS

Secondary metabolites are synthesized from primary metabolites with functional roles in defense, signaling, symbiosis, and so on which are not essential for vegetative growth (Collin, 2001). Plant secondary metabolites can be classified into four distinct groups, such as terpenes, phenolics, alkaloids, and glycosides.

3.3.4.1 TERPENES (TERPENOIDS)

The terpenes represent the largest group of secondary metabolites which are normally insoluble in water and biosynthesized either from acetyl CoA or intermediates of glycolysis. Structurally these are polymers of isoprene units which consist of the branched five-carbon isoprene skeleton and consequently often referred to as isoprenoid compounds. Terpenoids possess antitumor, anti-inflammatory, antibacterial, antiviral, antimalarial effects, promote transdermal absorption, prevent and treat cardiovascular diseases, and have hypoglycemic activities.

3.3.4.2 PHENOLICS

These compounds contain one or more phenol groups with simple structures containing one aromatic ring to complex polymeric substances. They are widespread in plants and contribute significantly to the color, taste, and flavor of many herbs, food, and drinks. Some phenolics are valuable pharmacologically for their anti-inflammatory activities such as quercetin or anti-hepato toxic properties such as silybin. According to their structure phenolics can be classified as simple phenolics, tannins, coumarins, flavonoids, and so on.

3.3.4.3 ALKALOID

These are often basic and physiologically active secondary metabolite containing nitrogen heterocycle as their structural unit. Some alkaloids such as colchicine and piperine are neutral as N is present as amide group in these. Alkaloids show wide spectrum of biological activities including antiviral, antibacterial, anti-inflammatory, immunomodulatory, and anticancer properties.

3.3.4.4 SAPONINS

Selectively referred to as triterpene glycosides are bitter-tasting usually toxic plant-derived organic chemicals that have a foamy quality when agitated in water. These surface-active properties distinguish these compounds from other glycosides. They are widely distributed but found particularly in soapwort. They are used in medicinal soaps, medicinal, fire extinguishers, speciously as dietary supplements, for the synthesis of steroids, and in carbonated beverages. Structurally, they are glycosides, sugars bonded to another organic molecule, usually a steroid or triterpene.

3.3.4.5 CARBOHYDRATES

Being the first product of photosynthesis, carbohydrates are the starting point for all phytochemicals. The most abundant single organic substance on earth is cellulose. Although carbohydrates are primary metabolites, they are incorporated in plenty of secondary metabolites through glycosidic linkages. Polymers of simple sugars and uronic acids produce mucilage and gums.

3.3.5 PLANT EXTRACTS AS BIOMATERIALS

Wound healing: Healing of chronic wounds for patients with complementary diseases is a challenge in skin tissue engineering and was managed by wound dressings based on collagen/gelatin and proposed variants loaded with bioactive compounds derived from plants (Gaspar-Pintiliescu et al., 2019).

Tissue engineering: Excellent bone repair scaffolds were prepared from plan extracts and nanohydroxyapatite and anionic collagen (Rajathurai et al., 2018).

The extracts from Mimosa pudica, Plumbago indica, Vitex trifolia, Glycyrrhiza glabra, Alstonia scholaris, Withania somnifera, and Aegle marmelos have been well explored for the anticancer property and the antioxidant activity of the plant extract ensured the decrease of the adverse side effects of chemo and radiotherapy (Rajathurai et al., 2018).

3.3.6 BIOMATERIALS BASED ON PLANT TISSUES

The tremendous developments in the field of tissue engineering opened up doors to many novel tools and techniques. Tissue engineering demands a precise architecture of engineered biomaterials capable of regenerating the affected tissues in an injured location. The approach of decellularization of tissues proffers the added advantage of avoidance of materials' processing steps as the biomimetic native structure can be preserved while removing the cellular components to obtain three-dimensional acellular scaffolds for tissue engineering applications (Rajathurai et al., 2018). Otherwise, decellularized tissues can be considered valuable substitute as tissue engineering scaffolds. Here, the decellularized tissues perform the role of biomimetic microenvironment aid in the cell and tissue growth. Decellularization comprises steps by which removal of native cells from tissues is achieved by the use of bleach and detergents leading to the elimination of protein or DNA. Decellularized matrices offer appropriate biochemical as well as morphological microenvironment for the adhesion of the cells as well as their proliferation and differentiation (Wu et al., 2015). In reality, on implantation to a host, decellularized matrices result in lower immune response compared to xenogeneic and allogeneic transplants, due to loss or alteration of immunogenicity pertaining to the intracellular components during the process of decellularization.

Literature highlights the use of various decellularized animal-derived tissues to make extracellular matrix (ECM) scaffolds with a conserved vascular architecture for nutrients as well as oxygen transport in the bone, skin, and vascular grafts. These days such acellular patches are commercially available. For example, Alloderm utilized in the breast reconstruction procedures is a pliable sheet of sterile and dehydrated tissue from the skin of cadaver from which the cells are removed. In the past decade decellularized whole organs like lungs, heart liver, kidney, pancreas of animal or human origin were availed with partial organ functionality after colonization by cells. But the promising outcomes do not wiped off the associated negative attributes like ethical concerns, expensive predisposition, variability of the donors (age of the donor, pathology, and explant site) limited availability, adverse host interactions, and the possibility of infections (Gaspar-Pintiliescu et al., 2019; Contessi Negrini et al., 2020).

All these undesirable facets of the animal-based decellularized tissues made the scientific community search for safer alternatives. Recent years have witnessed increased acceptance for plant-derived tissues (Phan et al., 2020) as an efficient alternative to animal sources. Due to their low cost, ready availability, ease of processing and application, cytocompatibility and lack of ethical issues underscore plant tissues' promising nature. The broad array of characteristics borne by various plants bring in exceptional prospect for the fabrication of tissue-specific scaffolds. This is based on the unique architecture, mechanical, or physical properties of particular plants and enables them to mimic a range of mammalian tissues (Scarrit, 2015), depending on the morphological, physical, and mechanical peculiarities of each plant.

Typically, decellularization of plant tissues can be achieved by treating plant samples with sodium dodecyl sulfate (SDS) for particular time interval on a shaker incubator and subjected to sonication, after which the treated plant material can be washed with distilled water followed by calcium chloride. Later these samples are incubated with amphotericin/streptomycin to avoid fungal contamination. Subsequently, these samples are disinfected in 70% v/v ethanol solution, washed and frozen at −20°C, freeze dried and UV radiated prior to in vitro cell culture-based studies (Contessi Negrini et al., 2020).

Various parts of the plants are decellularized for making scaffolds. By preserving their branched veins that resemble the mammalian vasculature, 2D scaffolds were prepared from the leaves of Artemisia annua. Anthurium, Ficus hispida, Spinacia. Decellularized spinach leaves showed cardiomyocytes proliferation highlighting the potential such scaffolds in cardiac tissue regeneration (Gershlak et al., 2017; Hickey et al., 2018). Alternatively, tubular scaffolds fabricated using decellularized vanilla and bamboo stems resulted in cellular proliferation. Decellularized apple hypanthium (the cuplike enlargement of the apple fruit), mushroom cap, and green onion bulb resulted in 3D scaffolds supporting mammalian cell growth and colonization. Porosity of such scaffolds enabled the nutrient transport while keeping in culture media and apple-based scaffold displayed angiogenesis (Lee et al., 2019; Contessi Negrini et al., 2020).

In yet another study that subjected decellularized celery, carrot and apple in cell culture, apple showed porous scaffolds with pores within the range 70–420 μm. They showed stability in phosphate-buffered saline up to 7 weeks at human body temperature. On coating with poly-L-lysine, apples supported 3T3-L1 preadipocytes adhesion, proliferation, and adipogenic differentiation, whereas carrots exhibited MC3T3-E1 pre-osteoblasts adhesion, proliferation, and osteogenic differentiation. Celery displayed L929 cells adhesion, proliferation, and guided anisotropic cells orientation (Contessi Negrini et al., 2020). Truly speaking, the pro-angiogenic traits borne by fruit/plant-based scaffolds by virtue of their cytocompatibility as well as the interconnected porous channels depict them as prospective candidates in the application of cell and tissue proliferation and growth.

Scientific community is in continuous search for novel and innovative products and processes. The turn of the new millennium has seen gigantic facelifts in the field of medicine by the advances in tissue engineering, genetic engineering, and regenerative medicine. Tissue engineering scaffolds has attracted wide acceptance in the past few years. Scaffolds prepared from a plethora of materials both synthetic and natural as well as composites prepared by proportionate combination of synthetic/natural materials brought in better efficiency as well as enhanced healing potential. Synthetic scaffold materials may result in undesirable immunological reactions. In fact, animal-based, plant-based, and microbial-based raw materials are used in the engineering of scaffolds because of their biological origin and natural disposition.

Plant-based polymers being natural bear biocompatibility, biodegradability, physicochemical-mechanical properties, as well as desirable scaffold architecture. The usage of plant-based materials eliminates the chances of transmission of infectious agents like viruses and prions to the host. Another noteworthy benefit of plant scaffolds is the ease with which they can be fabricated or manipulated. The nature of being inexpensive, renewable, pliable, as well as easy to process make plant-based biomaterials attractive candidates for the development of tissue engineering scaffolds as hydrogels, films, membranes, sponges, etc. Many times the processing and storage of raw materials of animal origin lead to undesirable outcomes related to processing and disposal compared to plant-based constituents. Plant-based constituents like proteins, polysaccharides, lignin, secondary metabolites, and decellularized tissues are proved to be efficient scaffold materials. The utilization of vegetal tissues from fruits and vegetables as well as leaves and stems to be modified as 3D scaffolds can be highlighted as an accessible, economical, and sustainable approach. Even though plants materials have their own share of positive and negative attributes, these drawbacks can be modulated into beneficial effect by cutting edge technology and multifarious approaches of physical/chemical modification as well as by transforming them into composite structures.

3.4 BIOMATERIALS BASED ON SEAWEED POLYMERS AND MARINE SOURCES

3.4.1 COLLAGEN AND GELATIN

The connective tissue matrix, which forms the framework of the skin, bones, joints, cornea, blood vessels, and placenta, contains collagen as the major organic phase. Collagen alone makes up about one-third of the human body's protein (Aberoumand, 2012).

Collagen is structured by three polypeptide helices (triple helix). Based on helical composition, collagen is categorized into several types, of which 90% of human body collagen falls into Type-I category. It is widely distributed in skin, bones, teeth, ligaments, tendons, and the placenta, where it mainly contributes toward the mechanical strength of the structures. Type- II collagen forms the basis of articular cartilage and hyaline cartilage (Horton et al., 1989). Type-III collagen is the second most abundant collagen in human tissues and is primarily responsible for the elastic properties of skin, blood vessels, and various internal organs.

Recently, collagen-based biocomposites have gained great momentum in biomedical applications, as collagen shields in ophthalmology, burns, and wound-healing sponges, collagen-liposome composite for sustained drug delivery, matrices for cell culture systems, surface coating material for metallic bone implants, and 3-D printed matrix for guided tissue regeneration. The unique characteristics of collagen such as absence of antigenicity and superior biocompatibility support cell adhesion and cell proliferation and a lack of cytotoxicity, qualify collagen as an excellent material for biomedical applications (Smethurst et al., 2007).

Collagen is the most commonly employed biopolymer for tissue engineering applications as it is a component of extracellular matrix of virtually all human tissues. The use of collagen as a biomaterial has been widely investigated globally, when cellular interaction of extracted collagen was first revealed (Huzella and Lengyel, 1932; Ehrmann and Gey, 1956). More recently, collagen was explored for its application in vascular medicine as functional coating for vascular grafts. Collagen provides receptor-ligand binding sites for endothelial cells on the graft surface as well as it reduces the porosity of grafts (Copes et al., 2019).

It is known that collagen fibril (25–30%) and Hydroxyapatite (HAp) (60–70%) are the main components of bone. Per se, collagen Type- I and hydroxyapatite are known to promote osteoblast differentiation, but together, are shown to stimulate the process of osteogenesis (Xie et al., 2004). Integration of collagen to ceramic devices imparts several advantages such as shape uniformity, improved adhesion properties (both particle and defect wall), and favors clot formation and stabilization. Most importantly, these composites possess much higher degradation rate of 2 months to maximum of a year, whereas polymeric scaffolds may take up to 2 years for complete degradation. Thus, composite structures of collagen and hydroxyapatite are more promising to elicit good bone tissue reaction, rather than collagen or HAp alone. The last two decades have seen continuous attempts on the development of HAp-collagen composites in various forms such as membranes, scaffolds, and gels for tissue regeneration applications. Such composites apparently retain the features of both collagen (viscoelasticity) and HAp (hardness). In effect, the presence of hydroxyapatite significantly enhances the tensile modulus and strength of the composite structure compared to the tropocollagen fibril matrix alone, even though the stiffening effect is strongly dependent on the thickness and distribution of HAp crystals. In response, the ductile properties of collagen help to increase the poor fracture toughness of hydroxyapatites. Rodrigues et al. (2003) fabricated a composite scaffold composed of hydroxyapatite sintered at 1100°C and Type-I collagen having osteoconductive and osteoinductive properties. The scaffold was shown to perform as an ideal matrix for the attachment and proliferations of human osteoblasts, which seemed to guide cells between adjacent particles. Apart from the mechanical and adhesion properties, the average porosity and pore diameter are crucial factors for tissue scaffolds. A patent obtained by Shoji and Corp (2011) explains the method for controlling the average pore diameter of an apatite/collagen porous body by optimizing environment temperature for solidifying the gel dispersion comprising fibrous apatite/collagen composite and collagen as a binder. In bone replacements, Type-I collagen-based implants are preferred over inert implants as the former exhibits better osteoblast adhesion properties. The Type-I collagen-based implants, which possess the characteristic aminoacid sequence (Arg-Gly-Asp), can be directly recognized by the cell membrane receptors such as integrins.

The functional performance of HAp-collagen composite scaffolds was extensively studied during the last couple of decades. Venugopal et al. (2008) observed significantly higher mineral deposition on Collagen-HAp composite nanofibrous scaffolds cultured with osteoblasts than that on Collagen nanofibrous scaffolds during 10 days of culture period. The superiority of porous HAp-collagen composite for bone regeneration in comparison to an established commercially available porous β-TCP was confirmed by Sotome et al. (2016). Also, collagen-HAp porous scaffold was successfully employed for cheekbone augmentation, which showed prominent ossification with low inflammation, confirming new bone formation over time (D'Agostino et al., 2016). The performance of Hydroxyapatite/collagen composite as a substitute for conventional corticocancellous autografts was demonstrated by Yoshida and Fujio (2016). Interestingly, Wang et al. (2016) in an in vivo experiment showed that a composite scaffold of Type-I collagen and hydroxyapatite (HA)/β-tricaleium phosphate (TCP) scaffold performed equally as well as Bio-Oss Collagen, a widely used bone graft in ridge preservation. Collagen was replaced by gelatin in many studies for the fabrication of three-dimensional nanofiber-Gelatin/apatite composite scaffolds, which mimic both nanoscale architecture and chemical composition of natural bone extra cellular matrix. (Liu et al. (2009) showed higher stability than other ratio compositions. The HAp-Collagen composites with bone-like orientation of HAp nanocrystals with c-axis regularly aligned along collagen fibrils are the ideal confirmation expected for tissue scaffolds (Itoh et al., 2004). As this is a unique conformational feature of bone matrix, more research inputs are needed for the fabrication of nanofibrous Collagen/HAp composite, which exactly mimics the complex nanostructured architecture of collagen matrix with c-axis orientation of nano-HAp particles.

Collagen-based devices such as sponges and membranes have been widely explored commercially for the treatment of burns and as wound dressing material (Chattopadhyay and Raines, 2014). These devices can be loaded with therapeutic medicines like growth factors so as to speed up the process of tissue regeneration and wound healing. Collagen-based materials are frequently used in orthopedic surgery as an osteogenic scaffold and filler material (Zhang et al., 2018). As an osteochondral scaffold, type I collagen-hydroxyapatite composite scaffolds have been widely explored to enhance bone and cartilage regeneration (Kon et al., 2011).

Collagen has been widely employed for dental treatment in different forms viz. films, 3D dermal matrix, and in combination with other polymers (Wang et al., 2020). Collagen is employed in the fabrication of most of the resorbable membranes used clinically for treating periodontal defects (e.g., Bio-Gide®, Osteohealth, USA; Cytoplast™ barrier membranes, Osteogenics Biomedical, USA) (Zhang et al., 2009). Collagen is proffered over several other biopolymers due to its superior characteristics such as optimum biodegradation rate, strong angiogenesity, fibroblasts chemotaxis, clot stabilization, and favorable tissue integration (Schwarz et al., 2008). Collagen scaffolds not only act as a substratum for mineralization, but also serve as the template for the ossification of bone matrices. The composite of collagen with hydroxyapatite and β-Tricalcium phosphate is well studied as they act complimentary to each other, that the brittleness of hydroxyapatite is counterfeited by the malleability and plasticity of collagen fibers (Lin et al., 2019).

Gelatin, the partially hydrolyzed collagen, can be one of the promising biomaterials for the regenerative medicine and is widely employed in orthopedic and dental therapy (Zhang et al., 2009). Gelatin, in comparison to collagen, possess low toxicity and angiogenicity in in vivo implantation experiments in animal models. Moreover, gelatin is comparatively inexpensive with similar cell adhesion and proliferation characteristics as that of collagen. Similarly to collagen, gelatin also exhibits wound healing and tissue regeneration properties (Fassina et al., 2010). The unique peptide sequence (Arg-Gly-Asp) of gelatin is said to be congenial for supporting to promote cell adhesion and migration (Dreesmann et al., 2007).

3.4.2 CHITINS

Chitin and its derivatives, including chitosan and chitosan oligomers, are collectively referred as "chitins," a name that has recently been coined. Chitin plays a crucial structural role in the cell walls of some plant-pathogenic fungi, including Zygomycets. Chitosan is generated by deacetylating chitin. Chitin and chitosan are biodegradable, nontoxic substances with a wide range of industrial uses. Chitosan is a polycationic polymer with degree of acetylation between 5 and 30%.

The biological effects of chitosan and its derivatives, including their antioxidant, antiallergic, anti-inflammatory, anticoagulant, anticancer, antibacterial, antihuman immunodeficiency virus, antihypertensive, anti-Alzheimer's, antidiabetic, antiobesity, and matrix metalloproteinases inhibitory activities, have been extensively studied for biomedical applications. The antibacterial property is the one that has been discussed the most in literature among these (Ardean et al., 2021). The antimicrobial activity of chitosan is thought to be caused by two main mechanisms: the first is that chitosan, which is polycationic in nature, interferes with bacterial metabolism by electrostatically stacking at the bacterial cell surface (Chung and Chen, 2008); the other is that chitosan prevents RNA transcription. Structurally, chitosan has three different reactive functional groups, including an amino/acetamido group and primary and secondary hydroxyl groups at the C-2, C-3, and C-6 positions. The primary factors of functionality in chitosan are the degree of acetylation and/or deacetylation of amino group, molecular weight, and chain length (Zhang et al., 2010). Chitosan sold commercially has a molecular weight range of around 1,00,000 to 10,00,000 Da.

Current research on the biocompatible natural polymers chitin and chitosan focuses on tissue engineering (bone, cartilage, skin, etc.), drug delivery, and wound healing. Because of their structural resemblance to glycosaminoglycans, the main component of bone's extracellular matrix, chitin, and chitosan are considered excellent scaffold materials for tissue engineering. Additionally, both chitin and chitosan possess good biocompatibility, non-antigenicity, biodegradability, antibacterial activity, and strong adsorption qualities. Chitin and chitosan are easily moldable into nanofibers, beads, gels, scaffolds, and other shapes. Additionally, the porous and interconnected network imparts osteoconductivity to chitosan scaffolds, which is congenial for guided tissue regeneration and bone healing. The biomineralization property of chitosan is well elucidated in several studies and hence chitosan scaffold is considered the universal template for mineralized tissue regeneration.

Tissue engineering structures based on chitin/chitosan ceramic nanocomposites loaded with growth factors is a recent area of research focus. Chitin/chitosan nanofibers can attract and support attachment of stem cells onto the scaffolds, thereby promoting cell adhesion, proliferation, and osteogenic differentiation after 7 days' culture in vitro (Chen et al., 2011). The mechanical strength of chitin-nanohydroxyapatite composite gels was ten times more than that of control chitin gels (Chang et al., 2013). Chitosan has been combined with tricalcium phosphate to form granulates, having MG63 cell proliferation capacity and higher alkaline phosphatase activity (Kowalczyk et al., 2021). An asymmetric chitosan guided bone regeneration membrane composed of a dense layer that protects the bone from the invasion of neighboring connective fibrous tissue and a loose layer that can promote cell adhesion was fabricated by Ma et al. (2016). Chitin from marine demosponge has been shown to be a promising and highly biocompatible biomaterial for stem cell-mediated tissue engineering (Mutsenko et al., 2017).

Chitin-based materials have been successfully fabricated into fibrous and tubular forms for application as a cell proliferation template for nerves and blood vessels (Machałowski et al., 2019; Lu et al., 2021). Furthermore, composite scaffolds made up of chitin/chitosan nanofibers blended with other polymers improve the biological and mechanical performances of the scaffold. Shalumon et al. (2009) reported the fabrication of a composite scaffold based on electrospun nanofibers of water-soluble carboxymethyl chitin (CMC-7%) and PVA (8%). The scaffold exhibited superior cell attachment and cell proliferation properties. Similarly, Peter et al. (2010) reported chitosan-gelatin/nanohydroxyapatite (nHAp) tissue engineering scaffold having superior biological responses. More recently, a novel biomimetic two-faced guided bone regeneration membrane with a chitin nanofiber face for bone regeneration and an antifouling polymeric face with 2-Methacryloyloxyethyl phosphorylcholine (MPC) for reducing the soft tissue migration was reported by Prajatelistia et al. (2021).

Among the various composites, HAp-chitosan polymer composites have attracted much attention, as chitosan shares a number of chemical and structural similarities with collagen. Chitosan can be easily reformed into injectable hydrogels, porous membranes, beads, scaffolds, sponges, and encapsulates without using toxic solvents. Moreover, chitosan's structure is similar to glycosaminoglycans, the major component of the extracellular matrix of bone and cartilage (Thein-Han and Misra, 2009). It is a copolymer of glucosamine and N-acetylglucosamine units, and hence shares several attributes of glycosaminoglycans and hyaluroic acid. In composites, chitosan and HAp act complementary to each other, that chitosan provides continuous matrix for retaining growth factors, in turn, HAp stimulates biomineralization and delivers mechanical strength to the scaffolds.

Numerous studies documented on chitosan-HAp composites suggest that hybrid hydroxyapatite/chitosan scaffolds and nano-hydroxyapatite/chitosan composite materials are ideal for bone filling applications as both chitosan and HAp exhibit osteoconductive and anti-inflammatory qualities (Thein-Han and Misra, 2009; Pangon et al., 2016). The preosteoblast affinity was improved when chitosan was used along with nano HAp in scaffolds (Xianmiao et al., 2009). Tsiourvas et al. (2016) reported superior mechanical and tissue regeneration properties for a 3D chitosan scaffold with bHAp content as high as 75% (w/w). Similar observations in mechanical properties and reduction in water sorption properties were observed for Chitosan/HAp composite rods intended for internal fixation of bone fracture (Hu et al., 2004). Uswatta et al. (2016) demonstrated excellent osteoblast attachment for a porous injectable spherical composite scaffold with chitosan and nano-hydroxyapatite (nHA). A recent report by Kara et al. (2019) demonstrated the bone regeneration properties of fish scale–chitosan composite structure.

In Wistar rats, an injectable composite of chitosan, nanohydroxyapatite, and collagen loaded with bone marrow mesenchymal stem cells was shown to be beneficial in stimulating ectopic bone formation, in vivo (Yu et al., 2013). He et al. (2015) demonstrated the osteogenic ability of nHA-Chitosan osteo-induced bone marrow mesenchymal stem cell composites in the rat model. Nano HAp–chitosan composite scaffold has also got application as a potential drug delivery platform for antibiotics in the treatment of osteomyelitis (Uskoković and Desai, 2014). Guo et al. (2015) demonstrated the superior bone generation property for HAp–chitosan composite scaffold in comparison to the chitosan fiber porous scaffold in rat calvarial defects. Similarly, nanohydroxyapatite (nHAp)–chitosan gel with unrestricted somatic stem cells (USSCs) also confirmed higher healing property in the calvarial bone in rat model (Guo et al., 2015).

The degree of deacetylation and molecular weight of chitosan largely determines the microstructure and reactivity of chitosan-based composites. According to Hidaka et al. (1999), chitosan membranes having lower DDA values in the range of 65–80% stimulate severe inflammatory reactions compared to chitosan with a higher DDA value of 94%. Currently, magnetic scaffolds are being in greater demand in tissue engineering, as the magnetic materials rooted within the scaffolds are known to stimulate bone healing. Toward this direction, paramagnetic bone scaffolds were fabricated by embedding super-paramagnetic iron oxide nanoparticles within bovine cortical bone hydroxyapatite/shrimp chitosan matrix which exhibited remarkable improvement in bone regeneration properties (Heidari et al., 2015).

3.4.3 GLUCOSAMINOGLYCANS

Glucosaminoglycans (GAGs) are linear polysaccharides made up of uronic acid (glucuronic acid or iduronic acid) or galactose and an amino sugar (*N*-acetyl-D-glucosamine, or *N*-acetyl-D-galactosamine). Hyaluronic acid, also known as hyaluronan, keratin sulfate, chondroitin sulfate, dermatan sulfate, heparin, and heparin sulfate are the main components of GAGs (HS). HA is a high-molecular-weight molecule with a typical molecular weight of 2–10 × 107 Da, and is not covalently bound to protein. Sulfate groups are absent in HA, whereas majority of other glycosaminoglycans are sulfated and are covalently bound to a protein core. Dermatan sulfate is a component of skin, blood vessel, cardiac valves, tendons, and lung. It is composed of repeated disaccharide units of *N*-acetyl galactosamine and iduronic acid. Chondroitin sulfate is primarily associated with cartilage and is composed of alternate units of *N*-acetyl-D- galactosamine and glucuronic acid. Keratan sulfates are the structural component of cornea, cartilage, and bone. It is a large molecule and can be hydrated to greater extent thereby providing a cushioning effect to joints. Keratan sulfate contains repeated units of sulfated galactose and *N*-acetylglucosamine and occurs as attached to cell surface or extracellular matrix proteins.

GAGs are usually regarded as the constituents of various connective and structural tissues. Marine organisms form a rich source of GAGs of which HA and CS have special relevance in tissue engineering. Molluscs, cartilaginous, and bony fishes are recognized as reservoirs of HA (Abdallah et al., 2020). HA occurs primarily as an extracellular matrix component, even though it is shown to be present intracellularly. It is present as a major component of fish eye vitreous humor. HA is also a key component of synovial fluid, where it is extensively hydrated to form a viscous gelatinous fluid that lubricates and protects joints. Being an extracellular component of skin, HA is well explored for antiaging therapy. CS is unique in properties that it imparts elasticity to the cartilage. CS is found in considerable quantities in shark cartilage, tunic of sea cucumber, ray/skate skin, sturgeon cartilage, squid, and many other bony fishes (Novoa-Carballal et al., 2017; Mou et al., 2018). CS is currently recommended as a SYSADOA (symptomatic slow-acting drug for osteoarthritis) by the European League Against Rheumatism in the treatment of knee and hand osteoarthritis (Verbruggen et al., 2002). The anti-inflammatory activity of CS has been well demonstrated in the cell culture systems and in vivo human experiments (Hochberg, 2013).

GTR scaffolds, particularly those impregnated with extracellular matrix components such as GAGs, have been increasingly studied in view of their superior cytocompatibility and unique biomedical properties. Cryogel scaffolds for cartilage tissue engineering have recently been attempted using HA and CS (Chen et al., 2018; Yu et al., 2017). An ECM-based cryogel, using methacrylated CS (MeCS) and methacrylated HA (MeHA), was documented by Han et al. (2016). In cell culture studies with rabbit chondrocytes, MeCS-based cryogels stimulated aggrecan gene expression and synthesis of GAGs , whereas in MeHA-based cryogels Type II collagen gene expression and collagen accumulation was observed.

GAGs have been extensively explored for the fabrication of scaffolds in skin engineering and wound-healing carriers. The commercially available skin substitutes such as Hyalomatrix®, Hyalofill®, or Integra® are all based on HA-ester and CS. Heparin is also a preferred GAG component in wound healing and skin regeneration scaffolds (Thönes et al., 2017; Cheng et al., 2017). In recent decades, GAGs have been the subject of several neural regeneration studies. It is evidently proven that HA hydrogels have great potential in peripheral nerve regeneration therapies (Thomas et al., 2017).

3.4.4 CARRAGEENAN

The synthetic bone grafts available at present are biocompatible and osteoconductive; however, very few of them are osteoinductive. Ideally, bone graft should have the capacity to support cell adhesion, cell proliferation, and osteogenic differentiation of loaded precursor cells or migrated endogenous stem cells. This can be achieved to a greater extent by coating the graft with various growth factors, proteins, and/or drugs (Ho-Shui-Ling et al., 2018).

Carrageenan present in diverse red seaweeds is a promising candidate having osteoinductive potential due to its similarity with glycosaminoglycans (GAGs) present in human bone and cartilage. The structural resemblance of carrageena with GAGs helps in enhanced cell adhesion and proliferation. Since it has abundant sulfate groups, carrageenan has the potential to mimic the charged proteins present in the extracellular matrix (Coenen et al. 2018). Apart from that, carrageenan poses both chondrogenic and osteogenic potential (Graceffa and Zeugolis, 2019). Among the three different carrageenan types identified presently, kappa (κ)-carrageenan and iota (ι)-carrageenan are preferred for tissue engineering applications. More commonly, carrageenan is administered in combination with chondroitin-4-sulfate and dermatan sulfate.

A more recent research by Cao et al. (2021) demonstrated that κ-carrageenan (0.5 and 2 mg/mL) increased both MC3T3-E1 pre-osteoblast adhesion, proliferation and osteogenic differentiation. Carrageenan also supported matrix mineralization and induced osteogenic gene expression suggesting the osteogenic inductive potential of k-carrageenan. The osteoinductive properties of k-carrgeenan-gelatin composite cryogels were demonstrated by Sharma et al. (2013).

3.4.5 *ALGINATE*

Alginate or alginc acid salts form the structural component of brown seaweeds and alginate in the commercial form are extracted from the different species such as Laminaria, Macrocystis, Sargassum, Ascophyllum, Lessonia, Eclonia, and Durvillea (Pawar and Edgar, 2012). Alginate can also be of bacterial origin, and can be produced by Azotobacter and Pseudomonas sp. Allgal alginate exhibits a wide range of molecular weights, whereas bacterial alginate are characterized by relatively larger molecular weight and high degree of polymerization. The monomeric units of alginate are D-mannuronate and L-guluronate. Alginate is widely employed in tissue engineering as media for cell cuter, cell transplantation, tissue regeneration, drug delivery, and as wound-healing and wound-dressing scaffolds due to its low toxicity, biodegradability, and biocompatibility. When compared to traditional gauze dressings, wound dressings made of alginate-based materials offer several advantages since the wound exudates may be easily evaporated, avoiding the introduction of pathogenic bacteria, and they also provide a moist environment that promotes faster healing of wounds. Alginate gels, when used in combination with chitin or chitosan, offer a favorable moist-healing environment for chronic wound dressing (Kamoun et al., 2017). The use of alginate and alginate-based composite materials was widely employed in the regeneration of dental tissues and may also be useful for the delivery of growth factors, to enhance the natural regenerative capacity of the dental pulp (Dobie et al., 2002). Recently, the regeneration efficacy of a novel xeno-free alginate-fibrin-platelet lysate hydrogel with human periodontal ligament stem cells was demonstrated by Qiu et al. (2022).

3.5 THE CLINICAL PERFORMANCE IN TISSUE ENGINEERING AND ORGANS

3.5.1 *SKIN TISSUE*

Skin tissues cover a large area of our body and therefore are exposed to many damaging factors. Damages to skin may occur due to extensive burns, accidents, diseases, cancer, etc. Commonly utilized regenerating bases like Integra and Alloderm are not found to be completely effective due to less efficient regeneration capacity and high cost. Patients with intense skin problems, burns, and severe diabetes have to rely on economically viable and biocompatible tissue engineered scaffolds, mainly obtained through natural sources to escape from life-threatening situations. Scaffolds are mainly designed and fabricated by bio-printing, lyophilization, and electrospinning.

Collagen, a component of tissue ECM, is one of the widely used skin scaffolds for repair and regeneration. It is extracted from tissues of animals like porcine and bovine skin and tendons, intestine, bladder, and tail. As animal-derived collagen has potential for pathogenic virus transmission, fish-based collagen is found to be an impressive alternate. To improve the integrity and mechanical properties of collagen scaffold chemical and enzyme-mediated crosslinking are done. Gelfoam (Pfizer), Helistat (Integra LifeSciences), Instat (Johnson & Johnson), and Biobrane (UDL Laboratories) are some commercially available and clinically relevant collagen scaffolds (Chattopadhyay and Raines, 2014). Certain other natural and marine-based polymer like chitosan is also incorporated into collagen to develop a sandwich scaffold seeded with keratinocytes and fibroblasts. A collagen-derived polymer Gelatin that has lower antigenicity than collagen also has its own fingerprint in scaffold application for skin repair. It has an advantage to integrate with other polymers to use as skin scaffold through enhanced binding with Arg-Gly-Asp amino acids that are recognized by cell integrin receptors (Sheikholeslam et al., 2018).

In recent days, apart from biopolymers derived from bovine or porcine sources, the clinical importance of marine-based polymer chitosan obtained from crustaceans in tissue engineering is widely discussed. Linking with collagen, gelatin, and fibrin, chitosan is the most promising skin scaffold used in the form of freeze-dried sponges and hydrogels. Chitopharm is a commercially available therapeutic chitosan scaffold used for skin regeneration. Electrospun chitosan scaffold shows immense spreading of blood vessels and improves cell adhesion (Ma et al., 2003). Another source of skin scaffold is silk obtained from either Bombyx mori cocoons or Nephila glands. Using the silk fibers, films, or foams or woven or nonwoven scaffolds are fabricated that can support fibroblast and keratinocyte binding and proliferation. Incorporating 5% chitosan in silk scaffold improves blood vessel formation and keratinocyte adhesion (Bhardwaj et al., 2015). As an advancement in treatment, keratin is directly conjugated with silk scaffold to emphasize regeneration. Natural biopolymers prove to deliver an improved cell response, while combination of polymers provides better control over chemical stability and mechanical properties. It is highlighted that not one material meets all the regeneration criteria for a skin substitute. Rather, a polymeric composite scaffold may allow for the generation of skin that meets all clinical requirements like wound size, the extent of burn, the patient's age, allied diseases, and the available constitution technique.

3.5.2 ARTICULAR CARTILAGE

A unique connective tissue, articular cartilage, covers the joints around chondrocytes and cartilage matrix. It has an important role in maintaining joint mobility and strength through mechanical load transmission between joints by frictionless means. Damage to the articular cartilage is usually due to sport-related injuries, trauma, tumors, and diseases. Cartilages show very poor self-regeneration capacity due to poor cell proliferative activity of chondrocytes, thereby poor vascularization and cell multiplication. The damage to articular cartilage leads to osteoarthritis in the future and rather than the repair with scar tissues, the repair through articulate cartilage formation is preferred to regain the joint function. To overcome this, cartilage tissue engineering is a better treatment methodology (Jeuken et al., 2016). For cartilage tissue engineering, chondrogenic progenitors (developed from mesenchymal stem cells) and factors and a biocompatible scaffold material are required. The biomaterial is selected based on the criteria like the similar mechanical properties seen in the cartilage and interconnected pores. Many natural biomaterials like gelatin, chitosan, silk fibroin, hyaluronan, collagen, and alginate have been used extensively in tissue engineering to foster the cartilage regeneration by providing satisfactory mechanical properties and bioactive environment (Duarte Campos et al., 2012).

3.5.3 TRACHEAL/AIRWAY

Tracheal tissue regeneration after severe tumor excision is the complicated part in permanent reconstruction due to the complexity in structure. The regeneration of columnar epithelia impregnated with goblet cells and cilia lining is a highly challenging aspect in tracheal regeneration. Many synthetic polymers like PLA, polycaprolactone, PLGA, etc. are widely standardized for the regeneration. Even then, involvement of some natural polymers like collagen and gelatin in combination with synthetic polymers is widely employed in the regeneration. A scaffold-based bioreactor system with poly 3-Caprolactone and type II collagen for tissue engineering of trachea was developed in which the scaffold was seeded with chondrocytes. Another approach in tracheal regeneration is the use of synthetic grafts containing collagen sponge conjugated with a spiral polypropylene stent in a mesh form embedded with gingival fibroblasts and adipose-derived stem cells. This approach limited risk of scaffold rejection by immune systems. Electrospun fibrillary scaffolds made with PCL and gelatin which are conjugated with decorin was also a promising approach in tracheal regeneration (Iqbal et al., 2018).

3.5.4 CARDIOVASCULAR TISSUE

Cardiovascular complications are the leading cause of death worldwide in comparison with cancer. Heart tissue engineering attracts considerable involvement in remodeling and reconstruction heart tissues after injury or cardiovascular damages. A noticeable application of heart tissue engineering is the development of biodegradable heart patches using silk protein fibroin obtained from Indian tropical tasar silkworm A. mylitta, where cells adhere on the scaffold and spread three dimensionally. Collagen–chitosan matrix-hydrogels are designed to improve the ventricular wall stability and the endothelial cells formed a better vascular structure. This hydrogel has an ability to minimize the dilation of heart upon myocardial infarction. Biosynthetic hydrogels comprising poly vinyl alcohol and alginate are also developed and the therapeutic importance in cardiac cell proliferation was analyzed and implemented clinically. Blending of natural polymers like alginate and gelatin to fabricate film for myocardial tissue engineering was highly focused currently (Liberski et al., 2016; Fang et al., 2020). Gelatin and fibrin combination and collagen-glycosaminoglycan gels matrices for reconstructing mitral valve tissue gain high significance in regeneration. Electrospinning enhances the porosity, optimal diameter of fibers, and cell seeding behavior.

3.5.5 BLADDER TISSUE

The urinary bladder is one of the organs that has unique anatomy, capable for expansion and contraction to withstand the urine pressure. The bladder is lined with a specialized multilayer system of epithelium called the urothelium to hold urine. Congenital disorders result in changes in bladder capacity, incontinence, and renal damage. In the history of urology, biomaterials application was started with the development of urethral catheters (Elsawy and de Mel, 2017). The initial biopolymer used for the reconstruction of the urinary bladder for therapeutic applications was gelatin sponge. Apart from the normal requirements of a good scaffold, bladder construct should act as a barrier to urine to avoid the toxicity of urine on underlying tissue. It should also possess an appropriate mechanical strength to balance the forces required for bladder filling and emptying. Polymers like collagen or silk, designed in a number of configurations and densities, seeded with stem cells are utilized clinically to reconstruct bladder (Duong et al., 2013). Chitosan is an advantageous polymer that has positive charge which helps for the immobilization of negatively charged polymers like gelatin and collagen along with growth factors. This immobilization property leads to controlling the stability of the regeneration. Silk fibroin patches are also an influential biomaterial-based bladder tissue engineering approach. The clinical benefit of bladder tissue engineering is more noticeable by incorporating synthetic polymers with bioscaffolds.

3.5.6 SPINAL CHORD

Spinal cord injury followed by recovery is the most complicated medical condition, as it leads to many pathological and physiological changes in humans. The injury may also result in loss of motor and sensory functions. At the site of spinal cord injury the regenerative biomaterials can fill injury site cavities, deliver drugs, and provide adsorption surface for newly formed cells at the site of spinal cord injury. Some biomaterials also inhibit apoptosis, inflammatory responses, and scar formation, which further induce neurogenesis and neural connections, axonal growth, and angiogenesis (Tian et al., 2015). As it is the most complicated regeneration, the selection of biomaterial is done based on certain criteria like biocompatibility, balance between smooth and mechanically stable materials to maintain the active peripheral tissues, guide axonal regeneration, interact with cell, and maintain cell functionality. Collagen is the most acceptable natural polymer as it is biodegradable, less immunogenic and supports the vascularization and neuronal attachments. Collagen scaffolds are also used to deliver drugs like neurotrophin-3 directly to the injury site. Neuragen®, NeuraWrapTM, NeuroMatrixTM, and NeuroFlexTM are in clinical use. Chitosan is another promising polymer that supports inter-neuronal connections and reduced glial scar (Kurakula et al., 2021). In many cases chitosan scaffold is seeded with stem cells and neurotrophic factors and drugs to hasten the spinal cord regeneration. The hydrophilic colloid, gelatin, is a best material for scaffold as it increases the neuroprotection, cell adhesion, and reduction in necrosis. The sea weed polymer, agarose, can also support cell growth and neurite outgrowth (Li et al., 2016). The use of bioloymers in spinal cord regeneration promises the patients with noncurable injury.

3.6 ADVANTAGES AND DISADVANTAGES

Biomaterials are biocompatible, biodegradable and possess antitoxic properties which have been beneficial in the synthesis of composite bone scaffolds compared to synthetic biomaterials (Barua et al., 2018). The utilization of protein- and polysaccharide-based biomaterials has some drawbacks, including the following: (i) Restricted tensile characteristics that prevent the creation of larger constructs and limit their implementations to load-bearing regions; (ii) industrial differences; and (iii) potential alloying elements from the proteins or polysaccharides prior to actual insertion, which may act as a source of immunogenicity. Disease transmission might occur while using scaffolds made from humans or animals. Particularly when employing animal-derived scaffolds, scaffolds show inadequate repeatability between batches. When utilizing imaging techniques, the propensity of collagenous scaffolds to autofluoresce might pose a serious issue and in addition to that many substances might interact with the scaffold (Raheem et al., 2021).

3.7 CHALLENGES/LIMITATIONS

The difficulty with tissue engineering is simulating an in vivo environment. Engineered tissues are being developed, including heart muscle and valves as well as the kidney, liver, nerve, gut, and pancreas. One of the difficulties in attempting to build cartilage or bone is the synthesis of scaffolds with acceptable mechanical properties. The implanted scaffold in these tissues needs to be strong enough to function from the time it is placed until the remodeling process is finished. The fact that the mending process is age-dependent presents an additional difficulty (Ghorai and Mishra, 2022). While the pace of mending slows down in the old, it speeds up in young people. Numerous substances featuring excellent mechanical characteristics lack significant porosity, and many materials that have shown promise in vitro frequently perform poorly when used in vivo due to low vascularization capability. One of the most crucial areas of tissue engineering that calls for the most in-depth study is methods to enhance vascularization. Vascularization can be enhanced by letting cells develop microcirculation in the scaffold before implantation. The control of cellular mechano-transduction as well as cell function depends critically on the mechanical characteristics of the substrate to which a cell adheres (Merckx et al., 2020).

3.8 CURRENT SCENARIO, FUTURE PERSPECTIVES, AND CONCLUSION

The contemporary developments in Tissue Engineering integrate contributions from the technological developments in the allied scientific fields including nanotechnology and material science. The design of structural scaffold with appropriate mechanical properties biocompatibility and biodegradability and disintegration rates is a key area of tissue engineering. Environmentally benign and sustainable biomaterials derived from plants and marine sources offer safer alternatives procreating impacts in cancer research and 3D bioprinting technologies enabling precise therapies.

Plant-derived proteins like soy protein, zein, wheat gluten, etc. are in the forefront for the fabrication of scaffolds preferred to animal components in view of their wide availability, structural diversity, and consistent qualities such as biocompatibility, mechanical and aqueous stability. These materials show specific solubility and film-forming properties which are useful for the easy blending with other synthetic biopolymers. Their limited solubility and irrelevant physico chemical properties limit their use as such and this disadvantage can be limited by converting to composites through blending plant proteins with synthetic polymers as well as crosslinking. These efficient strategies augment their biological responsiveness, water resistance, and mechanical properties. Hydrogels with soy protein are the recent candidates for electroactive micro sensors and actuators. Gladin is serving as a carrier by blending with PCL for various biomedical applications due to the presence of S–S bonds and cooperative hydrophobic interactions even when it possesses drawbacks like low water stability and immunogenic toxicity. The plant-derived protein, Glutenin, is well versed for the use in 3D scaffolds with promising adipogenic differentiation in adipose-derived mesenchymal stem cells.

Recombinant plant-derived proteins are a comparatively newer approach in Tissue Engineering and prevention therapy. The most exploited expression systems include bacteria like *Escherichia coli*, yeast like Pichiapastoris, and mammalian system as the Chinese Hamster Ovary cells. The important shortcomings of these biomaterials are expense, protein size, time of development, yield, growth conditions, posttranslational modifications, size of the proteins, and regulatory approval.

Plant-derived polysaccharides, such as starch, cellulose, hemicellulose, pectins, inulin, and gums, found immense usage as a mart biomaterial in tissue engineering, drug delivery, and regenerative medical applications. Starch is noted as a suitable biomaterial for drug release, wound healing, and bone tissue engineering. The interconnectivity and porosity of cellulose are well explored in biomedical drug delivery and food packaging applications. The multipurpose applications of hemicellulose in biomedical and food packaging fields are in view of the advantage of chemical modification of the hydroxyl and carboxylic groups. Pectin despite hypoglycemic and hypocholesterolemic properties are widely applied in tissue regeneration studies after modification as hydrogels or capsules. The easy water dispersion ability proffer plant based gums a prominent role for the design of hydrogels with potent applications as biomaterial. Lignin-based scaffolds find immense applications as a renewable material for drug encapsulation. Composites prepared from lignin found applications in anticancer and antioxidant activity studies with focus on wound healing as well.

The innate roles of plant secondary metabolites in defense, signaling, symbiosis, etc. are exploited in the design of sophisticated wound dressing materials and tissue repairing and of regeneration applications. A uniqueness of the plant extracts is they contain the terpenes, phenolics, alkaloids, and glycosides as chief components which can be useful as a potent lead for biologically active molecules. Most of these extracts perform as antitumor, anti-inflammatory, antibacterial, antiviral, antimalarial agents, promoters of transdermal absorption, preventives, and curatives of cardiovascular diseases and hepato toxicity. All of the above secondary metabolites alone or in tandem are competent as a biomaterial.

Decellularization plant tissues become an optimal material as their native biomimetic structure provides the microenvironment for cell and tissue growth. Due to their low cost, ready availability, ease of processing and application, cytocompatibility as well as lack of ethical issues resulted in increased acceptance for plant-derived tissues as an efficient alternative to animal sources. The wide choice of plants which can mimic a range of mammalian tissues underscores their prospect for the fabrication of tissue-specific scaffolds. The 2D scaffolds prepared from certain plant leaves are extensive scaffold in cardiac tissue regeneration.

Collagen and gelatin extracted from sea weeds and marine sources offer a noteworthy class of biomaterials in the field of diversified biomedical applications. Collagen-based shields are significant functional material in ophthalmology, burns, and wound-healing sponges whereas collagen–liposome composite is for sustained drug delivery, matrices for cell culture systems, and 3-D printed matrix for guided tissue regeneration. Composite formation of collagen with compounds such as hydroxyapatite was helpful in modifying the disadvantages and could mimic good bone tissue reaction. These are fabricated in various forms like membranes, scaffolds, and gels. Current research on tissue engineering institutes the potential applications of chitin and chitosan for repair and regeneration of bone, cartilage, skin, etc., and in drug delivery and wound healing. The very recent research points to the curative aspect of chitin/chitosan as their ceramic nanocomposites loaded with growth factors in stem cell therapy. Glucosaminoglycans found applications in view of their superior cytocompatibility and unique biomedical properties and have been extensively explored for the fabrication of scaffolds in skin engineering and wound-healing carriers. Carrageenan, present in diverse red seaweeds, is a promising candidate having osteoinductive, chondrogenic, and osteogenic potential. The alginate extracted from sea weeds have high degree of polymerization and are valuable biomaterials in tissue engineering for cell cuter, cell transplantation, tissue regeneration, drug delivery, and wound-healing and wound-dressing scaffolds. They are widely employed in the regeneration of dental tissues and also in human periodontal ligament stem cells as composite form. Their potential use for vectors in the delivery of growth factors is upcoming.

The clinical performance of all the above natural polymer-derived biomaterials is a matter of high priority to escape from life-threatening situations. The scaffolds are mainly designed with these materials and fabricated by bio-printing, lyophilization, and electrospinning. Plant-derived collagen is highly suitable for scaffolds and their mechanical properties could be tailored by chemical- and enzyme-mediated crosslinking. Chitosan can also be incorporated to develop effective sandwich scaffold seeded with keratinocytes and fibroblasts. Collagen-derived gelatin are noted for their skin repair due to lower antigenicity. Linking with collagen, gelatin, and fibrin, chitosan can be modified as freeze-dried sponges or gels for application toward skin scaffolds. The chitosan-incorporated silk scaffold improves blood vessel formation and keratinocyte adhesion. Many natural biomaterials like gelatin, chitosan, silk fibroin, hyaluronan, collagen, and alginate have been in extensive use for cartilage regeneration. The use of synthetic grafts impregnated with collagen is in constant trials and improvements for tracheal regeneration. Collagen, silk fiber, and gelatin are some of the biopolymers mixed with synthetic polymers that are in the advent for urinary bladder regeneration engineering. The development of biodegradable heart patches using silk protein fibroin, matrix-hydrogels of collagen–chitosan, and poly vinyl alcohol and alginate are important in the management of complicated cardiovascular diseases. Collagen is the most acceptable natural polymer in the repair, regeneration, and drug delivery of spinal cord as it is biodegradable, less immunogenic and supports the vascularization and neuronal attachments. The development of 3D bioprinting techniques, incorporating polymeric biomaterials as the bio-ink, is a very recent trend.

The natural versatility of ECM-like plant-derived biomaterials, their modifications, and development of new materials with novel applications are well appreciated. But there is an urge to develop novel biomaterials with reduced side effects, lower processing costs, and greater therapeutic efficacies. The recent research has focused on the precise manipulation and control of cells and cellular environments. In this regard, growing interest in search for new natural sources of biomaterials together with innovative fabrication techniques for scaffold will lead to potent and effective biomaterials and newer applications. The recent accomplishments with natural materials and the current arsenal of materials available will stimulate the search into Nature's pool for novel biomaterials. Fundamental understanding of the chemical and biological aspects of such materials will result in the emergence of new, innovative biomaterials with new biomedical application.

KEYWORDS

- **sustainability**
- **biotechnology**
- **biomaterials**
- **natural sources**
- **tissue engineering**
- **bioengineering**

REFERENCES

Abdallah, M. M.; Fernández, N.; Matias, A. A.; do Rosário Bronze, M. Hyaluronic Acid and Chondroitin Sulfate from Marine and Terrestrial Sources: Extraction and Purification Methods. *Carbohydr. Polym.* **2020,** *243*, 116441.

(a) Aberoumand, A. Comparative Study Between Different Methods of Collagen Extraction from Fish and Its Properties. *World Appl. Sci. J.* **2012,** *16* (3), 316–319; (b) Cao, W.; Jin, J.; Wu, G.; Bravenboer, N.; Helder, M. N.; Pathak, J. L. Zandieh-Doulabi, B. et al. κ-Carrageenan Stimulates Pre-Osteoblast Proliferation and Osteogenic Differentiation: A Potential Factor for the Promotion of Bone Regeneration? *Molecules* **2021,** *26* (20), 6131.

Afinjuomo, F.; Abdella, S.; Youssef, S. H.; Song, Y.; Garg, S. Inulin and Its Application in Drug Delivery. *Pharmaceuticals* **2021,** *14* (9), 855. https://doi.org/10.3390/ph14090855

Aliabadi, M.; Chee, B. S.; Matos, M.; Cortese, Y. J.; Nugent, M. J. D.; de Lima, T. A. M.; Magalhães, W. L. E.; de Lima, G. G. Yerba Mate Extract in Microfibrillated Cellulose and Corn Starch Films as a Potential Wound Healing Bandage. *Polymers* **2020,** *12* (12), 2807. https://doi.org/10.3390/polym12122807

Ardean, C.; Davidescu, C. M.; Nemeş, N. S.; Negrea, A.; Ciopec, M.; Duteanu, N.; Negrea, P.; Duda-Seiman, D.; Musta, V. Factors Influencing the Antibacterial Activity of Chitosan and Chitosan Modified by Functionalization. *Int. J. Mol. Sci.* **2021,** *22* (14), 7449.

Barros, A.; Quraishi, S.; Martins, M.; Gurikov, P.; Subrahmanyam, R.; Smirnova, I.; Duarte, A. R. C.; Reis, R. L. Hybrid Alginate-Based Cryogels for Life Science Applications. *Chemie Ingenieur Technik* **2016,** *88* (11), 1770–1778. https://doi.org/10.1002/cite.201600096

Barua E, Deoghare, A. B.; Deb P, Lala, S. D. Naturally Derived Biomaterials for Development of Composite Bone Scaffold: A Review. In *IOP Conference Series: Materials Science and Engineering*, Vol. 377, No. 1; IOP Publishing, 2018; p 012013.

Bhardwaj N, Sow, W. T.; Devi D, Ng, K. W.; Mandal, B. B.; Cho, N. J. Silk Fibroin-Keratin Based 3D Scaffolds as a Dermal Substitute for Skin Tissue Engineering. *Integr. Biol. (Camb).* **2015,** *7* (1), 53–63. DOI: 10.1039/c4ib00208c

Biazar, E.; Heidari Keshel, S.; Tavirani, M. R.; Jahandideh, R. Bone Reconstruction in Rat Calvarial Defects by Chitosan/Hydroxyapatite Nanoparticles Scaffold Loaded with Unrestricted Somatic Stem Cells. *Artif. Cells Nanomed. Biotechnol.* **2015,** *43* (2), 112–116.

Bostancı, N. S.; Büyüksungur, S.; Hasirci, N.; Tezcaner, A. Potential of Pectin for Biomedical Applications: A Comprehensive Review. *J. Biomater. Sci. Polym. Ed.* **2022,** 1–35. https://doi.org/10.1080/09205063.2022.2088525

Buck, E.; Maisuria, V.; Tufenkji, N.; Cerruti, M. Antibacterial Properties of PLGA Electrospun Scaffolds Containing Ciprofloxacin Incorporated by Blending or Physisorption. *ACS Appl. Biomater.* **2018,** *1* (3), 627–635. https://doi.org/10.1021/acsabm.8b00112

Burnett, M. J. B.; Burnett, A. C. Therapeutic Recombinant Protein Production in Plants: Challenges and Opportunities. *Plants, People, Planet.* **2020,** *2*, 121– 132. https://doi.org/10.1002/ppp3.10073

Cao, W.; Jin, J.; Wu, G.; Bravenboer, N.; Helder, M. N.; Pathak, J. L.; Zandieh-Doulabi, B.; Hogervorst, J. M.; Matsukawa, S.; Geonzon, L. C.; Bacabac, R. G. K-carrageenan Stimulates Pre-Osteoblast Proliferation and Osteogenic Differentiation: A Potential Factor for the Promotion of Bone Regeneration? *Molecules* **2021,** *26* (20), p.6131.

Chang, C.; Peng, N.; He, M.; Teramoto, Y.; Nishio, Y.; Zhang, L. Fabrication and Properties of Chitin/Hydroxyapatite Hybrid Hydrogels as Scaffold Nano-Materials. *Carbohydr. Polym.* **2013,** *91* (1), 7–13.

Charbe, N. B.; Tambuwala M, Palakurthi, S. S.; Warokar A, Hromić-Jahjefendić A, Bakshi H, Zacconi F, Mishra V, Khadse S, Aljabali, A. A.; El-Tanani M. Biomedical Applications of Three-Dimensional Bioprinted Craniofacial Tissue Engineering. *Bioeng. Transl. Med.* **2022,** e10333.

Chattopadhyay, S.; Raines, R. T. Review Collagen-Based Biomaterials for Wound Healing. Biopolymers **2014,** *101*, 821–833. DOI: 10.1002/bip.22486

Chen, C. H.; Kuo, C. Y.; Chen, J. P. Effect of Cyclic Dynamic Compressive Loading on Chondrocytes and Adipose-Derived Stem Cells Co-cultured in Highly Elastic Cryogel Scaffolds. *Int. J. Mol. Sci.* **2018,** *19* (2), 370.

Chen, F. M.; Liu X. Advancing Biomaterials of Human Origin for Tissue Engineering. *Progr. Polym. Sci.* **2016,** *53*, 86–168.

Chen, L.; Zhu, C.; Fan, D.; Liu, B.; Ma, X.; Duan, Z. et al. A Human-Like Collagen/ Chitosan Electrospun Nanofibrous Scaffold from Aqueous Solution: Electrospun Mechanism and Biocompatibility. *J. Biomed. Mater. Res.Part A* **2011,** *99* (3), 395–409.

Cheng, L.; Ji, K.; Shih, T.-Y.; Haddad, A.; Giatsidis, G.; Mooney, D. J.; Orgill, D. P.; Nabzdyk. C. S. Injectable Shape-Memorizing Three-Dimensional Hyaluronic Acid Cryogels for Skin Sculpting and Soft Tissue Reconstruction. *Tissue Eng. Part A* **2017,** *23* (5–6), 243–251.

Chung, Y. C.; Chen, C. Y. Antibacterial Characteristics and Activity of Acid-Soluble Chitosan. *Bioresour. Technol.* **2008,** *99* (8), 2806–2814.

Coenen, A. M.; Bernaerts, K. V.; Harings, J. A.; Jockenhoevel, S.; Ghazanfari, S. Elastic Materials for Tissue Engineering Applications: Natural, Synthetic, and Hybrid Polymers. *Acta Biomater.* **2018,** *79*, 60–82.

Collin, H. Secondary Product Formation in Plant Tissue Cultures. *Plant Growth Regul.* **2001,** *34*, 119–134. https://doi.org/10.1023/A:1013374417961

Contessi Negrini, N.; Toffoletto, N.; Farè, S.; Altomare, L. Plant Tissues as 3D Natural Scaffolds for Adipose, Bone and Tendon Tissue Regeneration. *Front. Bioeng. Biotechnol.* **2020,** *8*. https://doi.org/10.3389/fbioe.2020.00723

Copes et al.Colagen-based Tissue Engineering Strategies for Vascular Medicine. *Front. Bioeng. Biotechnol.* **2019.**

D'Agostino, A.; Trevisiol, L.; Favero, V.; Gunson, M. J.; Pedica, F.; Nocini, P. F.; Arnett, G. W. Hydroxyapatite/Collagen Composite Is a Reliable Material for Malar Augmentation. *J. Oral Maxillofacial Surg.* **2016,** *74* (6), 1238-e1.

Das, D.; Ara, T.; Dutta, S.; Mukherjee, A. New Water Resistant Biomaterial Biocide Film Based on Guar Gum. *Bioresour. Technol.* **2011,** *102* (10), 5878–5883. https://doi.org/10.1016/j.biortech.2011.02.034

Dobie, K.; Smith, G.; Sloan, A. J.; Smith, A. J. Effects of Alginate Hydrogels and TGF-β1 on Human Dental Pulp Repair In Vitro. *Connect. Tissue Res.* **2002,** *43* (2–3), 387–390.

Dreesmann, L.; Ahlers, M.; Schlosshauer, B. The Pro-Angiogenic Characteristics of a Cross-Linked Gelatin Matrix. *Biomaterials* **2007,** *28* (36), 5536–5543.

Duarte Campos, D. F.; Drescher, W.; Rath, B.; Tingart, M.; Fischer, H. Supporting Biomaterials for Articular Cartilage Repair. *Cartilage* **2012,** *3* (3), 205–221. DOI: 10.1177/1947603512444722. PMID: 26069634; PMCID: PMC4297118.

Duong, D. T.; Chung, Y. G.; Gil, E. S.; Seth, A.; Franck, D.; Cristofaro, V.; Sullivan, M. P.; Di Vizio, D.; Gomez, P.; Adam, R. M.; Kaplan, D. L.; Estrada, C. R.; Mauney, J. R. Bladder Tissue Regeneration Using Acellular Bi-Layer Silk Scaffolds in a Large Animal Model of Augmentation Cystoplasty, *Biomaterials* **2013,** *34* (34), 8681–8689. ISSN 0142-9612. https://doi.org/10.1016/j.biomaterials.2013.08.001.

Ehrmann, R. L.; Gey, G. O. The Growth of Cells on a Transparent Gel of Reconstituted Rat-Tail Collagen. *J. Natl. Cancer Inst.* **1956,** *16*, 1375–1403.

Elsawy, M. M.; de Mel A. Biofabrication and Biomaterials for Urinary Tract Reconstruction. *Res Rep Urol.* **2017,** *9*, 79–92. DOI: 10.2147/RRU.S127209. PMID: 28546955; PMCID: PMC5436783.

Fang, Y.; Zhang, T.; Song, Y.; Sun, W. Assessment of Various Crosslinking Agents on Collagen/Chitosan Scaffolds for Myocardial Tissue Engineering. *Biomed Mater.* **2020,** *15* (4), 045003. DOI: 10.1088/1748-605X/ab452d. PMID: 31530754.

Fassina, L.; Saino, E.; Visai, L.; Avanzini, M. A.; De Angelis, M. G. C.; Benazzo, F. et al. Use of a Gelatin Cryogel as Biomaterial Scaffold in the Differentiation Process of Human Bone Marrow Stromal Cells. In *2010 Annual International Conference of the IEEE Engineering in Medicine and Biology*, August; IEEE, 2010; pp 247–250.

Gaspar-Pintiliescu, A.; Stanciuc, A.-M.; Craciunescu, O. Natural Composite Dressings Based on Collagen, Gelatin and Plant Bioactive Compounds for Wound Healing: A Review. *Int. J. Biol. Macromol.* **2019,** *138*, 854–865. https://doi.org/10.1016/j.ijbiomac.2019.07.155

Gershlak, J. R.; Hernandez, S.; Fontana, G.; Perreault, L. R.; Hansen, K. J.; Larson, S. A.; Binder, B. Y. K.; Dolivo, D. M.; Yang, T.; Dominko, T.; Rolle, M. W.; Weathers, P. J.; Medina-Bolivar, F.; Cramer, C. L.; Murphy, W. L.; Gaudette, G. R. Crossing Kingdoms: Using Decellularized Plants as Perfusable Tissue Engineering Scaffolds. *Biomaterials* **2017,** *125*, 13–22. https://doi.org/10.1016/j.biomaterials.2017.02.011

Ghorai, S. M.; Mishra, S. Tissue Engineering in Reconstruction and Regeneration of Visceral Organs. In *Tissue Engineering*; Apple Academic Press, 2022; pp 233–274.

Gopinath, V.; Kamath, S. M.; Priyadarshini, S.; Chik, Z.; Alarfaj, A. A.; Hirad, A. H. Multifunctional Applications of Natural Polysaccharide Starch and Cellulose: An Update On Recent Advances. *Biomed. Pharmacother.* **2022,** *146*, 112492. https://doi.org/10.1016/j.biopha.2021.112492

Graceffa, V.; Zeugolis, D. I. Carrageenan Enhances Chondrogenesis and Osteogenesis in Human Bone Marrow Stem Cell Culture. *Eur. Cell Mater* **2019,** *37*, 310–332.

Guo, Y. P.; Guan, J. J.; Yang, J.; Wang, Y.; Zhang, C. Q.; Ke, Q. F. Hybrid Nanostructured Hydroxyapatite–Chitosan Composite Scaffold: Bioinspired Fabrication, Mechanical Properties and Biological Properties. *J. Mater. Chem. B* **2015,** *3* (23), 4679–4689.

Han, M.-E.; Kim, S.-H.; Kim, H. D.; Yim, H.-G.; Bencherif, S. A.; Kim, R.-I.; Hwang, N. S. Extracellular Matrix-Based Cryogels for Cartilage Tissue Engineering. *Int. J. Biol. Macromol.* **2016,** *93*, 1410–1419.

He, Y.; Dong, Y.; Cui, F.; Chen, X.; Lin, R. Ectopic Osteogenesis and Scaffold Biodegradation of Nano-Hydroxyapatite-Chitosan in a Rat Model. *PLoS One* **2015,** *10* (8), e0135366.

Heidari, F.; Bahrololoom, M. E.; Vashaee, D.; Tayebi, L. In Situ Preparation of Iron Oxide Nanoparticles in Natural Hydroxyapatite/Chitosan Matrix for Bone Tissue Engineering Application. *Ceram. Int.* **2015,** *41* (2), 3094–3100.

Hickey, R. J.; Modulevsky, D. J.; Cuerrier, C. M.; Pelling, A. E. Customizing the Shape and Microenvironment Biochemistry of Biocompatible Macroscopic Plant-Derived Cellulose Scaffolds. *ACS Biomater. Sci. Eng.* **2018,** *4* (11), 3726–3736. https://doi.org/10.1021/acsbiomaterials.8b00178

Hidaka, Y.; Ito, M.; Mori, K.; Yagasaki, H.; Kafrawy, A. H. Histopathological and Immunohistochemical Studies of Membranes of Deacetylated Chitin Derivatives implanted Over Rat Calvaria. *J. Biomed. Mater. Res.* **1999,** *46* (3), 418–423.

Hochberg, M.; Chevalier, X.; Henrotin, Y.; Hunter, D. J.; Uebelhart, D. Symptom and Structure Modification in Osteoarthritis with Pharmaceutical-Grade Chondroitin Sulfate: What's the Evidence? *Curr. Med. Res. Opin.* **2013,** *29* (3), 259–267.

Horton, W. A.; Campbell, D.; Machado, M. A.; Chou, J. Type II Collagen Screening in the Human Chondrodysplasias. *Am. J. Med. Genet.* **1989,** *34* (4), 579–583.

Ho-Shui-Ling, A.; Bolander, J.; Rustom, L. E.; Johnson, A. W.; Luyten, F. P.; Picart, C. Bone Regeneration Strategies: Engineered Scaffolds, Bioactive Molecules and Stem Cells Current Stage and Future Perspectives. *Biomaterials* **2018,** *180*, 143–162.

Hu, Q.; Li, B.; Wang, M.; Shen, J. Preparation and Characterization of Biodegradable Chitosan/Hydroxyapatite Nanocomposite Rods via In Situ Hybridization: A Potential Material as Internal Fixation of Bone Fracture. *Biomaterials* **2004,** *25* (5), 779–785.

Huzella, T.; Lengyel, J. Orientation de la croissance des cultures de tissus sur la trame fibrillaire artificielle coagulée de la solution de "collagène A" (Nageotte) par les forces de la cristallisation. *Compt. Rend. Soc. Biol.* **1932,** *109*, 515–518.

Iqbal, N.; Khan, A. S.; Asif, A. et al. Recent Concepts in Biodegradable Polymers for Tissue Engineering Paradigms: A Critical Review. *Int. Mater. Rev.* **2018,** *64* (2), 91–126. ISSN 0950-6608. https://doi.org/10.1080/09506608.2018.1460943

Itoh, S.; Kikuchi, M.; Koyama, Y.; Takakuda, K.; Shinomiya, K.; Tanaka, J. Development of a Hydroxyapatite/Collagen Nanocomposite as a Medical Device. *Cell Transpl.* **2004,** *13* (4), 451–462.

Jahangirian, Azizi, Rafiee-Moghaddam, Baratvand, Webster. Status of Plant Protein-Based Green Scaffolds for Regenerative Medicine Applications. *Biomolecules* **2019,** *9* (10), 619. https://doi.org/10.3390/biom9100619

Jelkmann, M.; Leichner, C.; Menzel, C.; Kreb, V.; Bernkop-Schnürch, A. Cationic Starch Derivatives as Mucoadhesive and Soluble Excipients in Drug Delivery. *Int. J. Pharma.* **2019,** *570*, 118664. https://doi.org/10.1016/j.ijpharm.2019.118664

Jeuken, R. M.; Roth, A. K.; Peters, R. J. R. W.; Van Donkelaar, C. C.; Thies, J. C.; Van Rhijn, L. W.; Emans, P. J. Polymers in Cartilage Defect Repair of the Knee: Current Status and Future Prospects. *Polymers (Basel)* **2016,** *8* (6), 219. DOI: 10.3390/polym8060219. PMID: 30979313; PMCID: PMC6432241.

Jing, L.; Sun, J.; Liu, H.; Wang, X.; Huang, D. Using Plant Proteins to Develop Composite Scaffolds for Cell Culture Applications. *Int. J. Bioprint.* **2020,** *7* (1). https://doi.org/10.18063/ijb.v7i1.298

Kamoun, E. A.; Kenawy, E. R. S.; Chen, X. A Review on Polymeric Hydrogel Membranes for Wound Dressing Applications: PVA-Based Hydrogel Dressings. *J. Adv. Res.* **2017,** *8* (3), 217–233.

Kara, A.; Tamburaci, S.; Tihminlioglu, F.; Havitcioglu, H. Bioactive Fish Scale Incorporated Chitosan Biocomposite Scaffolds for Bone Tissue Engineering. *Int. J. Biol. Macromol.* **2019,** *130*, 266–279.

Koev, T. T.; Harris, H. C.; Kiamehr, S.; Khimyak, Y. Z.; Warren, F. J. Starch Hydrogels as Targeted Colonic Drug Delivery Vehicles. *Carbohydr. Polym.* **2022,** *289*, 119413. https://doi.org/10.1016/j.carbpol.2022.119413

Kon, E.; Delcogliano, M.; Filardo, G.; Busacca, M.; Di Martino, A.; Marcacci, M. Novel Nano-Composite Multilayered Biomaterial for Osteochondral Regeneration: A Pilot Clinical Trial. *Am. J. Sports Med.* **2011,** *39*, 1180–1190. DOI: 10.1177/0363546510392711

Kowalczyk, P.; Podgórski, R.; Wojasiński, M.; Gut, G.; Bojar, W.; Ciach, T. Chitosan-Human Bone Composite Granulates for Guided Bone Regeneration. *Int. J. Mol. Sci.* **2021,** *22* (5), p.2324.

Kurakula, M.; Gorityala, S.; Patel, D. B.; Basim, P.; Patel, B.; Kumar Jha, S. Trends of Chitosan Based Delivery Systems in Neuroregeneration and Functional Recovery in Spinal Cord Injuries. *Polysaccharides* **2021,** *2*, 519–537. https://doi.org/10.3390/polysaccharides2020031

Lee, J.; Jung, H.; Park, N.; Park, S.-H.; Ju, J. H. Induced Osteogenesis in Plants Decellularized Scaffolds. *Sci. Rep.* **2019,** *9* (1). https://doi.org/10.1038/s41598-019-56651-0

Li G, Che, M. T.; Zhang K, Qin, L. N.; Zhang, Y. T.; Chen, R. Q.; Rong, L. M.; Liu S, Ding Y, Shen, H. Y.; Long, S. M.; Wu, J. L.; Ling, E. A.; Zeng, Y. S. Graft of the NT-3 Persistent Delivery Gelatin Sponge Scaffold Promotes Axon Regeneration, Attenuates Inflammation, and Induces Cell Migration in Rat and Canine with Spinal Cord Injury. *Biomaterials* **2016,** *83*, 233–248. DOI: 10.1016/j.biomaterials.2015.11.059. Epub 2015 Dec 31. PMID: 26774562.

Liberski, A.; Latif, N.; Raynaud, C.; Bollensdorff, C.; Yacoub, M. Alginate for Cardiac Regeneration: From Seaweed to Clinical Trials. *Glob. Cardiol. Sci. Pract.* **2016,** *2016* (1), e201604. DOI: 10.21542/gcsp.2016.4. PMID: 29043254; PMCID: PMC5642828.

Lin, H. K.; Pan, Y. H.; Salamanca, E.; Lin, Y. T.; Chang, W. J. Prevention of Bone Resorption by ha/β-tcp+ Collagen Composite After Tooth Extraction: A Case Series. *Int. J. Environ. Res. Public Health* **2019,** *16* (23), 4616.

Liu, H.; Chen, T.; Dong, C.; Pan, X. Biomedical Applications of Hemicellulose-Based Hydrogels. *Curr. Med. Chem.* **2020,** *27* (28), 4647–4659. https://doi.org/10.2174/0929867327666200408115817

Liu, X.; Smith, L. A.; Hu, J.; Ma, P. X. Biomimetic Nanofibrous Gelatin/Apatite Composite Scaffolds for Bone Tissue Engineering. *Biomaterials* **2009,** *30* (12), 2252–2258.

Lu, C. F.; Wang, B.; Zhang, P. X.; Han, S.; Pi, W.; Kou, Y. H.; Jiang, B. G. Combining Chitin Biological Conduits with Small Autogenous Nerves and Platelet-Rich Plasma for the Repair of Sciatic Nerve Defects in Rats. *CNS Neurosci. Therap.* **2021,** *27* (7), 805–819.

Ma, L.; Gao, C.; Mao, Z.; Zhou, J.; Shen, J.; Hu, X.; Han, C. Collagen/Chitosan Porous Scaffolds with Improved Biostability for Skin Tissue Engineering. *Biomaterials* **2003,** *24* (26), 4833–4841. DOI: 10.1016/s0142-9612(03)00374-0. PMID: 14530080.

Ma, S.; Adayi, A.; Liu, Z.; Li, M.; Wu, M.; Xiao, L.; Sun, Y.; Cai, Q.; Yang, X.; Zhang, X.; Gao, P. Asymmetric Collagen/Chitosan Membrane Containing Minocycline-Loaded Chitosan Nanoparticles for Guided Bone Regeneration. *Sci. Rep.* **2016,** *6* (1), 1–10.

Machałowski, T.; Wysokowski, M.; Żółtowska-Aksamitowska, S.; Bechmann, N.; Binnewerg, B.; Schubert, M. et al. Spider Chitin: The Biomimetic Potential and Applications of Caribena Versicolor Tubular Chitin. *Carbohydr. Polym.* **2019,** *226*, 115301.

Merckx, G.; Tay, H.; Lo Monaco, M.; van Zandvoort, M.; De Spiegelaere, W.; Lambrichts, I.; Bronckaers, A. Chorioallantoic Membrane Assay as Model for Angiogenesis in Tissue Engineering: Focus on Stem Cells. *Tissue Eng. Part B: Rev.* **2020,** *26* (6), 519–539.

Mohammadinejad, R.; Maleki, H.; Larrañeta, E.; Fajardo, A. R.; Nik, A. B.; Shavandi, A.; Sheikhi, A.; Ghorbanpour, M.; Farokhi, M.; Govindh, P.; Cabane, E.; Azizi, S.; Aref, A. R.; Mozafari, M.; Mehrali, M.; Thomas, S.; Mano, J. F.; Mishra, Y. K.; Thakur, V. K. Status and Future Scope of Plant-Based Green Hydrogels in Biomedical Engineering. *Appl. Mater. Today* **2019,** *16*, 213–246. https://doi.org/10.1016/j.apmt.2019.04.010

Morganti, P.; Fusco, A.; Paoletti, I.; Perfetto, B.; Del Ciotto, P.; Palombo, M.; Chianese, A.; Baroni, A.; Donnarumma, G. Anti-Inflammatory, Immunomodulatory, and Tissue Repair Activity on Human Keratinocytes by Green Innovative Nanocomposites. *Materials* **2017,** *10* (7), 843. https://doi.org/10.3390/ma10070843

Mou, J.; Li, Q.; Qi, X.; Yang, J. Structural Comparison, Antioxidant and Anti-Inflammatory Properties of Fucosylated Chondroitin Sulfate of Three Edible Sea Cucumbers. *Carbohydr. Polym.* **2018,** *185*, 41–47.

Mutsenko, V. V.; Bazhenov, V. V.; Rogulska, O.; Tarusin, D. N.; Schütz, K.; Brüggemeier, S.; Gossla, E.; Akkineni, A. R.; Meißner, H.; Lode, A.; Meschke, S. 3D Chitinous Scaffolds Derived from Cultivated Marine Demosponge *Aplysina aerophoba* for Tissue Engineering Approaches Based on Human Mesenchymal Stromal Cells. *Int. J. Biol. Macromol.* **2017,** *104*, 1966–1974.

Nechita, P.; Mirela, R.; Ciolacu, F. Xylan Hemicellulose: A Renewable Material with Potential Properties for Food Packaging Applications. *Sustainability* **2021,** *13* (24), 13504. https://doi.org/10.3390/su132413504

Novoa-Carballal, R.; Pérez-Martín, R.; Blanco, M.; Sotelo, C. G.; Fassini, D.; Nunes, C.; Coimbra, M. A.; Silva, T. H.; Reis, R. L.; Vázquez, J. A. By-Products of *Scyliorhinus canicula, Prionace glauca* and *Raja clavata*: A Valuable Source of Predominantly 6S Sulfated Chondroitin Sulfate. *Carbohydr. Polym.* **2017,** *157*, 31–37.

Pangon, A.; Saesoo, S.; Saengkrit, N.; Ruktanonchai, U.; Intasanta, V. Hydroxyapatite-Hybridized Chitosan/Chitin Whisker Bionanocomposite Fibers for Bone Tissue Engineering Applications. *Carbohydr. polym.* **2016,** *144*, 419–427.

Pascoli, M.; de Lima, R.; Fraceto, L. F. Zein Nanoparticles and Strategies to Improve Colloidal Stability: A Mini-Review. *Front. Chem.* **2018,** *6*. https://doi.org/10.3389/fchem.2018.00006

Pawar, S. N.; & Edgar, K. J. Alginate derivatization: A review of chemistry, properties and applications. Biomaterials, 33(11), 3279-3305.

Peng, C. A.; Kozubowski, L.; Marcotte, W. R. Advances in Plant-Derived Scaffold Proteins. *Front. Plant Sci.* **2020,** 11. https://doi.org/10.3389/fpls.2020.00122

Peter, M.; Ganesh, N.; Selvamurugan, N.; Nair, S. V.; Furuike, T.; Tamura, H.; & Jayakumar, R. Preparation and Characterization of Chitosan–Gelatin/Nanohydroxyapatite Composite Scaffolds for Tissue Engineering Applications. *Carbohydr. Polym.* **2010,** *80* (3), 687–694.

Phan, N. V.; Wright, T.; Rahman, M. M.; Xu, J.; Coburn, J. M. In Vitro Biocompatibility of Decellularized Cultured Plant Cell-Derived Matrices. *ACS Biomater. Sci. Eng.* **2020,** *6* (2), 822–832. https://doi.org/10.1021/acsbiomaterials.9b00870

Prajatelistia, E.; Sanandiya, N. D.; Nurrochman, A.; Marseli, F.; Choy, S.; & Hwang, D. S. Biomimetic Janus Chitin Nanofiber Membrane for Potential Guided Bone Regeneration Application. *Carbohydr. Polym.* **2021,** *251*, 117032.

Qiu, G.; Huang, M.; Liu, J.; Ma, T.; Schneider, A.; Oates, T. W.; Lynch, C. D. et al. Human Periodontal Ligament Stem Cell Encapsulation in Alginate-Fibrin-Platelet Lysate Microbeads for Dental and Craniofacial Regeneration. *J. Dentistry* **2022,** *124*, 104219.

Raeisi, F.; Raeisi, E. Mini Review of Polysaccharide Nanoparticles and Drug Delivery Process. *AANBT.* **2020,** *1* (2), 33–34. https://dormaj.org/index.php/AANBT/article/view/35

Raheem, A. A.; Hameed, P.; Whenish, R.; Elsen, R. S.; Jaiswal, A. K.; Prashanth, K. G.; Manivasagam, G. A Review on Development of Bio-Inspired Implants Using 3D Printing. *Biomimetics.* **2021,** *6* (4), 65.

Rajathurai, S.; Kannabiran, P.; Parameswaran, S. Ocular Toxicity in Human Subjects Through Accidental Exposure to Latex of *Euphorbia umbellata* (Pax) bruyns. *Ancient Sci. Life* **2018,** *37* (4), 222. https://doi.org/10.4103/asl.asl_77_19

Ramji, K.; Shah, R. N. Electrospun Soy Protein Nanofiber Scaffolds for Tissue Regeneration. *J. Biomater. App.* **2014,** *29* (3), 411–422. https://doi.org/10.1177/0885328214530765

Reddy, N.; Yang, Y. Potential of Plant Proteins for Medical Applications. *Trends Biotechnol.* **2011,** *29* (10), 490–498. https://doi.org/10.1016/j.tibtech.2011.05.003

Richter, A. P.; Brown, J. S.; Bharti, B.; Wang, A.; Gangwal, S.; Houck, K.; Cohen Hubal, E. A.; Paunov, V. N.; Stoyanov, S. D.; Velev, O. D. An Environmentally Benign Antimicrobial Nanoparticle Based on a Silver-Infused Lignin Core. *Nat. Nanotechnol.* **2015,** *10* (9), 817–823. https://doi.org/10.1038/nnano.2015.141

Rodrigues, C. V. M.; Serricella, P.; Linhares, A. B. R.; Guerdes, R. M.; Borojevic, R.; Rossi, M. A.; Duarte, M. E. L.; Farina, M. Characterization of a Bovine Collagen–Hydroxyapatite Composite Scaffold for Bone Tissue Engineering. *Biomaterials* **2003,** *24* (27), 4987–4997.

Scarrit, M. E. A Review of Cellularization Strategies for Tissue Engineering of Whole Organs. *Front. Bioeng. Biotechnol.* **2015,** *3*. https://doi.org/10.3389/fbioe.2015.00043

Schwarz, F.; Rothamel, D.; Herten, M.; Wüstefeld, M.; Sager, M.; Ferrari, D.; Becker, J. Immunohistochemical Characterization of Guided Bone Regeneration at a Dehiscence-Type Defect Using Different Barrier Membranes: An Experimental Study in Dogs. *Clin. Oral Implants Res.* **2008,** *19* (4), 402–415.

Sell, S. A.; Wolfe, P. S.; Garg, K.; McCool, J. M.; Rodriguez, I. A.; Bowlin, G. L. The Use of Natural Polymers in Tissue Engineering: A Focus on Electrospun Extracellular Matrix Analogues. *Polymers* **2010,** *2* (4), 522–553.

Shalumon, K. T.; Binulal, N. S.; Selvamurugan, N.; Nair, S. V.; Menon, D.; Furuike, T. et al. Electrospinning of Carboxymethyl Chitin/Poly (Vinyl Alcohol) Nanofibrous Scaffolds for Tissue Engineering Applications. *Carbohydr. Polym.* **2009,** *77* (4), 863–869.

Sharma, A.; Bhat, S.; Vishnoi, T.; Nayak, V.; Kumar, A. Three-Dimensional Supermacroporous Carrageenan-Gelatin Cryogel Matrix for Tissue Engineering Applications. *BioMed Res. Int.* **2013,** *2013*.

Sheikholeslam, M.; Wright, M. E. E.; Jeschke, M. G.; Amini-Nik, S. Biomaterials for Skin Substitutes. *Adv Healthc Mater.* **2018,** *7* (5). DOI: 10.1002/adhm.201700897. Epub 2017 Dec 22. PMID: 29271580; PMCID: PMC7863571.

Shoji, D.; Hoya Corp. Apatite/Collagen Composite Powder, Formable-to-Any-Shape Artificial Bone Paste, and Their Production Methods. U. S. Patent Application 12/989,107, 2011.

Smethurst, P. A.; Onley, D. J.; Jarvis, G. E.; O'Connor, M. N.; Graham Knight, C.; Herr, A. B.; Ouwehand, W. H.; Farndale, R. W. Structural Basis for the Platelet-Collagen Interaction: The Smallest Motif Within Collagen That Recognizes and Activates Platelet Glycoprotein VI Contains Two Glycine-Proline-Hydroxyproline Triplets. *J. Biol. Chem.* **2007,** *282* (2), 1296–1304.

Sotome, S.; Ae, K.; Okawa, A.; Ishizuki, M.; Morioka, H.; Matsumoto, S.; Nakamura, T.; Abe, S.; Beppu, Y.; Shinomiya, K. Efficacy and Safety of Porous Hydroxyapatite/Type 1 Collagen Composite Implantation for Bone Regeneration: A Randomized Controlled Study. *J. Orthopaedic Sci.* **2016,** *21* (3), 373–380.

Thein-Han, W. W.; Misra, R. D. K. Biomimetic Chitosan–Nanohydroxyapatite Composite Scaffolds for Bone Tissue Engineering. *Acta Biomaterialia* **2009,** *5* (4), 1182–1197.

Thomas, R. C.; Vu, P.; Modi, S. P.; Chung, P. E.; Clive Landis, R.; Khaing, Z. Z.; Hardy, J. G.; Schmidt, C. E. Sacrificial Crystal Templated Hyaluronic Acid Hydrogels as Biomimetic

3D Tissue Scaffolds for Nerve Tissue Regeneration. *ACS Biomater. Sci. Eng.* **2017,** *3* (7), 1451–1459.

Thönes, S.; Kutz, L. M.; Oehmichen, S.; Becher, J.; Heymann, K.; Saalbach, A.; Knolle, W.; Schnabelrauch, M.; Reichelt, S.; Anderegg, U. New E-Beam-Initiated Hyaluronan Acrylate Cryogels Support Growth and Matrix Deposition by Dermal Fibroblasts. *Int. J. Biol. Macromol.* **2017,** *94*, 611–620.

Tian, L.; Prabhakaran, M. P.; Ramakrishna, S. Strategies for Regeneration of Components of Nervous System: Scaffolds, Cells and Biomolecules. *Regen Biomater*. **2015,** *2* (1), 31–45. DOI: 10.1093/rb/rbu017. Epub 2015 Jan 13. PMID: 26813399; PMCID: PMC4669026.

Tsiourvas, D.; Sapalidis, A.; Papadopoulos, T. Hydroxyapatite/Chitosan-Based Porous Three-Dimensional Scaffolds with Complex Geometries. *Mater. Today Commun.* **2016,** *7*, 59–66.

Urade, R.; Sato, N.; Sugiyama, M. Gliadins from Wheat Grain: An Overview, from Primary Structure to Nanostructures of Aggregates. *Biophys. Rev.* **2017,** *10* (2), 435–443. https://doi.org/10.1007/s12551-017-0367-2

Usković, V.; Desai, T. A. In Vitro Analysis of Nanoparticulate Hydroxyapatite/Chitosan Composites as Potential Drug Delivery Platforms for the Sustained Release of Antibiotics in the Treatment of Osteomyelitis. *J. Pharm. Sci.* **2014,** *103* (2), 567–579.

Uswatta, S. P.; Okeke, I. U.; Jayasuriya, A. C. Injectable Porous Nano-Hydroxyapatite/Chitosan/Tripolyphosphate Scaffolds with Improved Compressive Strength for Bone Regeneration. *Mater. Sci. Eng.: C* **2016,** *69*, 505–512.

Venugopal, J.; Low, S.; Choon, A. T.; Sampath Kumar, T. S.; Ramakrishna, S. Mineralization of Osteoblasts with Electrospun Collagen/Hydroxyapatite Nanofibers. *J. Mater. Sci.: Mater. Med.* **2008,** *19* (5), 2039–2046.

Verbruggen, G.; Goemaere, S.; Veys, E. M. Systems to Assess the Progression of Finger Joint Osteoarthritis and the Effects of Disease Modifying Osteoarthritis Drugs. Clin. Rheumatol. **2002,** *21* (3), 231–243.

Wang, H.; Liu, Y.; Cai, K.; Zhang, B.; Tang, S.; Zhang, W.; Liu, W. Antibacterial Polysaccharide-Based Hydrogel Dressing Containing Plant Essential Oil for Burn Wound Healing. *Burns Trauma* **2021,** *22* (9). DOI: 10.1093/burnst/tkab041

Wang, R.; Bao, B.; Bao, C.; Wang, S.; Ur Rahman, S.; Hou, C.; Elango, J.; Wu, W. Resveratrol and Celastrol Loaded Collagen Dental Implants Regulate Periodontal Ligament Fibroblast Growth and Osteoclastogenesis of Bone Marrow Macrophages. *Chem. Biodiversity* **2020,** *17* (9), e2000295.

Wang, T.; Li, Q.; Zhang, G. F.; Zhou, G.; Yu, X.; Zhang, J.; Wang, X. M.; Tang, Z. H. Comparative Evaluation of a Biomimic Collagen/Hydroxyapatite/β-Tricaleium Phosphate Scaffold in Alveolar Ridge Preservation with Bio-Oss Collagen. *Front. Mater. Sci.* **2016,** *10* (2), 122–133.

Wu, Q.; Bao, J.; Zhou, Y.; Wang, Y.; Du, Z.; Shi, Y.; Li, L.; Bu, H. Optimizing Perfusion-Decellularization Methods of Porcine Livers for Clinical-Scale Whole-Organ Bioengineering. *BioMed Res. Int.* **2015,** *2015*, 1–9. https://doi.org/10.1155/2015/785474

Xianmiao, C.; Yubao, L.; Yi, Z.; Li, Z.; Jidong, L.; Huanan, W. Properties and In Vitro Biological Evaluation of Nano-Hydroxyapatite/Chitosan Membranes for Bone Guided Regeneration. *Mater. Sci. Eng.: C* **2009,** *29* (1), 29–35.

Xie, J.; Baumann, M. J.; McCabe, L. R. Osteoblasts Respond to Hydroxyapatite Surfaces with Immediate Changes in Gene Expression. *J. Biomed. Mater. Res. Part A* **2004,** *71* (1), 108–117.

Xu, H.; Cai, S.; Sellers, A.; Yang, Y. Intrinsically Water-Stable Electrospun Three-Dimensional Ultrafine Fibrous Soy Protein Scaffolds for Soft Tissue Engineering Using Adipose Derived Mesenchymal Stem Cells. *RSC Adv.* **2014,** *4* (30), 15451. https://doi.org/10.1039/c3ra47547f

Yoshida, M.; Fujio, K. Extreme Lateral Interbody Fusion Using Bone Marrow Aspirate Combined with a Porous Hydroxyapatite/Collagen Composite. *Glob. Spine J.* **2016,** *6* (1_suppl), s-0036.

Yu, C. C.; Chang, J. J.; Lee, Y. H.; Lin, Y. C.; Wu, M. H.; Yang, M. C.; Chien, C. T. Electrospun Scaffolds Composing of Alginate, Chitosan, Collagen and Hydroxyapatite for Applying in Bone Tissue Engineering. *Mater. Lett.* **2013,** *93*, 133–136.

Yu, X.; Qian, G.; Chen, S.; Xu, D.; Zhao, X.; Du, C. A Tracheal Scaffold of Gelatin-Chondroitin Sulfate-Hyaluronan-Polyvinyl Alcohol with Orientated Porous Structure. *Carbohydr. Polym.* **2017,** *159*, 20–28.

Zhang, D.; Wu, X.; Chen, J.; Lin, K. The Development of Collagen Based Composite Scaffolds for Bone Regeneration. *Bioact. Mater.* **2018,** *3*, 129–138. DOI: 10.1016/j.bioactmat.2017.08.004

Zhang, S.; Huang, Y.; Yang, X.; Mei, F.; Ma, Q.; Chen, G.; Ryu, S.; Deng, X. Gelatin Nanofibrous Membrane Fabricated by Electrospinning of Aqueous Gelatin Solution for Guided Tissue Regeneration. *J. Biomed. Mater. Res. Part A* **2009,** *90* (3), 671–679.

Zhang, Y.; Reddy, V. J.; Wong, S. Y.; Li, X.; Su, B.; Ramakrishna, S.; Lim, C. T. Enhanced Biomineralization in Osteoblasts on a Novel Electrospun Biocomposite Nanofibrous Substrate of Hydroxyapatite/Collagen/Chitosan. *Tissue Eng. Part A* **2010,** *16* (6), 1949–1960.

CHAPTER 4

Mechanical Properties and Applications of Biomaterials for Bones

SUBIN P. GEORGE and RAJNANDINI DAS

Department of Engineering Design IIT Madras, India

ABSTRACT

Biomaterials are needed to repair, heal, or replace damaged bones and joints in surgeries. They are critical in restoring the lost functionality of the affected body parts. Orthopedic biomaterials have evolved over the past few decades owing to advances in Engineering that have made better biocompatible materials and superior design procedures that customize them to people. The mechanical properties of biomaterials are critical in their integration with the external biological environment. The stiffness of the implant plays a major role in this integration. When alloy metal implants were used at the beginning of the 20th century, the abrupt stiffness mismatch was a significant problem that contributed to stress shielding and then loosening. Many designers and manufacturers jointly worked to reduce this mismatch and came up with many novel implants that are better off in terms of integrating with the physiological environment around them. A lot of research in this field is still going to develop and manufacture better bio-implants that alter the physiology of the body to the least.

4.1 INTRODUCTION

Biomaterials have found their applications in the field of orthopedics in recent years, including the repair and replacement of damaged bones and joints. This can be achieved by using artificial prostheses like hip joints,

Application of Engineering Principles and Practices in Biotechnology.
Ann Rose Abraham, Leonardo Sepúlveda Torre, Tamara Tatrishvili, and A. K. Haghi (Eds.)

knees, elbows, etc., or by regenerating parts using stem cells from the patient's body. This chapter will aim to explain in brief biomaterials used in bone replacements and their application along with the study of mechanical properties of biomaterials which will help us understand better how they work and how they can be improved. The mechanical properties and application of biomaterials for bone research include a basic introduction to the bone, describing its role in supporting and protecting our bodies, looking at factors that affect bone health, and discussing treatments for bone disease.

A biomaterial is used in biological systems to meet medical objectives, whether remedial (to treat, enhance, heal, or replace a physiological tissue function) or to detect disease. The main purpose of any biomaterial is to replace what has been lost due to injury or illness. In some cases, though, we can use these materials to study biological processes, such as cell growth and migration. Biomaterials is a nearly fifty-year-old scientific discipline. With numerous organizations investing significant amounts of money in producing new technologies, it has experienced continuous and brisk expansion throughout its history. The fields of chemistry, biology, regenerative medicine, and materials science are all involved in biomaterials science.

The application of biomaterials for bone tissue engineering has attracted considerable attention because of their high potential for clinical application, especially for those needing total joint replacements. Implants' mechanical properties and physical characteristics are critical to implant success and must be understood before any clinical implementation. However, differences in mechanical properties between various biomaterials affect their biocompatibility and ability to stimulate osseointegration. In addition, numerous physical factors also affect how a material will respond within an individual patient's body, including patient-specific variables such as age, health status, smoking habits (for metallic components), and genetic background (for most allograft applications). Most of these physical factors can be considered independent variables that contribute toward a material's success when used therapeutically.

There are two kinds of materials used for bone replacement: implantable biomaterial and synthetic biomaterial. In recent years, synthetic bone replacements have grown in popularity. Orthopedic surgeons and manufacturers are interested in synthetic materials that promote bone healing and can be quickly invaded or replaced by new bone. These biomaterials are currently only employed in a few surgical procedures. Due to its numerous advantages over allogeneic or xenogeneic bone transplants, this therapeutic approach avoids many difficulties. Certainly, they lessen the number of transfusions required, and the amount of blood lost as a result of transplant intake.

On the one hand, disease transmission is not an issue when synthetic biomaterials are used. Patients are more accepting of them as a result. On the other hand, they ensure that there is enough material to fill or replace the missing bone, preventing a second surgical procedure with possible morbidities such as pain, infection concerns, and site embrittlement (Peppas and Langer, 1994)

Biomaterials come in various chemical components and properties, resulting in various biomaterials. Each category includes different materials with specific physical characteristics that determine their suitability for use in different applications. The most common biomaterials in orthopedics and traumatology include calcium carbonates, phosphocalcic ceramics, composite materials, biopolymers, bio verres, and calcium sulfates (Park and Lakes, 2007).

4.1.1 WHY BIOMATERIALS?

Biomaterials are important because in the current medical field it is possible to create artificial material which has similarities with bones. Using biomaterial, we can achieve new innovative ways to produce tools and implants to replace damaged parts of the human body such as bones, cartilage, heart valves, etc. There are many reasons why biomaterials have become an increasingly common part of modern medicine. This can be attributed to two factors:

- Advances in technology
- Increasing consumer demand

The most common type of biomaterial is a synthetic material with properties similar to those found in animals, plants, or humans. Examples of these can be seen in both medical and nonmedical applications. In medicine, biomaterials are used as replacements for damaged body parts such as fractured bones or damaged teeth. An example would be dental implants which replace missing teeth with durable artificial roots that are made from titanium, a metal not naturally found in our bodies. Nonmedical applications exist too; synthetically produced leather or wood could be used to make shoes or furniture which look similar to their natural counterparts but contain key differences that prevent them from decaying like real wood would over time.

The technological advancements that allow us to use biological molecules, cells, or tissue structures (and even living organisms) within a synthetic structure help us better understand how they function and provide clues about how they could be used in future products. For example, synthetic bone grafting material made from calcium phosphate-based ceramics works by taking advantage of our natural affinity for calcium-ions that bind together like glue. Also, according to a market report published by Transparency Market Research, one key development expected to drive growth in global bone biomaterials is the increasing demand for innovative healthcare devices.

4.1.2 HISTORY OF BIOMATERIALS

The first biomaterials were naturally occurring materials derived from living tissues. Bone, wood, horn, ivory, and tortoise shell have all been used to repair or replace body parts. One of the earliest recorded examples of biomaterials was dentures. Dentures were originally made from real teeth that belonged to soldiers who died in battle. Later on, dentures were commonly made out of cow bone; they were held together with pins that passed through holes drilled into each tooth—very medieval! Once plastic became more widely available after World War II (for example, with synthetic resins such as Bakelite), dentists began replacing teeth with artificial ones made from plastic. Tissue engineering is an interdisciplinary field concerned with integrating natural and/or synthetic biological components into tissues, which then become functional substitutes for those damaged by injury or disease. This can be accomplished by using natural materials such as collagen or hyaluronic acid that can be taken from one part of your body and implanted elsewhere without causing harm.

The first noncellular substances were introduced into the anatomy millennium ago. The "Kennewick Man" is a human whose remains were discovered close to Kennewick, Washington, in the United States (despite some debate). Archeologists characterize this man as a tall, robust, energetic person. He carried a spearpoint buried in his hip and journeyed through what is currently southern Washington. It seemed to have repaired itself and was no longer getting in the way of his efforts. This inadvertent implantation demonstrates the body's capacity to handle the introduction of foreign things. According to researchers, despite having no similarities to modern biomaterials, the spear tip was the same foreign material transplant that was "tolerated." The earliest known use of biomaterials was by the ancient Egyptians, who used sutures made of animal sinew.

The term Biomaterials (sometimes referred to as biocompatible materials) was coined by Jean Poiseuille, who identified it as a subset of materials engineering. Biomaterials is an area that covers many specialties such as chemistry, tissue engineering, material science, mechanical engineering, bioengineering, biomechanics, and biomedical engineering. The field includes research on topics such as 3D printing technology for producing scaffolds for cell growth; biodegradable polymers used to grow replacement skin; patches containing neurotransmitters to stimulate nerve re-growth; pacemakers; functional electrical stimulation devices for amputees; hip replacements that last for decades instead of years through controlled release of drug compounds at physiologic levels; stem cells which can be used to regenerate healthy tissue. Though they may seem like they were developed solely to help patients who have lost certain body parts due to injury or disease, biomaterials are also finding important applications in other fields such as medicine (surgery), sports (athletic wear), food science, and technology, cosmetics, cosmetic surgery, and consumer products.

4.2 BONE BIOLOGY

Bones are living tissues with their own blood vessels and are made up of a variety of cells, proteins, minerals, and vitamins. Because of this structure, they may continue to develop, transform, and mend themselves throughout their lifetimes. About 300 soft bones are present when we are born. Cartilage develops and is gradually replaced by hard bone during childhood and adolescence. Some of these bones eventually fuse together, resulting in a 206-bone adult skeleton.

The main purpose of bones is to

- Assist the body's structural integrity.
- Ensure that important organs are protected.
- Make a marrow-friendly atmosphere (where blood cells are produced).
- Serve as a mineral storage facility (such as calcium).
- Bone is made up of:
- The hard, dense cortical bone is the outermost layer of the bone.
- A network of trabeculae known as cancellous bone is less dense and lightweight than cortical bone.

4.2.1 STRUCTURE OF BONE

In order to understand how bone biology plays a role in fracture and disease, it is important to know what bones are made of and what happens when bones break. Bone tissue is made up of two main components, collagen and calcium phosphate, with other minerals and vitamins making up smaller percentages of the whole. The collagen helps the bones remain strong, flexible, and durable, while the calcium phosphate makes bones resistant to acidity, which allows them to maintain their shape even after death.

An essential component of bones is the bone matrix, composed of both compact and porous bone and forms the hard underpinning framework of bones. The bone matrix is composed of rigid protein fibers, primarily collagen, that stiffen and become inflexible during the mineralization of calcium crystals. Blood arteries and nerves are interspersed throughout the bone matrix, which also contains specialized bone cells that are actively involved in metabolic processes. The bone matrix is responsible for the basic structure of bones (Fig. 4.1). The spongy bone in the core and the compact bone on the perimeter should be noted. The osteon is the functional unit of a compact bone (Weiner and Traub, 1992).

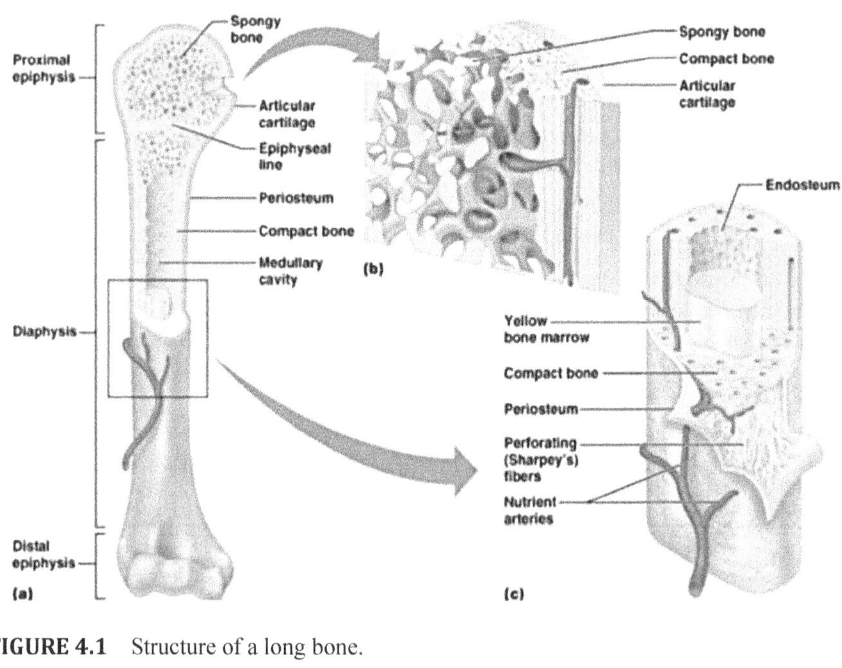

FIGURE 4.1 Structure of a long bone.

Source: Reprinted with permission from Asadi et al., 2016

All cells, tissues, organs, and organ systems have specific jobs to perform that are unique to each one. Bone tissue is no different; it has a specialized structure that helps serve as an efficient storage system for calcium and provides structure for muscles, tendons, ligaments, and other body parts. It also has mechanical properties that allow it to withstand high compressive forces. While natural bone's biological engineering has been perfected over millions of years through evolution, sometimes nature takes unexpected turns. One example is osteoporosis, which affects more than 200 million people worldwide.

4.2.2 MATERIALS OF NATURAL BONE

Bone comprises the protein collagen and calcium-containing mineral hydroxyapatite, the stiff fibrous component of ligaments and tendons. Collagen fibers act as a scaffold for forming hydroxyapatite crystals, which results in hardness.

The protein molecules that form collagen fibers are densely woven into a cable shape. The fibers spontaneously merge, resembling pre-programmed girders. These connect the hydroxyapatite crystals and control how the stacked sheets of atoms within the crystals are oriented, enhancing the material's strength (Zimmermann and Ritchie, 2015).

4.2.3 BONE FRACTURE

When the continuity of bone tissue is wholly or partially broken, it is called a bone fracture. Each bone in the body has the potential to fracture. High-force impact or stress is responsible for a substantial portion of bone fractures. Conversely, a fracture could come from a medical condition that weakens the bones. Cancer and osteoporosis are a couple of them. These are referred to in medicine as pathological fractures (Fazzalari, 2011). There are numerous ways in which a bone might fracture.

- A closed fracture is a bone break when there is no rupture to the skin and no impact on the surrounding tissue.
- On the contrary, a complex fracture frequently results in more severe injuries and will have an impact on the surrounding tissue.

There are numerous additional types of fractures, such as avulsion fracture, when a ligament or muscle pushes on the bone, and comminuted fracture, which happens when a bone is broken into numerous fragments due to impact. The spongy bone of the spine is most frequently affected by compression fractures or crush fractures; a greenstick fracture occurs when the bone fractures on one side but does not shatter because of the flexibility of the remaining bone; an oblique fracture occurs when a bone's long axis is broken in the opposite direction, a longitudinal fracture is a break along the length of a bone, etc.

Strong, highly resilient, healthy bones can withstand considerable stress. However, they could fracture or break with a significant amount of pressure. Physical harm, excessive use, and health issues like osteoporosis that weaken the bones are the leading causes of bone fractures. A person's risk of breaking a bone may also increase due to other factors. As a person ages, their likelihood of getting a bone-weakening condition increases.

4.2.4 BONE DISEASES

The physiological systems that regulate skeleton growth and maintenance can be disturbed in a number of ways, resulting in a range of bone illnesses and disorders. These include issues that might arise at or before birth, such as genetic anomalies and developmental disorders, as well as illnesses that harm the skeleton later in life, such as osteoporosis and Paget's disease of bone. Several illnesses impact bone indirectly by interfering with mineral metabolism, in addition to those that affect bone directly (Boyce et al., 1999).

Bone illnesses make it simple to shatter bones. The following are examples of several types of bone problems:

4.2.4.1 LOW BONE DENSITY AND OSTEOPOROSIS

Osteoporosis is a condition marked by bone loss and a higher risk of fractures due to minor stresses. The most prevalent metabolic bone disease, osteoporosis, primarily affects postmenopausal women over 50. The prevalence of osteoporosis in women over 60 is estimated to be one-fourth of all females. In these women, fractures are the leading cause of disease and mortality.

4.2.4.2 PAGET'S DISEASE OF BONE MAKES THEM WEAK

With Paget's disease (pronounced "PAJ-its"), the body's regular recycling system malfunctions, gradually replacing old bone with new bone tissue.

Bones can deform and become brittle with time. The most frequently affected areas are the spine, head, pelvis, and legs. As people age and if they have relatives who have the condition, they are more likely to develop Paget's bone disease. The illness has, however, grown less frequent in recent years, and when it develops, it is less severe for unknown reasons.

4.2.4.3 BONE CANCER

The uncontrolled growth of bone cells is a condition known as bone cancer. Only approximately 3600 new instances of primary bone cancer are detected each year in the United States, for example. Most cancers that affect the bones have spread (metastasized) from other body parts via the blood or lymphatic systems. Primary bone cancer can arise from various forms of bone tissue. Osteosarcoma arises from the cells that make up the bone, whereas Ewing sarcoma arises from immature nerve tissue within the bone. Both groups have the greatest impact on males between the ages of 10 and 20. Chondrosarcoma is a kind of cartilage cancer that affects predominantly persons over 50. More than half of all cases of primary bone cancer, including those that were previously deadly, may now be successfully treated.

Other bone illnesses, such as those caused by poor diet, genetics, or other issues, slow bone development or regeneration.

4.2.4.4 RICKETS

Rickets is a condition characterized by a lack of epiphyseal plate mineralization. Rickets can be handed down the generations or acquired. Acquired rickets is the most common cause of rickets in the globe (nutritional). The signs and symptoms range from asymptomatic to irritability, growth retardation, and abrupt death. The key variables that impact bone development and mineralization are vitamin D, calcium, and phosphorus. Rickets and/or osteomalacia can be caused by a lack of mineralization. The enlargement of the epiphyseal plates and a deficiency in mineralization define rickets. However, osteomalacia is a problem with the mineralization of the bone matrix. In most cases, rickets and osteomalacia coexist in youngsters. Adults acquire osteomalacia once the epiphyseal plate fuses, whereas children only have rickets (Dahash and Sankararaman, 2020).

4.2.5 NEED OR ADVANTAGE OF BIOMATERIALS IN BONE ENGINEERING

The significance of biomaterials in bone regeneration engineering has been redefined at the convergence of stem cell science, systems biology, and progressive material science research. Half of all chronic illnesses in persons over 50 are related to the bone and its diseases, which continue to be a significant clinical concern worldwide. The health of this age group is seriously threatened by several conditions, including infection, large bone defects brought on by fracture nonunion, trauma, removal of bone tumors, and spinal abnormalities. There are currently no viable alternatives for bone transplants due to the unexplored regeneration potential of bone abnormalities and the limited efficacy of available treatments. Due to the untapped ability of bone defects to regenerate new bone tissue and the current efficacy of therapeutic approaches, there are currently no suitable alternatives to bone transplants.

Biomaterials can overcome some crucial limitations by providing new options for controlling skeletal growth. For example, advanced biomaterials have been used to successfully treat traumatic fractures of bones. Some of these materials include living cells that promote bone healing or synthetic scaffolds that support new bone formation in a similar way to natural bone. This is particularly important because many current methods for fixing broken bones rely on external fixators, which are often uncomfortable for patients, cause damage to surrounding tissues, and can result in infections or other complications. Traditional biomaterial scaffolds also do not usually provide an optimal environment for tissue regeneration, resulting in low success rates in treatments such as joint replacements. Advanced engineering methods allow researchers to create replacement joints from scratch by carefully selecting specific materials with certain mechanical properties. Another benefit of biomaterials is their ability to replicate conditions found inside human bodies.

The advantage of using biomaterials to repair bones is that it can reduce stress fractures, infections, and complications during surgeries. Bioengineering techniques provide an option for overcoming issues related to bone weakness. Traditional forms of treatment for bone diseases such as osteoporosis or arthritis, which are limited to drugs or physical therapy, fail to target underlying causes of diseased tissue and lack long-term effects. Biomedical engineers have developed biosynthetic implants that offer a new method for treating these conditions by supporting weak bones with synthetic materials.

Using advanced engineering techniques allows researchers to design various forms of implants that are extremely similar to their natural counterparts. For example, engineered biomaterials have been used to develop prosthetic devices such as kneecaps that flex and bend with walking motions. Other projects involve developing bones or joints completely from scratch by carefully selecting materials based on their mechanical properties so they can interact with surrounding tissue appropriately.

4.3 CLASSIFICATION OF BIOMATERIALS

Depending on the synthetic material implanted in the human body, the tissue responds in various ways. The tissue's reaction to the implant surface determines the method of tissue contact. In general, three terminologies may be used to define or classify a biomaterial in terms of tissue reactions. These are bioinert, bioresorbable, and bioactive, all of which have been thoroughly discussed (Yu et al., 2015).

Bioinert biomaterials: When implanted in the human body, bioinert materials like stainless steel, titanium, alumina, partially stabilized zirconia, and ultra-high molecular weight polyethylene have finite contact with the tissue around them. Most of the time, a fibrous capsule forms surrounding bioinert implants, and tissue integration is required for the implant's bio functionality.

Bioactive biomaterials: The term "bioactive" describes a biomaterial that interacts with the surrounding bone and, in certain circumstances, soft tissue after being implanted in the human body. As a result of their implantation into living bone, a time-dependent kinetic modification of the surface occurs.

Bioresorbable biomaterials: When a substance is introduced into the human body, it disintegrates (resorb), and new tissue (such as bone) progressively replaces it. Two examples of bioresorbable materials are polylactic-polyglycolic acid copolymers and tricalcium phosphate [Ca3(PO4)2]. Other typical materials used in the previous three decades include calcium carbonate, calcium oxide, and gypsum (Heness and Ben, 2013).

Tissue engineering, or the repair or replacement of injured cells, tissues, or organs, uses biomaterials as scaffolds. The classification of biomaterials is an important topic for understanding how different materials work within biomedical applications. Depending on the application of biomaterials, there are three main classes of biomaterials: biomatrices, bio prostheses, and implantable devices:

- **Biomatrices** is a biological material that helps stimulate cell growth to encourage tissue repair or regeneration after an injury.
- **Bio prostheses** are artificial replacements for body parts such as bones, joints, and tendons. These can be made from either synthetic or natural materials, but they are generally considered permanent implants.
- **Implantable devices** include cardiac pacemakers and artificial heart valves; these too are often permanent implants.

4.3.1 BIOMATRICES

Biomatrices are biological materials that help stimulate cellular growth to encourage tissue repair or regeneration after an injury. Common Biomatrices include Chitosan scaffolds, hydroxyapatite, dextran gel, alginate hydrogel, and agarose hydrogel; each of these can be used to develop functional material for drug delivery systems, 3D cell culture applications, and wound management. A key component of any biomatrix is cell proliferation for cell seeding. Biomatrices must possess properties that are similar to those found naturally in our bodies.

Biometrics is used to understand how much force is needed to break a certain type of bone which can be used in trauma cases where you want to see how much pressure was applied or when trying to determine if an accident may have contributed to someone's death. You can even use it to look at nonfatal injuries such as car accidents. It is critical to gather as much information about an injury or disease by merely looking at a small piece of tissue that has been affected. For example, DNA testing can tell you what type of cell is involved (i.e., osteoclast vs. osteoblast). The knowledge gained from biometrics helps us better understand how we repair ourselves after an injury or what happens when things go wrong with these processes. For example, osteoporosis is one of those diseases that affects our bones and their ability to repair themselves properly, which leads to weaker bones over time. We are still not exactly sure why people get osteoporosis, but we do know that our genetics do play a big part in whether someone will develop it or not. Understanding bone biology allows us to better understand why something like osteoporosis arises and, ideally, identify strategies to prevent it from occurring in the first place!

4.3.2 BIOPROSTHESES

Bioprostheses are artificial replacements for body parts such as bones, joints, and tendons. These can be made from synthetic or natural materials, but they are generally considered permanent implants.

Bioprostheses for bones and joints heal damage caused by trauma, cancer, or congenital anomalies. Natural materials such as bone can be used for implantation. Synthetic replacements made from materials such as steel or titanium, known as metal prostheses, have been successfully used for over a century; however, metal implants are often rejected by host tissue and can cause inflammation: Bone bio-prostheses are not without their complications. Due to degenerative conditions, they are susceptible to infection and may fail over time. For example, hip replacement surgery requires patients to replace artificial hips periodically because they lose resiliency over time. This is where osteoinductive biomaterials come into play. Osteoinductive biomaterials are synthetic polymers (materials composed of long chains of molecules) that stimulate new bone growth when implanted in damaged areas. Osteoinductive biomaterials work by mimicking specific properties found in healthy human bone tissue.

4.3.3 IMPLANTABLE DEVICES

Implants are used to mend broken bones. The process begins with removing fragments from both sides of the break; that is called debridement. Next, implants are placed either within or on top of bones. Plates, screws, nails, and other devices are often attached to those implants to connect two pieces of bone for support until healing occurs. Because implant materials can all be made radiolucent (not visible under X-ray), they do not interfere with imaging after healing is complete. An MRI or CT scan can detect bone fracture and soft tissue injuries such as ligament tears. Long bones such as legs and arms take at least six weeks to heal; some fractures may require longer treatment before they are fully healed.

4.4 ECHANICAL PROPERTIES OF BIOMATERIALS

Mechanical properties are essential characteristics of any material, especially for medical devices or implants used in or on the human body. Bone, for example, has specific mechanical properties that allow it to function as an ideal scaffold for tissue growth and repair; thus, scientists and bioengineers are constantly working to incorporate the mechanical properties of synthetic materials with the bone to create implants and devices that can be integrated into the human body without being rejected or causing injury to the host tissue cells. Any material designated for biomedical use must meet three requirements. The substance must be biocompatible, meaning that the body should not view it as an external substance. Second, the substance must be biodegradable (for in-graft only); it must disintegrate or dissolve harmlessly in the organism's body, enabling it to return to regular functioning. The material must be mechanically sound and have similar or better mechanical stability when substituting load-bearing structures to guarantee the graft's good durability. Here are some of the mechanical properties of biomaterials and how they can be controlled and improved.

4.4.1 ELASTIC MODULUS

Modulus is a measure of stiffness. The stress–strain ratio within the proportional limit is described as elastic modulus. When tensile or compressive loads are applied, the material's stiffness within the elastic range is reflected. It is therapeutically significant since the chosen biomaterial has identical deformability to the original material. High elastic modulus and minimal deflection are required for these force-bearing materials. As a material's elastic modulus rises, its resistance to fracture decreases. The elastic modulus of the biomaterial should be similar to that of bone. This is because the material only supports the load if its elastic modulus exceeds the bones. Still, if the elastic modulus of the bone is less than that of the material, the load is carried solely by the bone. Human trabecular bone modulus ranges from 10 to 3000 MPa, whereas strength, which is linearly and highly correlated with modulus, ranges from 0.1 to 30 MPa (Kokubo, 2008).

4.4.2 HARDNESS

The force per unit area of penetration or indentation is the definition of hardness, a measure of plastic deformation. One of the essential factors for comparing material attributes is hardness. It is employed to determine whether biomaterials are suitable for usage in clinical situations. Like bone, biomaterials should be as hard as possible. It penetrates the bone if it is higher than the biomaterial. Increased hardness lessens abrasion (Kokubo, 2008).

4.4.3 FRACTURE TOUGHNESS

The maximum stress that a substance can withstand before breaking is defined as strength. Because of their fragility, strength is a crucial mechanical attribute for biomaterials (bioceramics). When brittle materials, such as bioceramics, are subjected to tensile loading instead of compressive loading, cracks quickly spread. Several methods are available for determining a material's tensile strength, including the Weibull approach, biaxial flexural strength test, and bending flexural test. In bioceramics, defects affect the biomaterial's dependability and strength during production and implantation. Thermal sintering and heating processes are two of the many ways bioceramics might develop defects. In summary, bioceramics do not require great strength; good dependability is crucial.

Fracture toughness in ceramics is required to control crack propagation. It is advantageous to evaluate biomaterials' usability, functionality, and long-term clinical success. High fracture toughness materials improved clinical performance and dependability compared to low fracture toughness materials. It can be evaluated using various techniques, including indentation strength, indentation fracture, single edge precracked beam, single edge notched beam, and double cantilever beam (Rodgers et al., 2015).

4.4.4 FATIGUE

When a material fails due to repeated/cyclic loading and unloading, it is said to have experienced fatigue (tensile or compressive stresses). Cyclic load is also crucial because it is applied to biomaterials during service life. Under this cyclic loading condition, microcracks or other defects may develop at the matrix-filler contact. A significant crack expansion or collapse could result from this minor fracture, which can induce chronic plastic deformation. The development of microcracks during the cyclic load is influenced by several elements, such as the mating surface sliding with friction, residual pressures at grain boundaries, progressive wear, and tension resulting from shear (Kokubo, 2008).

4.5 APPLICATION OF BIOMATERIALS IN IMPLANTS-DESIGN CONSIDERATIONS

Skeletal structure gives locomotion capability, structural stiffness, and shape to the human body. The stiffness distribution in the bone has always been a wonder to the scientific community because of the biological adaptation of the stiffness to different parts. Bones that are thicker or stiffer in the outer region (cortical bone) and less dense in interior structure are called cancellous bone.

This gives optimum or least weight to the skeletal structures with the best possible stiffness distribution to withstand the strength considerations of the static and dynamic Loading. This is why the skeletal structure contributes only 15% of the total body weight. When designing a biomaterial the designer has to take into account these aspects and bring the stiffness of the Artificial structure as close as possible to that of the biological one. The mismatch in stiffness yields to a phenomenon called stress shielding that further gives rise to unnatural load distribution and hence implant dysfunction.

The stiffness of any component comprises Geometry and Material properties. So when bio-mimicking is done the designer has to take care of both these dimensions. The shape of any bone implant itself can have an external shape as well as internal details. For example, a recently developed hip implant stem by Altair Engineering has an external shape as shown in Figure 4.2. This external shape fits into the medullary canal of the femur and the top portion takes up the load from the acetabulum socket. The lattice structure shown promotes bone in-growth along with the additional advantage of weight reduction.

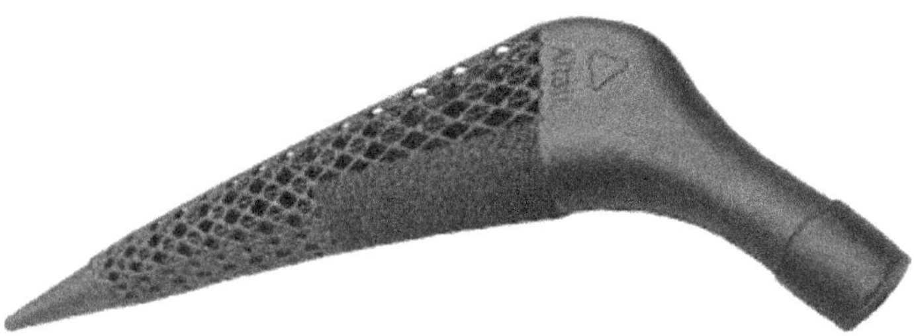

FIGURE 4.2 Hip implant stem by Altair Engineering

Image courtesy: EOS-printed TI 6AL-4V solid-lattice hip prosthesis, Altair inspire.

So bioengineers work on both the structural dimension and the material properties to design and manufacture better bio implants. Considerations in the geometry are affected by extracting the anatomical features of the operation site. Usually, standard sizes of implants are available for surgery. But a lot of work in customizing the implant is also done to develop implants that best fit the anatomy of any patient. Those are devices for patients affected by major bone losses due to revision, infection, or trauma, or for oncologic cases treatment.

Powder manufacturing Technology is employed in making the desired geometry of the structure with the expected internal architecture.

4.5.1 *OPTIMIZATION IN THE DESIGN OF IMPLANTS*

The stiffness that is a combination of geometry and material property has to be optimum for a particular implant construct for the best physiological functioning. Or in other words, the distribution of materials in the implant structure should give the least weight to the structure as well as transfer the load with the best strength considerations. In the design procedure, the porosity in a site of an implant is modeled as stiffness-based elasticity moduli. The optimization algorithm proceeds by minimizing the stress shielding taking care of the critical strength considerations like failure strength at a given porosity. Porous architecture is a design that is now widely adopted to meet these goals. The porous structure is made with repeating patterns that can be manufactured using powder metallurgy. The size of each repeating unit has to be fixed by means of a design framework. Lattice structure (Rodgers et al., 2015) is such a self-repeating unit that has gained popularity in this field, owing to its advantages. A lattice structure is a 3D open-cellular structure of repeating unit cells. Unit cells are built up of struts connected to nodes. Due in part to the lattice's high stiffness-to-weight ratio, negative Poisson ratio, low thermal expansion coefficient, and rapid heat dissipation, these characteristics are advantageous to sectors of the economy like aerospace, transportation, and medicine (Chunze et al., 2014). Researchers claim that this structure promotes better bone ingrowth compared to the solid structure thus bonding an integration in a better way.

4.6 CONCLUSION

Biomaterials have gone a long way in their features to benefit the operated patients, especially in terms of postsurgical functionality, with the advent of modern design and manufacturing techniques. The goal of any biomaterial is to restore the operated site to normal physiological function as closely as possible. Implants have evolved from a very stiff solid heavy structure to a less stiff, porous architecture with less weight and thus promoting better

Osseointegration. Compared to present implants, porous implants may have improved implant fixation, service life, and mechanical qualities.

KEYWORDS

- **biomaterials**
- **orthopedic implants**
- **stress shielding**
- **stiffness**
- **osseointegration**
- **implant design**

REFERENCES

Peppas, N. A.; Langer, R. New Challenges in Biomaterials. *Science***1994,** *263* (5154), 1715–1720.

Park, J.; Lakes, R. S. *Biomaterials: An Introduction*; Springer Science & Business Media, 2007.

Weiner, S.; Traub, W. Bone Structure: From Ångstroms to Microns. *FASEB J.***1992,** *6* (3), 879–885.

Asadi, S. Syndrome Raine, A Rare Autosomal Recessive Dysplasia Sclerotic Osteoarthritis, the First Reports of a New Mutation of Tabriz City in IRAN. *J. Genet. Syndr. Gene Ther.* **2016,** *7* (296), 2.

Zimmermann, E. A.; Ritchie, R. O. Bone as a Structural Material. *Adv. Healthc. Mater.* **2015,** *4* (9), 1287–1304.

Fazzalari, N. L. Bone Fracture and Bone Fracture Repair. *Osteoporos. Int.* **2011,** *22* (6), 2003–2006.

Boyce, B. F.; Hughes, D. E.; Wright, K. R.; Xing, L.; Dai, A. Recent Advances in Bone Biology Provide Insight into the Pathogenesis of Bone Diseases. *Lab. Invest.* **1999,** *79* (2), 83–94.

Dahash, B. A.; Sankararaman, S. Rickets, 2020.

Yu, X.; Tang, X.; Gohil, S. V.; Laurencin, C. T. Biomaterials for Bone Regenerative Engineering. *Adv. Healthc. Mater.* **2015,** *4* (9), 1268–1285.

Heness, G.; Ben, N. B. Biomaterials-Classifications and Behavior of Different Types of Biomatrials. *Mater. Forum*, **2013,** 27.

Tetsuka, H.; Shin, S. R. Materials and Technical Innovations in 3D Printing in Biomedical Applications. *J. Mater. Chem. B* **2020,** *8* (15), 2930–2950.

Kokubo, T., Ed. *Bioceramics and their Clinical Applications*; Elsevier, 2008.

Fischer, H.; Marx, R. Fracture Toughness of Dental Ceramics: Comparison of Bending and Indentation Method. *Dent. Mater.* **2002,** *18* (1), 12–19.

Rodgers, G. W.; Van Houten, E. E.; Bianco, R. J.; Besset, R.; Woodfield, T. B. Optimizing Porous Lattice Structures for Orthopaedic Implants. *Annu. Int. Conf. IEEE Eng. Med. Biol. Soc.* **2015,** *2015,* 450–3.

Chunze, Y.; Liang, H.; Ahmed, H.; Philippe, Y.; David, R. Advanced Lightweight 316L Stainless Steel Cellular Lattice Structures Fabricated via Selective Laser Melting. *Mat. Design* **2014,** *55,* 533–541.

CHAPTER 5

Role of Biodegradable Polymeric Nanohydrogel in Bone Regeneration: An Engineering Conception

RUBY VARGHESE[1,2], NAMITHA BINU[2], and YOGESH B. DALVI[2]

[1]*Department of Chemistry, School of Sciences, Jain Deemed to be University, Bangalore, Karnataka, India*

[2]*Pushpagiri Institute of Medical Sciences and Research Centre, Thiruvalla, Kerala, India*

ABSTRACT

Bone exhibits an immense capability for endogenous self-healing. Nevertheless, bone regeneration without an external intervention has its limitations. Conventional methods for treating bone defects like autografts, allografts, and xenografts are widely used, but their usefulness is limited by their disadvantages and limiting clinical use. Current strategies, including several biomaterials, cellular therapies, and scaffolds, are developed to facilitate the vascularization, and engraftment of the constructs ultimately recreating a bone tissue that resembles native bone but the desired therapeutic effect is not fully achieved. Presently, nanogel has emerged as innovative dispersion of hydrogel nanoparticles based on 3-D crosslinked polymeric networks with uniformity, tuneability, encapsulation capacity, receptiveness to the stimuli, and easy synthesis with minimal toxicity. This review will be focusing on the composition and defects of the bone, discussion on the conventional treatment strategies for bone defects, the role of Bone tissue engineering in bone regeneration, and the role of hydrogel polymers in the synthesis of bone regeneration with special reference to biodegradable nanogels and its

Application of Engineering Principles and Practices in Biotechnology.
Ann Rose Abraham, Leonardo Sepúlveda Torre, Tamara Tatrishvili, and A. K. Haghi (Eds.)

current status. Finally, future prospective of biodegradable nanogels in bone regeneration will be outlined.

5.1 INTRODUCTION

Bone is a connective tissue that together with cartilage forms a rigid and strong exoskeleton. The architecture of bone provides maximum strength for the least weight. Most bone has a cortex, cancellous zone with thin interconnecting narrow trabeculae with a rigid and impenetrable outer shell of compact bone. The extracellular matrix (ECM) of bone is a biphasic system:

a. one-third part constitutes organic matter, i.e., Type-I collagen
b. one-third part constitutes inorganic matter/bone-salt such as Hydroxyapatite (HA) like calcium salt (Bai et al., 2018).

Predominantly type-I collagen constitutes of the collagenous extracellular organic matrix and is called osteoid which undergoes mineralization due to the accumulation of calcium HA while the non-collagenous portion is specific to dental hard connective tissue which consists of proteins and proteoglycans. The net weight of bone is 60% inorganic material, 25% inorganic material, and 5% water. By volume, bone comprises: (a) 36% inorganic material, (b) 36% organic material, and (c) 28% water (Mohamed, 2008).

Bone is mainly composed of four types of cells and they are bone lining cells, osteocytes, osteoclasts, and osteoblasts. Integrated endocrine and paracrine control of these cells are important in maintaining bone mass by providing a precise balance between bone formation and bone resorption. Bone lining cells, Osteoblasts, and Osteoclasts are present on the bone surfaces while Osteocytes are present in the interiors of the bone (Mohamed, 2008).

Bone lining cells: It is considered post proliferative osteoblasts. It prevents osteoclast resorptive activity by covering the bone surfaces and can be reactivated to become osteoblasts.

Osteocytes: These are present in the interiors of bone and are the most mature differentiated state of the osteoblast lineage. They are widespread and hence detect stress induced in bone and are thus regarded as the main mechanoreceptors of bone. It secretes paracrine factors such as Insulin-like growth factor-1 (IGF-1) and expresses c-fos in response to mechanical stress (Lean et al., 1996; Peake et al., 2000). Osteocytes are always in communication with osteoblasts.

Osteoblasts: Osteoblasts are fibroblast-like cells of primitive mesenchymal stem cells that originated from pluripotent stem cells from an adherent part of the bone marrow. The major function of osteoblasts is the synthesis of components for the ECM matrix and promoting mineralization of the organic matrix. The process of mineralization is associated with matrix calcification and is carried out by matrix vesicles (Anderson, 1969; Nair and Jagannathan, 2013), extracellular organelles found in osteoid.

Matrix vesicles contain Alkaline Phosphatase (ALPase), Adenosine Triphosphatase (ATPase), and Inorganic pyrophosphatase as well as protein activator, e.g., Plasminogen activator. It contributes to the HA crystal formation via enzymatic deposition of Calcium and Phosphate (Anderson and Reynolds, 1973; Hasegawa et al., 2017). Many transcription factors [Core binding factor α-1 (Cbfa-1)] and Secreted molecules factor [Bone Morphogenetic Proteins (BMPs) and Indian hedgehog (Ihh)] are involved in the osteoblast differentiation.

Osteoclasts: Osteoclasts are derived from macrophage–monocyte lineage. They are large mononucleated phagocytic cells. Osteoclasts express enzymes such as tartrate-resistant acid phosphatase (TRAP), calcitonin receptors, vacuolar proton ATPase, and vitronectin receptors (Lee et al., 1995). The major function of Osteoclasts is the maintenance of blood-calcium homeostasis and bone resorption. Various genes are involved in Osteoclast differentiation like Transcription control (Osteopetrosis (op/op), PU.1, c-fos, Nuclear factor-kappa B (NF-κB), c-Src, and Microphthalmia (mi)) and Secreted molecules factor (Macrophage colony-stimulating factor (M-CSF), Osteoprotegerin, and Receptor activator of NF-κB and its ligand Receptor activator of NF-κB (RANK)).

5.2 OSTEOCLAST–OSTEOBLAST RELATIONSHIP

Osteoblast and Osteoclast maintain a balance during growth and resorption. It is achieved by cycles of resorption of old bones by osteoclasts which are followed by osteoblasts-induced bone formation (Khosla, 2001) (Fig. 5.1).

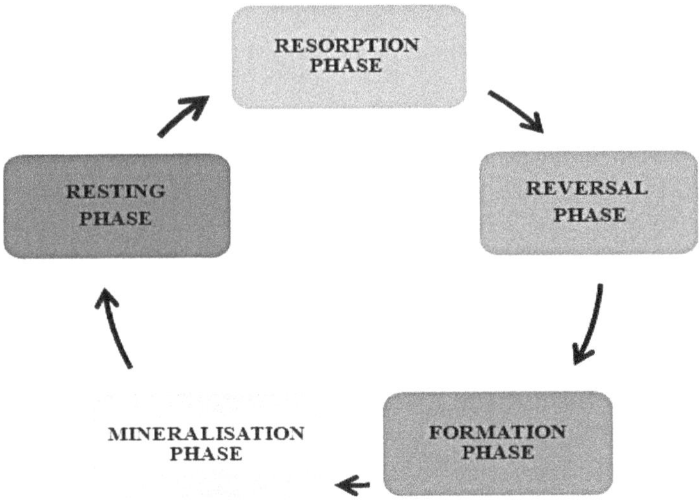

FIGURE 5.1 Osteoclast–osteoblast relationship.

5.3 BONE DAMAGE AND TREATMENT STRATEGIES

In recent years, the cost of treating bone-related ailments like infection, trauma, or tumor is immoderate. This graph seems to be escalating as the global orthobiologic market is estimated to be $ 5.5 billion worth and continues to increase with an anticipated growth of 7.03% by 2020. Orthobiologics (e.g., bone grafts, etc.) are substance developed from materials found in our body and that uses biomaterials and cell-based therapies for better recuperation.

Bone damages can be distinguished into various categories like bone fractures, aging, hereditary, and infection. One of the major causes of bone injuries is bone fractures which can affect any part of the body such as the clavicle, femur, skull, tibia, radius, scapula, humerus, etc. Aging-related ailments such as osteoporosis, bone infection (osteomyelitis), bone tumors, and hereditary diseases such as hereditary bone marrow failure and Hereditary multiple exostoses (HME) increase the risk of bone fractures. As bone formation is a dynamic process, the release of various cytokines and growth factors by the body itself can stimulate self-healing to an extent, but once the bone defects get out of order, there is a firm requirement for extraneous intervention to promote bone regeneration to restore normal functioning and synthesis of bone cells (Carrington, 2005; Baroli, 2009; Wijewardena et al., 2011; Bai et al., 2018).

5.4 CURRENT CLINICAL TREATMENTS

Current Clinical Treatments include autografts, allografts, and xenografts which use metal implants (e.g., bone nails), osteoconductive materials (e.g., Calcium phosphate), Hydroxyapatite, etc. These conventional treatment strategies failed due to the inability to integrate with surrounding tissue around the wound site/bone defect/bone injury site, limited mechanical strength, poor water-soluble resistance, slow degradation time, poor recuperating time, host rejection, high risk of disease transmission, and infection (Lee et al., 2009).

Bone tissue engineering (BTE) is an exciting approach to combat the limitations of conventional clinical treatments of bone disease. BTE uses scaffolds by incorporating growth factors, nanoparticles, and cells to promote bone repair and regeneration (Puppi et al., 2010). These scaffolds provide support and structural integrity, a suitable and healthy environment for cell adhesion, migration, and proliferation, induce the slow release of the bioactive molecule, and help in recapitulating bone activity.

Scaffolds are made up of natural polymers (Chitosan, Gelatin, Collagen, etc.), synthetic polymers [Poly (lactic acid) (PLA) and Poly (D, L-lactide-co-glycolide) (PLGA)], and inorganic composite materials (Ceramic). Though scaffolds demonstrate as an ideal replacement for traditional treatment strategies, they all have corresponding disadvantages, thus limiting their clinical use (Table 5.1).

TABLE 5.1 Drawbacks of Natural/Synthetic Polymers and Inorganic Composite Materials.

S. no.	Drawbacks of natural/synthetic polymers and inorganic composite materials
1	A high degree of variability
2	Complex structure
3	Costly process
4	Less stable
5	Immunogenic
6	Difficult in maintaining structural integrity
7	Cytocompatibility varies
8	Weak mechanical properties
9	Biodegradability varies
10	Costly synthesis process

One of the major drawbacks in the design of polymeric scaffolds is that the structure, characteristics of cells, and surrounding tissues are rarely considered. Therefore, the scaffolds usually display poor integration with native bone tissues. Thus materials used in constructing these scaffolds need to achieve optimal mechanical and biological performance to promote bone regeneration and thereby be used in rectifying bone defects (Bai et al., 2018).

To encourage advancement in BTE by promoting bone regeneration, hydrogel-based cell delivery and drug delivery have emerged as impending solutions in tissue engineering and regenerative medicine (Bai et al., 2018). Hydrogel is a 3D cross-linked hydrophilic polymer that mimics the ECM of the bone. Due to meshy networks or crosslinked polymers, bioactive molecules can be easily incorporated and can control their release. It is very well absorbable and can integrate surrounding tissue without any immunogenic reaction. Hydrogels can be fabricated using either natural or synthetic polymers. Optimized hydrogel formulations need to meet the following parameters:

1. Continuous improvement in the preparative method is required.
2. Cytocompatible and nonimmunogenic
3. Mimic ECM to promote cell adhesion, migration, and proliferation
4. Biodegradable
5. Strong structural stability and mechanical integrity
6. For a successful configuration, matrix modification is required which can thereby enhance biocompatibility, osteoinductive, osteoconductive, and osteogenic ability of bone, and finally stimulates bone repair.
7. Injectable capability with patient acquiescence and simplifying the administration process to reduce the pain (Lee et al., 2007).

Various hydrogel structures (Hydrogel microbeads; Hydrogel nanoparticles (nanogels), Hydrogel fibers, Hydrogel-based growth factors, and stem-cell delivery) can be constructed via multiple fabrication techniques.

In this review, we will focus on Biodegradable nanogels that have attracted interest in the scientific world by stimulating bone regeneration.

5.5 NANO HYDROGEL IN BONE REGENERATION

Nanogels (Hydrogel nanoparticles/nano hydrogel/polymeric nanogels/macromolecular micelles) are a group of multitudinous polymer-based material with adaptive properties and have been tremendously explored in the field of nanotechnology, drug delivery, diagnostic agent, pharmacology, gene delivery, etc (Fig. 5.2) (Neamtu et al., 2010). These are 3-D structures based on cross-linked polymeric networks with hydrophilic/amphiphilic macromolecular chains and are formed by chemical (covalent crosslinking) or physical (crosslinking with noncovalent bonds by hydrogen bonds, hydrophobic and electrostatic interaction) method.

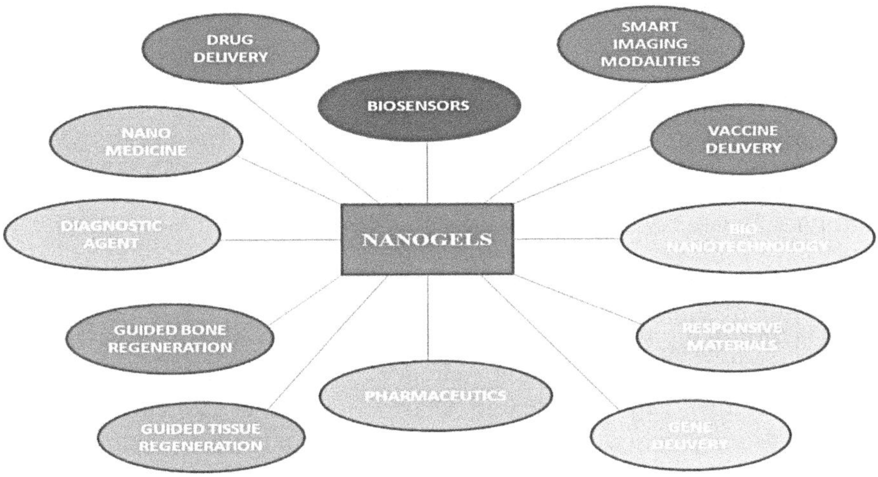

FIGURE 5.2 Multitudinous application of Nanogel.

It has immense capacity to retain water which allows it to swell without disturbing the actual structure. This property is attributed to the presence of various hydrophilic functional groups such as –OH, –CONH, $–CONH_2$, and $–SO_3H$. High water content or retention of water correlates with fluid-like properties for bioactive molecules relevantly smaller than the pore size. Hence, Nanogels are promising and innovative biomedical systems and are called next generation of drug delivery systems due to their high diversified drug encapsulation capacity, uniformity, tunability, ease of preparation, cytocompatibility, stability in the serum, and receptiveness to external stimuli (Fig. 5.3) (Neamtu et al., 2010).

Usually, Nanogels are synthesized through an emulsion polymerization (like the inverse emulsion polymerization method and distillation–precipitation polymerization), which copolymerizes a rapidly stirred solution at elevated temperature to acquire stable dispersions. Nanogels are biocompatible with better mechanical properties, and thus have a great advantage in the application of bone repair and regeneration (Fig. 5.4).

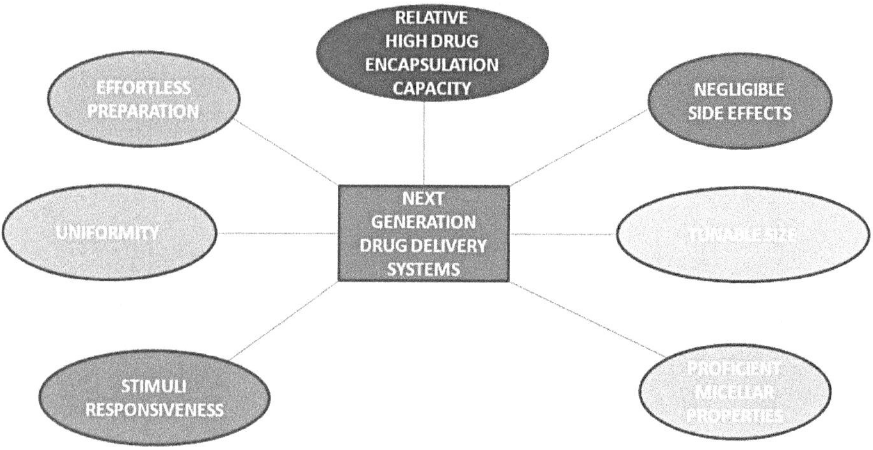

FIGURE 5.3 Parameters to develop an optimized Nanogel.

The following studies will provide a brief description of the synthesis and utilization of biodegradable nanogels. A previous study showed that Type-I collagen nanogel released MG-63 osteoblasts like cells in surgically created diaphyseal defects of New Zealand White rabbits which aided in the migration and proliferation of osteoblasts leading to bone healing (Themistocleous et al., 2007). Kato and colleagues displayed the release of PGE-2, a bone anabolic agent by Cholesterol-bearing pullulan (CHP)-nanogel which induced bone formation in ICR mice (Kato et al., 2007). Further, in another study, W9 peptide was released using CHP nanogel which prevented bone loss in a murine model (Alles et al., 2007). Release of BMP-2 stimulated osteoblast and bone formation was observed in surgically created calvarial defect in ICR mice; in this study nanogel-crosslinking hydrogel was used (Hayashi et al., 2009). In another study nanogel-based scaffold constituting EP4A and a low dose of BMP-2 was implanted on the calvarial defect created in ICR mice. A control and optimal dose of BMP-2 has been released which in turn stimulated bone formation and prevented bone loss (Kamolratanakul et al., 2011).

Fujioka-Kobayashi et al. (2012) showed successful delivery of BMP-2 and FGF-8 via Cholesteryl group and acrolyl group bearing pullulan nanogel using combination therapy. Nanogel stimulated bone regeneration in C5BL/6N mice (Fujioka-Kobayashi et al., 2012). Miyahara et al. (2012) demonstrated that when Wistar rats were treated with Cholesteryl bearing

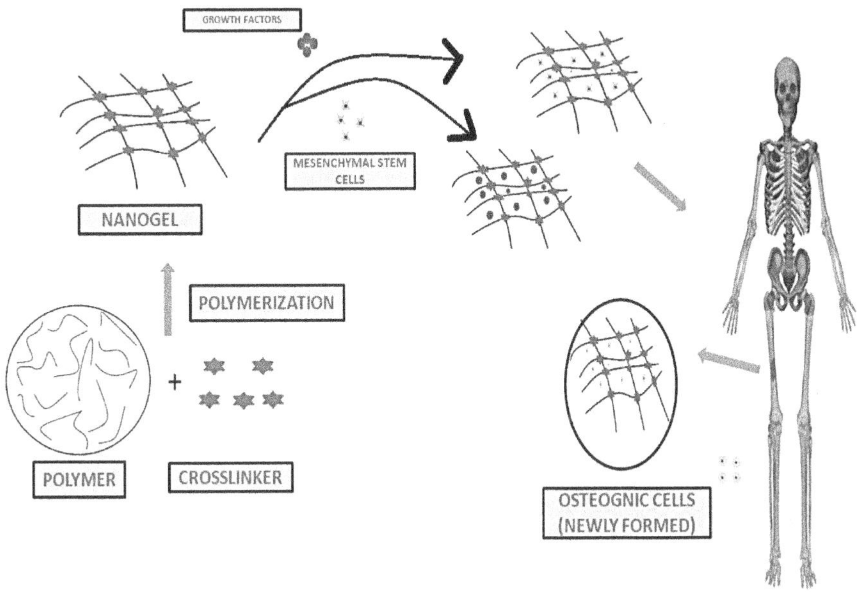

FIGURE 5.4 Pictorial representation of nanogel in bone repair and regeneration.

pullulan nanogel (Acrolyl group-modified Cholesteryl - bearing pullulan) showed a significant bone healing as compared to the control group (untreated) and Collagen membrane group. Interestingly, the histological evaluation suggested that surgically created parietal bone defect was not at all observed in CHP-the nanogel group, and both animals from the CHP-nanogel group and control group looked the same. However, to avoid rapid release of drugs, it is recommended to design nanoscale structured band type, mesh, cross-linking agent, etc. Young and his colleagues developed PEG nanogel using inverse polymerization. PEG nanogel carried QK, a pro-angiogenic peptide. Here, the cross-linking density was controlled by changing the mole fraction of the crosslinker to adjust the release of QK (Young et al., 2017).

In an in vitro study, controlled release of lithium was done by PHB-PAA nanogel (biodegradable polyhydroxy butyrate (PHB) matrix-polyacrylic acid (PAA) nanogels incorporated hybrid solid-gel nano-composite) to stimulate bone regeneration (Larsson et al., 2014). Sato et al. (2018) created NanoCliP-FD gel with dOBs (directly converted osteoblasts) which significantly promoted bone regeneration in bone defect lesions surgically created in NOG/SCID mice. The combination of the NanoCliP-FD gel and dOBs can act as a potent feasible therapeutic modality for bone diseases. Table 5.2 illustrates some more potential work by various researchers in the development of nanogel for bone repair and regeneration.

Biodegradable nanogels have demonstrated remarkable success in delivering controlled release of proteins, and growth factors and thereby induced bone growth. Designing tunable hydrogels provided strong mechanical integrity and stability. These parameters are imperative in developing efficacious treatments for bone repair and regeneration.

TABLE 5.2 Nanogels in Bone Tissue Engineering.

S. no.	Nanogel	Details	Animal	Reference
1	Type-I collagen nanogel	MG-63 osteoblasts like cells aided in migration and proliferation of osteoblasts leading to bone healing in surgically created diaphyseal defects	New Zealand White rabbit	Themistocleous et al., 2007
2	Cholesterol-bearing pullulan (CHP)-nanogel	Delivered PGE-2, a bone anabolic agent; induces bone formation	ICR mice	Kato et al., 2007
3	Polysaccharide-based nanogel (Cholesterol-bearing pullulan)	Delivered W9; prevention of bone loss	Murine model	Alles et al., 2009
4	Nanogel-crosslinking hydrogel (cholesterol-bearing pullulan nanogel (CHPA/Hydrogel)-crosslinking hydrogel)	Delivered BMP-2; stimulate osteoblast and induce bone formation in a surgically created calvarial defect	ICR mice	Hayashi et al., 2009
5	Nanogel-based scaffold [Acrylate group-modified cholesterol-bearing pullulan (CHPA)/PEG hydrogel]	Release of EP4A (EP4 receptor antagonist) in combination with a low dose of BMP-2; Regeneration of bone cells at calvarial defect; regeneration of bone marrow tissue	ICR mice	Kamolratanakul et al., 2011
6	Cholesteryl group and acrolyl group bearing pullulan nanogel	Delivered BMP-2 and FGF-8; bone regeneration	C5BL/6N mice	Fujioka-Kobayashi et al., 2012

TABLE 5.2 (Countinued)

S. no.	Nanogel	Details	Animal	Reference
7	Cholesteryl-bearing pullulan nanogel (Acrolyl group-modified cholesterol-bearing pullulan)	Delivered PGDF-BB at surgically created parietal bone defect; aiding in Guided bone regeneration	Wistar rats	Miyahara et al., 2012
8	PHB-PAA nanogel (Biodegradable polyhydroxy butyrate (PHB) matrix- polyacrylic acid (PAA) nanogels incorporated hybrid solid-gel nanocomposite)	Controlled release of lithium; inhibits bone loss; stimulates bone regeneration	In vitro	Larsson et al., 2014
9	Poly(organophosphazene); compact BMP-2/D-NPs complex formation by dual complex	BMP-2; bone regeneration	C5BL/6 mice	Seo et al., 2015
10	Nanoclik [Acrolyl group-modified cholesterol-bearing pullulan(CHOPA) nanogels were crosslinked by pentaerythritol (mercaptoethyl) polyoxyethylene)]	Carrier for peptide therapeutics; W9-bone resorption peptide used; aided in the inhibition of bone loss	C5BL/6J mice	Sato et al., 2015
11	p(N-isopropylacrylamide-co-butyl methylacrylate) (PIB) nanogels were combined with boron-containing mesoporous bioactive glass (B-MBG) scaffolds	Potential bone tissue engineering biomaterial able to treat defects of irregular shapes and deformities	Wistar rats	Chen et al., 2015
12	3D-printed microstructure incorporated with hybrid nano hydrogel-GelMA [cell-laden hydrogels incorporated with methacrylate gelatin (GelMA)+ RGNPs (cyclic peptide containing cell adherent arg-gly-asp (RGD) sequence conjugated to the surface of GNP)+ PLA]	Human Adipose-Derived Stem cells; stem cell differentiation and bone tissue regeneration	In vitro	Heo et al., 2017
13	PIB nanogel (with strontium loaded mesoporous bioactive glass)	Stimulate bone regeneration at surgically created femur bone defect	Rats	Zhang et al., 2017

TABLE 5.2 (Countinued)

S. no.	Nanogel	Details	Animal	Reference
14	Peptide Amphiphile Nanogel	Reduces the requirement of BMP-2; achieved high spine fusion rates with improved ease of delivery in posterolateral spine fusion rat model	Sprague Dawley rats	Hsu et al., 2017
15	Nanogel tectonic porous 3d scaffold (nanogel-crosslinked porous (NanoClip) Freeze dried (Fd) gel	Regeneration therapy of bone disease; Direct reprogramming of fibroblast to osteoblasts and regeneration	NOG/SCID mice	Sato et al., 2018

5.6 CONCLUSION

The concept of nanogel registered a noteworthy evolution, but before the transition from clinical trial to the current clinical application, there is an urgent need for a more detailed study on their pharmacodynamics, metabolism, and pharmacokinetics with more in vivo studies supported by relevant clinical data. At that point, nanogels can be considered bioactive' delivery carriers with improved efficiency of medical care and benefit to the patients.

KEYWORDS

- **bone repair and regeneration**
- **bone tissue engineering**
- **nanohydrogel**
- **osteoblast**
- **osteoclast osteogenesis**

REFERENCES

Alles, N.; Soysa, N. S.; Hussain, M. A.; Tomomatsu, N.; Saito, H.; Baron, R.; Morimoto, N.; Aoki, K.; Akiyoshi, K.; Ohya, K. Polysaccharide Nanogel Delivery of a TNF-α and RANKL Antagonist Peptide Allows Systemic Prevention of Bone Loss. *Eur. J. Pharm. Sci.* **2009,** *37* (2), 83–88.

Anderson, H. C.; Reynolds, J. J. Pyrophosphate Stimulation of Calcium Uptake into Cultured Embryonic Bones. Fine Structure of Matrix Vesicles and their Role in Calcification. *Devel. Biol.* **1973.**

Anderson, H. C. Vesicles Associated with Calcification in the Matrix of Epiphyseal Cartilage. *J. Cell Biol.* **1969,** *41,* 59–72

Bai, X.; Gao, M.; Syed, S.; Zhuang, J.; Xu, X.; Zhang XQ. Bioactive Hydrogels for Bone Regeneration. *Bioact. Mater.* **2018,** *3* (4):401–417.

Baroli, B. From Natural Bone Grafts to Tissue Engineering Therapeutics: Brainstorming on Pharmaceutical Formulative Requirements and Challenges. *J. Pharm. Sci.* **2009,** *98* (4), 1317–1375.

Carrington, J. L. Aging Bone and Cartilage: Cross-Cutting Issues. *Biochem. Biophys. Res. Commun.* **2005,** *328* (3), 700–708.

Chen, X.; Zhao, Y.; Geng, S.; Miron, R. J.; Zhang, Q.; Wu, C.; Zhang, Y. In Vivo Experimental Study on Bone Regeneration in Critical Bone Defects Using PIB Nanogels/Boron-Containing Mesoporous Bioactive Glass Composite Scaffold. *Int. J. Nanomed.* **2015,** *10,* 839.

Fujioka-Kobayashi, M.; Ota, M. S.; Shimoda, A.; Nakahama, K. I.; Akiyoshi, K.; Miyamoto, Y.; Iseki, S. Cholesteryl Group- and Acryloyl Group-Bearing Pullulan Nanogel to Deliver BMP2 and FGF18 for Bone Tissue Engineering. *Biomaterials* **2012,** *33* (30), 7613–7620.

Hasegawa, T.; Yamamoto, T.; Tsuchiya, E.; Hongo, H.; Tsuboi, K.; Kudo, A.; Abe, M.; Yoshida, T.; Nagai, T.; Khadiza, N.; Yokoyama, A. Ultrastructural and Biochemical Aspects of Matrix Vesicle-Mediated Mineralization. *J. Dent. Sci. Rev.* **2017,** *53* (2), 34–45.

Hayashi, C.; Hasegawa, U.; Saita, Y.; Hemmi, H.; Hayata, T.; Nakashima, K.; Ezura, Y.; Amagasa, T.; Akiyoshi, K.; Noda M. Osteoblastic Bone Formation is Induced by Using Nanogel-Crosslinking Hydrogel as Novel Scaffold for Bone Growth Factor. *J. Cell. Physiol.* **2009,** *220* (1), 1–7.

Heo, D. N.; Castro, N. J.; Lee, S. J.; Noh, H.; Zhu, W.; Zhang LG. Enhanced Bone Tissue Regeneration Using a 3D Printed Microstructure Incorporated with a Hybrid Nano Hydrogel. *Nanoscale* **2017,** *9* (16), 5055–5062.

Hsu, W.; Weiner, J.; Chun, D.; Lee, S.; McClendon, M.; Freshman, R.; Cook, R.; Schallmo, M.; Singh, S.; Yun, J.; Yun, C. Peptide Amphiphile Nanogel as an Improved BMP-2 Carrier for Spinal Arthrodesis. *Glob. Spine J.* **2016,** *6* (1 Suppl), s0036.

Kamolratanakul, P.; Hayata, T.; Ezura, Y.; Kawamata, A.; Hayashi, C.; Yamamoto, Y.; Hemmi, H.; Nagao, M.; Hanyu, R.; Notomi, T.; Nakamoto, T. Nanogel-Based Scaffold Delivery of Prostaglandin E2 Receptor–Specific Agonist in Combination with a Low Dose of Growth Factor Heals Critical-Size Bone Defects in Mice. *Arthritis Rheum.* **2011,** *63* (4), 1021–1033.

Kato, N.; Hasegawa, U.; Morimoto, N.; Saita, Y.; Nakashima, K.; Ezura, Y.; Kurosawa, H.; Akiyoshi, K.; Noda, M. Nanogel-Based Delivery System Enhances PGE2 Effects on Bone Formation. *J. Cell. Biochem.* **2007,** *101* (5), 1063–1070.

Khosla S. Minireview: The OPG/RANKL/RANK System. *Endocrinology* **2001,** *142,* 5050–5055.

Larsson, M.; Bergstrand, A.; Mesiah, L.; Van Vooren, C.; Larsson, A. Nanocomposites of Polyacrylic Acid Nanogels and Biodegradable Polyhydroxybutyrate for Bone Regeneration and Drug Delivery. *J. Nanomater.* **2014,** *2014,* 1–9.

Lean, J. M.; Mackay, A.; Chow, J.; Chambers, T. Osteocytic Expression of mRNA for c-fos and IGF-I; An Immediate Early Gene Response to An Osteogenic Stimulus. *Am. J. Physiol.* **1996,** *270,* 937–945

Lee, K.; Chan, C. K.; Patil, N.; Goodman, S. B. Cell Therapy for Bone Regeneration—Bench to Bedside. *J. Biomed. Mater. Res. B Appl. Biomater.* **2009,** *89* (1):252–263.

Lee, S. H.; Shin, H. Matrices and Scaffolds for Delivery of Bioactive Molecules in Bone and Cartilage Tissue Engineering. *Adv. Drug Deliv. Rev.* **2007,** *59* (4–5), 339–359.

Lee, S. K.; Goldring, S. R.; Lorenzo, J. A. Expression of the Calcitonin Receptor in Bone Marrow Cell Cultures and in Bone: A Specific Marker of the Differentiated Osteoclast that is Regulated by Calcitonin. *Endocrinology* **1995,** *136,* 4572–4581.

Miyahara, T.; Nyan, M.; Shimoda, A.; Yamamoto, Y.; Kuroda, S.; Shiota, M.; Akiyoshi, K.; Kasugai, S. Exploitation of a Novel Polysaccharide Nanogel Cross-Linking Membrane for Guided Bone Regeneration (GBR). *J. Tissue Eng. Regen. Med.* **2012,** *6* (8), 666–672.

Mohamed, A. M. An Overview of Bone Cells and their Regulating Factors of Differentiation. *Malays. J. Med. Sci.* **2008,** *15* (1), 4–12.

Nair, A.; Jagannathan, N. The Role of Matrix Vesicles in Mineralization of Bone-Review. *Ann. Romanian Soc. Cell Biol.* **2013,** *18* (2), 28–33.

Neamtu, I.; Rusu, A. G.; Diaconu, A.; Nita, L. E.; Chiriac, A. P. Basic Concepts and Recent Advances in Nanogels as Carriers for Medical Applications. *Drug Deliv.* **2017,** *24,* 539–557.

Peake, M. A.; Cooling, L. M.; Magnay, J. L.; Thomas, P. B.; El Haj, A. J. Selected Contribution: Regulatory Pathways Involved in Mechanical Induction of c-fos Gene Expression in Bone Cells. *J. Appl. Physiol.* **2000,** *89* (6), 2498–2507.

Puppi, D.; Chiellini, F.; Piras, A. M.; Chiellini, E. Polymeric Materials for Bone and Cartilage Repair. *Prog. Polym. Sci.* **2010,** *35* (4), 403–440.

Sato, T.; Alles, N.; Khan, M.; Nagano, K.; Takahashi, M.; Tamura, Y.; Shimoda, A.; Ohya, K.; Akiyoshi, K.; Aoki, K. Nanogel-Crosslinked Nanoparticles Increase the Inhibitory Effects of W9 Synthetic Peptide on Bone Loss in A Murine Bone Resorption Model. *Int. J. Nanomed.* **2015,** *10,* 3459.

Sato, Y.; Yamamoto, K.; Horiguchi, S.; Tahara, Y.; Nakai, K.; Kotani, S. I.; Oseko, F.; Pezzotti, G.; Yamamoto, T.; Kishida, T.; Kanamura, N. Nanogel Tectonic Porous 3D Scaffold for Direct Reprogramming Fibroblasts into Osteoblasts and Bone Regeneration. *Sci. Rep.* **2018,** *8* (1), 15824.

Seo, B. B.; Choi, H.; Koh, J. T.; Song, S. C. Sustained BMP-2 Delivery and Injectable Bone Regeneration Using Thermosensitive Polymeric Nanoparticle Hydrogel Bearing Dual Interactions with BMP-2. *J. Control. Release* **2015,** *209,* 67–76.

Themistocleous, G. S.; Katopodis, H. A.; Khaldi, L.; Papalois, A.; Doillon, C.; Sourla, A.; Soucacos, P. N.; Koutsilieris, M. Implants of Type I Collagen gel Containing MG-63 Osteoblast-like Cells can Act as Stable Scaffolds Stimulating the Bone Healing Process at the Sites of the Surgically-produced Segmental Diaphyseal Defects in Male Rabbits. *In Vivo* **2007,** *21* (1), 69–76.

Wijewardena, A.; Vandervord, E.; Lajevardi, S. S.; Vandervord, J.; Jackson, C. J. Combination of Activated Protein C and Topical Negative Pressure Rapidly Regenerates Granulation Tissue over Exposed Bone to Heal Recalcitrant Orthopedic Wounds. *Int. J. Low. Extrem. Wounds* **2011,** *10* (3), 146–151.

Young, D. A.; Pimentel, M. B.; Lima, L. D.; Custodio, A. F.; Lo, W. C.; Chen, S. C.; Teymour, F.; Papavasiliou, G. Design and Characterization of Hydrogel Nanoparticles with Tunable Network Characteristics for Sustained Release of a VEGF-mimetic Peptide. *Biomater. Sci.* **2017,** *5* (10), 2079–2092.

Zhang, Q.; Chen, X.; Geng, S.; Wei, L.; Miron, R. J.; Zhao, Y.; Zhang, Y. Nanogel-based Scaffolds Fabricated for Bone Regeneration with Mesoporous Bioactive Glass and Strontium: In Vitro and in Vivo Characterization. J. *Biomed. Mater. Res. A* **2017,** *105* (4), 1175–1183.

PART 3

BIOTECHNOLOGY AND BIO-BASED ROUTES TO SUSTAINABLE COMPOSITES

CHAPTER 6

Coir-Reinforced Biocomposites: Engineering Properties and Applications

P. H. VAISAKH[1], SNEHA SARA VARGHESE[1], TRESSIA ALIAS PRINCY PAULOSE[1], and H. AKHINA[2]

[1]*Post Graduate and Research Department of Chemistry, Bishop Moore College, Mavelikara, Kerala, India*

[2]*School of Energy Materials, Mahatma Gandhi University, Kottayam, Kerala, India*

ABSTRACT

Nowadays, novel composites are developed using sustainable natural fibers (such as coir) primarily because they are more environmentally friendly than synthetic fibers, with low density, low cost, high stiffness, medium strength, and high elongation.

In this chapter, coir is successfully used as reinforcement (as short fiber, long fiber, tangled or compressed mat, etc.). As the mechanical and interfacial properties of coir along with the matrix are significantly enhanced by surface modification, it is shown that it can be widely applied as a reinforcement material when combined with structural materials and polymers.

6.1 INTRODUCTION

Recent years have seen a rise in consumers' strict knowledge of new products made from sustainable sources. The consumer has been drawn to environmentally friendly items as a result of green marketing, new recycling regulations, social pressure, and changes in cognitive values.

Application of Engineering Principles and Practices in Biotechnology.
Ann Rose Abraham, Leonardo Sepúlveda Torre, Tamara Tatrishvili, and A. K. Haghi (Eds.)

The development and redesign of composite materials in particular aims to enhance, adapt, and offer new products in a sustainable and ethical manner. Whenever two or more basic materials (metal, ceramic, and polymer) are combined and treated, a composite is created. This new content has qualities that are greater than those of the individual components that constituted the composite. Modern composites were developed using natural fibers primarily because they are more environmentally friendly than synthetic fibers (Oladele et al., 2022). They are reusable, somewhat strong, and stiff, without irritating the skin, although they do have drawbacks including quality differences and poor heat stability. As a result, numerous studies on the potential of natural fibers as reinforcement in polymer and ceramic-based composites have been conducted, and some are still ongoing. Results from various cases have demonstrated that among other qualities looked at, the biofiber-based composites exhibit good stiffness. Composites made of coir fiber have been researched in this area with encouraging outcomes. Animal or plant sources make up the majority of natural fibers. The first is primarily made of cellulose, whereas the latter is made of proteins. However, natural fibers are frequently referred to as vegetable fibers in the composites field (Peças et al., 2018).

6.1.1 NATURAL FIBER-REINFORCED COMPOSITES (NFRC)

The thermosetting or thermoplastic polymers are embedded with natural fibers to create natural fiber-reinforced composites (NFRCs), which are also known as "green composites," "ecocomposites," and "biocomposites" (Mohammed et al., 2015). The NFRCs are made up of reinforcing material and a polymer matrix that can either be derived from natural biopolymers or petroleum (in the form of fibers or particles). NFRCs can be divided into three types based on the proportion of natural materials employed as the reinforcing medium: green, semi-green, and hybrid composites (Kanitkar et al., 2017). Green composites are those in which the polymer and reinforcing elements (such as polylactic acid and hemp) are both derived from natural or renewable sources (Witayakran et al., 2017). More natural components make up the semi-green composites, which are made of both natural and synthetic polymers. The hybrid composites, like a composite construction comprised of glass or carbon fibers, are constructed from a single polymeric matrix and two or more distinct synthetic or man-made fibers. A 100% bio-based composite is being developed, but it is challenging because natural fibers have some undesirable qualities, such as high moisture absorption, difficult and drawn-out extraction processes, and low thermal stability, which frequently have a negative impact on the final mechanical properties of composite materials (Väisänen et al., 2017). As a result, there is currently a viable and significant effort being made to build composites that allow for the addition of various amounts of natural fibers to polymeric matrices. These composites (natural fiber) have a minimal bio-based component. The NFRCs are cost-effective, renewable, biodegradable, and ecologically friendly (Safri et al., 2018). In the automobile industry, for instance, these composites might eventually take the place of steel, which could cut the overall weight of a vehicle by around 25% and the need to use almost 250 million barrels of oil. The NFRCs can be utilized in the creation of ceilings, columns, doors, and window frames, among other things (Shinoj et al., 2011). Additionally, in recent years, in addition to the virgin natural fibers, the widely accessible short and non-spinnable waste natural fibers as well as recycled plastic materials have been used in the fabrication of the NFRCs. For situations where composites with strong mechanical qualities are not required, bio-based green composites can be made using, for instance, waste oil plum fibers, wood flour and fibers, recyclable polymers (such polyolefins), and short fibers of cotton, flax, sisal, jute, and hemp (e.g., panels, gardening products, and packaging) (Mukherjee et al., 2011).

6.1.2 CLASSIFICATION OF COMPOSITES BASED ON THE NATURE OF NATURAL FIBER

Plant, animal, and mineral fibers are the three categories into which natural fibers are separated based on origin. The fiber is extracted from plant fiber, a type of natural resource. The plant fiber comes in both short and long fiber forms, and when it mixes with the polymer matrix, it has a high level of stiffness and strength. The geometry of a plant fiber affects its stiffness and strength. Animal body parts such as skin and hair are used to make animal fiber. Because they are created with the fewest surface flaws, mineral fibers are the strongest fibers that have ever been discovered. Asbestos is the material used most frequently. Chemically speaking, cellulose, hemicellulose, lignin, pectin, and ash make up natural fibers. The chemical makeup of each fiber is unique. The number of chemical components in a fiber affects its qualities, and the amount of cellulose in a fiber affects its strength and stiffness (Gaurav et al., 2019). Some characteristics of vegetable fiber, including moisture absorption, heat breakdown, and biodegradation, are controlled by the presence of hemicelluloses. Thermal stability in natural fibers is caused by the lignin concentration. In this chapter, we will be discussing coir-reinforced composites, its engineering properties and applications.

6.2 COIR

Natural fiber known as coir is obtained from the coconut fruit's husk. The pith, a corky tissue, and coir fiber make up the husk. India has the second-highest availability of this fiber in the world, behind the Philippines. Water, fibers, and trace amounts of soluble substances make up its composition. When compared to other natural fibers, coir is more durable due to its high lignin content. Natural fibers, such as those found in coir-based composites, are finding increased use in automobiles as well as in trains, buses, and other forms of public transportation as the emphasis on fuel efficiency grows. A fantastic opportunity exists to manufacture coir-based composites for a variety of uses in architecture and construction, including boards and blocks like reconstituted wood, flooring tiles, etc. In addition to significantly enhancing the quality of life for those involved in coir production, value-added innovative applications of natural fibers and coir-based composites would also secure an international market for less expensive alternatives (Verma et al., 2013).

The three countries producing the most coir are India, Vietnam, and Sri Lanka, with yearly yields of 580, 382, and 161 thousand tons, respectively (Food and Agriculture Organization of the United Nations, 2015). There are two different forms of coir fibers, brown fiber and white fiber, depending on the coconut's age. When coconut fiber is removed, it comes out of older coconuts as brown fiber and young coconuts as white fiber. White or light brown is typically the color of white coir fiber. White coir fiber is typically spun into yarn for coir mat and rope because it is smooth and fine. Due to its prolonged growing period, brown coir fiber is often thicker, stronger, and more abrasion resistant than white coir fiber. The coir fiber-reinforced cementitious composite can therefore use brown fiber as monofilament reinforcement (CFRC).

6.2.1 COMPOSITION AND PROPERTIES OF COIR FIBERS

The advantages of coir fibers include their low price, high lignin content, low density, availability, strong elongation at break, and low elastic modulus. The creation of fiber-reinforced composites requires an understanding of this composition (Sudhakara et al., 2013). The chemical, physical–mechanical, thermal, and microstructural properties will be covered in this section.

6.2.1.1 CHEMICAL COMPOSITION

Chemically, lignin, hemicellulose, and cellulose make up the majority of coir fibers. Coir fibers typically contain between 32 and 50% cellulose, 0.15 and 15% hemicellulose, 30–46% lignin, and about 3–4% pectin. This highlights the fact that cellulose and lignin make up the majority of plant fibers. The origin of the coconut plant from which the fibers were extracted or the method of extraction may be responsible for the variations in coir fiber characteristics.

6.2.1.2 PHYSICAL AND MECHANICAL COMPOSITION

The qualities of the components that make up a composite and how those materials interact determine a lot of its properties. A material's physical characteristics include its diameter, density, and weight increase due to water absorption, whereas its mechanical characteristics include its tensile, flexural, and impact strengths. The density, young's modulus, and tensile strength of coir fibers are 1.1–1.5 g/cm^3, 2–8 GPa, and 105–593 MPa, respectively; 15–51% elongation at break and 10–180% at water absorption. The source of the fiber, the pretreatment, and the extraction techniques may affect how these qualities vary.

Many researchers have looked into coconut fibers for a variety of reasons. While the diameter of coconut fibers is around the same and the magnitudes of tensile strength are significantly different, there is a significant variance in other aspects. Coir fiber's tensile strength ranges from 80 to 304 MPa, while its tensile modulus ranges from 0.9 to 6.2 GPa. Of all natural fibers, coconut fiber is the most ductile. As demonstrated by (Munawar et al., 2007), coconut fibers can withstand tension 4–6 times greater than other fibers. Coir fiber's strain at failure ranges from 12.5 to

83.7%, which is higher than flax's (1.23%–3.3%), jute's (1%–1.8%), sisal's (2.07%–7.0%), and hemp's (1%–3.5%). The large MFA and low cellulose content of the coir fiber may be the primary causes of the coir fiber's low tensile strength, low tensile modulus, and high strain at failure. Due of these qualities, coir fiber can effectively replace steel fiber in cementitious materials to increase ductility. The kind of species, location, and plant maturity are claimed to affect the fiber diameters of the various individual cells. The length to diameter ratio of the fiber affects its flexibility and ability to rupture, and thus affects the products that may be manufactured from it. The cell wall thickness and the origin of the fiber both affect the form and size of the center hollow hole, or lumen. The hollow chamber reduces the bulk density of the fiber, acting as an acoustic and thermal insulator. Abiola (C.O.P.D et al., 2008) conducted an experimental evaluation of the mechanical characteristics (load–extension curves, stress–strain curves, Young's modulus, yield stress, and stress and strain at breaks), and the outcomes were confirmed by finite element method using the commercial program ABAQUS. The outer coconut fiber had a stronger elongation characteristic than the inner coconut fiber, which could allow it to absorb or withstand higher stretching energy than the inner coconut fiber. The author discovered that the inner coconut fiber had a higher mechanical strength than the outer fiber.

6.2.1.3 CHEMICAL PROPERTIES

The three main components of coconut fibers are cellulose, hemicellulose, and lignin. The various characteristics of coconut fibers are impacted by these compositions. The composition of fibers is altered by pretreatment, which also affects their final properties and those of composites. Sometimes it makes fibers behave better, but other times its impact is unfavorable. Ramakrishna and Sundararajan (2005) studied the variation in chemical composition and tensile strength of four natural fibers (coconut, sisal, jute, and hibiscus cannabinus fibers) when subjected to alternate wetting and drying and continuous immersion for 60 days in three mediums. They also investigated the chemical composition of coconut fibers (water, saturated lime and sodium hydroxide). All examined fibers underwent a chemical composition change (continuous immersion was shown to be crucial), losing strength. However, coconut fibers were said to be the best at maintaining a sizable portion of their original tensile strength under all test conditions.

6.2.1.4 THERMAL PROPERTIES OF COIR FIBERS

Thermogravimetric analysis (TGA) can be used to look at the thermal stability of any material. The greatest temperature at which a fiber can withstand decomposition is referred to as the fiber's thermal stability. The disintegration of a fiber's hemicellulose/pectin and cellulose/lignin concentration is linked to thermal degradation of the fiber. Morandim–Giannetti claims that cellulose Agnelli degrades between 240 and 350°C, lignin between 280 and 500°C, and hemicellulose between 200 and 260°C. It has been discovered that alkali treatment of fibers and hybridization of fiber composites both significantly increase the thermal stability of the corresponding material. It has also been observed that adding coir fibers lowers the heat conductivity of composite specimens.

6.2.1.5 FUNCTIONAL GROUP ANALYSIS OF COIR FIBERS

A Fourier transform infrared spectroscopy (FTIR) machine can be used to determine the functional groups of natural fiber and natural fiber composites utilizing the attenuated total reflectance (ATR) method. Raw coir fiber has been shown to have many functional groups, including hydroxyl (OH), carboxyl (COOH), carbonyl (C=O), and methylene because it contains cellulose, hemicellulose, and lignin (CH_2). However, given that fiber treatment lowers the lignin concentration of the fibers, these functional groups and their detection can be changed by any type of fiber treatment (Adeniyi et al., 2019).

6.2.1.6 MICROSTRUCTURAL PROPERTIES OF COIR FIBERS

Numerous studies have looked into the coir fibers' microstructural characteristics, which can be seen using a scanning electron microscope (SEM). The coir fiber typically has a cylindrical shape (diameter of around 10–460 m) with a lacuna in the center surrounded by 200–300 elementary fibers (Fig. 6.1). According to Yan et al. (2016), an elementary fiber is a hollow, cylindrical structure made up of individual fiber cells with lengths of around 1 mm and diameters of 10–20 m. One coir fiber's lacuna area ranged from 4000 to 20,000 m^2, according to Tran et al. reported the SEM image analysis and SEM–computer tomography (CT) scans.

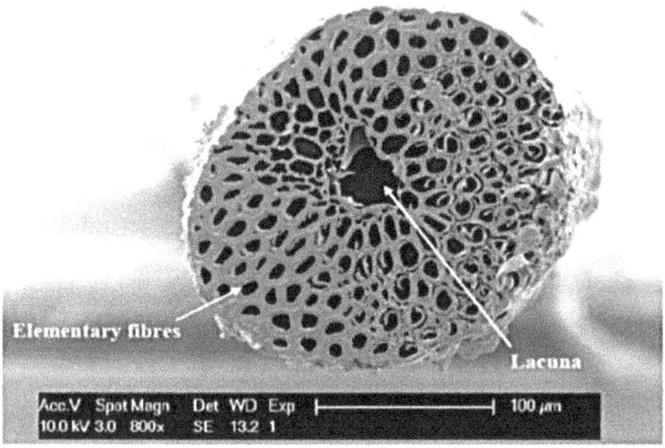

FIGURE 6.1 Cross section of coir fiber.

Source: Reprinted with permission from Wang et al., 2022

The overall porosity of the fiber was estimated to be between 21 and 31%. This high porosity means that coconuts may float, as well as their extensive habitation in practically all tropical and subtropical climates. Figure 5.2 displays the coir fiber surface in the fiber direction. On the surfaces, there are little circular perforations known as pits. The pits are responsible for carrying out the water or general nutrient exchange since the lignification of the cell membrane renders the cell less permeable. Tylosis, also known as globular protrusions, are typically present in the pit. The protoplast of the neighboring parenchymatous cells overgrows to produce a new wall material, or tylosis, when under stress or when pathogens invade. Typically, cellulose, hemicellulose, pectin, suberin, and lignin make up the tylosis. The pit membrane is stretched and forced into the vessel as tylosis develops. Tylosis simultaneously protrudes into xylem vessels via pit. Tylosis has the ability to fully plug plant vessels and prevent diseases from invading them further. Tylosis limits water exchange in the case of coir fiber by filling the surface pits. When under stress or when pathogens infiltrate, the protoplast of the adjacent parenchymatous cells overgrows to form additional wall material, called tylosis. Typically, the tylosis is composed of cellulose, hemicellulose, pectin, suberin, and lignin. Tylosis progresses by stretching and pulling the pit membrane into the vessel. Tylosis concurrently protrudes from the pit into xylem vessels. Tylosis has the power to completely clog plant vessels, keeping pathogens from spreading farther within. By filling the surface pits, tylosis restricts water exchange in the case of coir fiber.

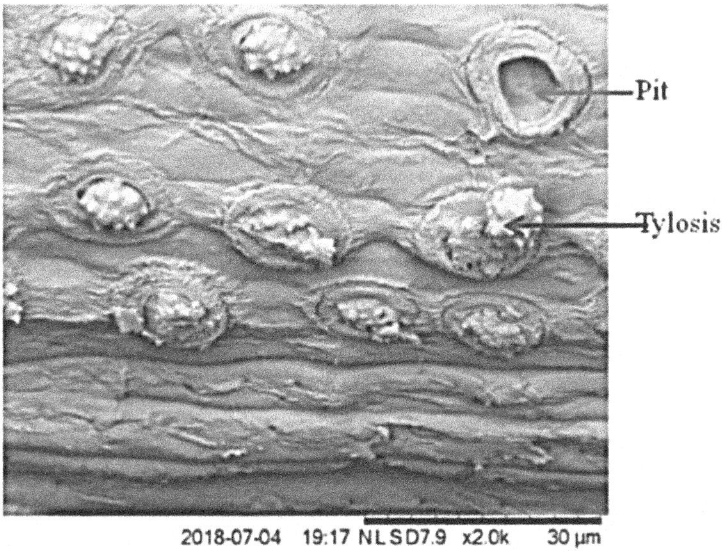

FIGURE 6.2 Coir surface along fiber direction under SEM.
Source: Reprinted with permission from Wang et al., 2022.

6.2.2 EXTRACTION AND TREATMENT OF COIR FIBERS

Large quantities of various leftovers, with coir shells as one of their main components, are obtained during the manufacturing of coconut fruits. In addition to the common use of coir wastes in heating, these shells can be used to extract coir fibers, leaving behind coir shell particles that are helpful in polymer reinforcements (Essabir et al., 2016). Before being used as a polymer reinforcement, coir fibers can be crushed, ground, and cut into a variety of sizes. Coconut husks can be used to obtain coir fibers by mechanical or water retting methods (defibering or decortication). Since cellulose and hemicellulose, the two primary components of cellulosic fibers, have hydroxyl groups that are strongly polarized, these fibers are typically hydrophilic in nature. Due to their propensity to absorb moisture from the environment and their weak interfacial interaction with the hydrophobic polymer matrix, this restricts the usage of these fibers in industrial applications. It has been found that chemically treating fibers can help to get around these issues and encourage strong fiber-matrix bonding. Improvements in interfacial adhesion between fiber and resin have been made using a variety of techniques, including enzymatic treatment, steam explosion (Zhang and Hu, 2014), physical treatment techniques such as plasma and corona discharge, and chemical methods such as acid or alkali treatment and coupling agent modification (silane and maleated polypropylene).

Polyester, polypropylene, low-density polyethylene, starch, wheat gluten, high-density polyethylene, epoxy, polylactide, magnesium phosphate cement, bakelite, etc. are just a few of the matrix materials that coir is compatible with. It has been found that the mechanical properties of coir-based composite are highly impacted by the type, size, percentage, and chemical treatment of the fibers as well as the type of compatibilizer. The interfacial interaction between fiber and matrix material is directly impacted by the mechanical capabilities and surface qualities of coir, which researchers investigated using various chemical treatments. On coir, they have effectively used treatments such as NaOH, $NaHCO_3$, plasma, silane, $KMnO_4$, sodium chlorite, and acetylated, and they have seen that these treatments greatly improve the surface qualities of the fiber. However, many researchers favor the 4–10% NaOH treatment, which increases coir's surface roughness and mechanical characteristics. In addition, compatibilizer is important in coir-reinforced composites; nevertheless, the choice and content of compatibilizer is greatly influenced by the matrix material. Due of its medium strength, coir is sometimes unable to significantly increase the tensile strength of the composite, but it can greatly increase its tensile modulus, flexural modulus, energy absorption, and ductility.

6.2.3 MECHANICAL PROPERTIES OF COIR-BASED COMPOSITES

Coir is a strong, durable, biodegradable fiber that can endure exposure to saltwater, hot water, and heat. Thermoplastic and thermosetting plastics, as well as cement-type materials, are all highly compatible with coir. When exposed to water or soil for an extended period of time, the acetylation treatment of the fiber helps the composite keep its mechanical qualities. According to Rout et al. (2001), 25% weight of untreated coir can be added to the polyester matrix to achieve the best mechanical qualities. In comparison to the impact strength of the Polyester matrix, which was 15 J/m, the impact strength significantly increased and was measured at 967 J/m. These qualities of composite are further enhanced by the chemical treatment of fiber. Improved bonding of short coir with natural rubber is seen after toluene diisocyanate and alkali treatments. For coir-based natural rubber composite, potassium permanganate treatment of alkali-treated short coir is not acceptable. Compared to good interfacial connections, the weak interfacial bonds of short coir and natural rubber gum dissipate more energy. The short coir-based polypropylene composite was successfully created by Lai et al. (2005), who also emphasized that the coir has exceptional potential to replace the synthetic fibers in thermoplastic composites. More fiber content was found to increase the mechanical characteristics. The mechanical properties of the recycled polymer composite are worse than expected, but they become better when 2% styrene maleic anhydride is added as a bonding agent. Li et al. (2007) examined several flexural characteristics of coir mesh-based coir-based cement composite. The flexural strength is increased by 44% with the addition of three layers of coir mesh, or 1.8% of the overall weight. After applying a wetting agent, a further improvement was seen (Albatex FFC). On a short coir-based polypropylene composite, Santos et al. (2009) looked at the effects of vinyl triethoxysilane and maleic anhydride coupling agents. By adding a coupling agent, the elastic modulus was found to be greatly raised, and vinyltriethoxysilane was shown to be superior than maleic anhydride. From 10% to 50% more fiber, there is a modest rise in elastic modulus. Long coir fibers may be a good choice to increase the strength and stiffness of tropical soil. He noted that the NaOH content must be less than 8% because a larger percentage greatly decreases the tensile strength. Both the tensile strength and the modulus of the composite were greatly improved by the addition of NaOH-treated fiber. Short coir fiber-reinforced polypropylene composites with varying fiber and compatibilizer percentages were created by Bettini et al. (2010) and have a length of about 827 mm. The mechanical properties were greatly improved by the compatibilizer (maleic anhydride grafted polypropylene), but its proportion had little effect. The percentage of fiber increases impact and tensile strength while decreasing the percentage of elongation. The mechanical characteristics of coir-based and abaca-reinforced polypropylene composites were examined by Haque et al. (2010). Abaca-reinforced polypropylene composite did not perform as well as coir-reinforced polypropylene composite. They used 3-mm long fibers that were treated with benzene diazonium and 5% NaOH solution. Tensile strength rises as coir percentage rises up to 10% before beginning to fall. Wheat gluten's characteristics were improved by adding coir. Using glycerol as a thermoplasticizer, Ramirez et al. (2011) created a coir fiber composite based on cassava starch. The composite's mechanical characteristics were found to be superior than the matrix. Without treatment, a composite with 30% fiber content had a tensile strength of 1.56 MPa and a Young's modulus of 14.56 MPa, while an annealed composite had a tensile strength of 3.24 MPa and a Young's modulus of 59.81 MPa. Experimental research on the silane-treated coir-reinforced high density polyethylene was conducted by Arrakhiz et al. (2012). Young's modulus and tensile strength both appeared to grow by 50% and 70%, respectively. The suitability of coir and polyester composite for storage tank applications was looked into by Yousif and Ku (2012). They discovered that the material in question can be utilized to store diesel, oil filters, freshwater, and saltwater for a long time. The impact of coir and compatibilizer fraction on the fatigue properties of polypropylene and coir composite was calculated by Antunes et al. (Diani and Gall, 2006). The fatigue qualities were improved by adding compatibilizer; however, adding more compatibilizer had negative effects. A study comparing glass fiber-reinforced plastics and natural fiber-reinforced plastics was reported by Wambua et al. (2003). They came to the conclusion that polypropylene with coir reinforcement can be a good option for impact applications.

Coir's potential to improve the flexural qualities of magnesium phosphate cement. At room temperature and with a 3% fiber loading, the flexural strength was reported to grow from 5.98 to 7.31 MPa after 7 days of curing and from 11.66 to 13.49 MPa after 28 days. Coir, jute, and polyester were used to create a hybrid composite by Singh et al. They discovered that while increasing the amount of coir enhanced the percentage of elongation and ductility, adding jute to the composite increased its mechanical strength. Bensalah et al. (2021) investigated the results of submerging coir that had been treated with NaOH at a concentration of about 6.4% in a Bakelite matrix. The highest mechanical properties are found in Bakelite with a 30% fiber loading; the flexural modulus increases by about 8.2%, or from 7.6 to 8.22 GPa, but the flexural strength decreases by about 2.8% and the strain increases dramatically, improving the ductility of the composite. The damping factor grows along with an increase in coir percentage.

6.2.4 APPLICATION OF COIR FIBER-BASED COMPOSITES

It is clear from the aforementioned mechanical characteristics that coconut fibers are the most ductile and energy-absorbing material. The development of composite materials with coconut fibers has the potential to be employed in a variety of applications. It was discovered that numerous researchers had already looked into a variety of coconut fiber-reinforced composites, with good and affordable outcomes. Engineers employ mature coir fiber-reinforced polymer matrix composites for a variety of reasons, including those related to the automotive industry, building, aeronautical engineering, etc. Coir-based composites are widely used in automobiles and railroad coaches due to the rising demand for fuel efficiency. Coir fibers may be handled more easily than synthetic fibers since they are non-toxic, lightweight, affordable, and environmentally friendly. Because of their widespread availability, adaptability, renewability, cost-effectiveness, and biodegradability as lingocellulosic-based fibers, coir fibers are employed as reinforcement in many polymer's matrix composites. It is an extra agro-industrial non-food feedstock that has been utilized to create a wide range of products and is regarded as a feedstock for creating eco-friendly composite materials. Because of its low thermal conductivity and high bulk density, coconut coir is one of the most intriguing items made from agricultural waste. As a result, adding coconut coir made products lighter and reduced the heat conductivity of composites. The environmental and energy problems will be resolved by the development of composite materials for building applications employing coconut coir with low thermal conductivity.

For the creation of frequently used materials like ceilings, partition boards, and car interiors, Amoako et al. (2018) study's and recommendation of coir fiber-reinforced recycled waste polyethylene-based composites was conducted. These waste products were altered to be used as possible engineering materials since they were harming the environment. For usage in making helmets, roofing sheets, and post boxes, coir fiber-reinforced polyester composites have been thoroughly studied by numerous researchers. Recent research on the manufacturing of engineered materials has continued to center on this activity. The incorporation of bio-based/natural reinforcement elements into composites now being produced is the result of the search for biodegradable/eco-friendly materials. Numerous products, including recreational goods, aviation components, maritime equipment, building materials, and transportation supplies, are made using these composites. For the manufacture of yarn, ropes, brushes, mats, rugs, mattresses, sacking, caulking boats, geo-textiles, insulation panels, and packaging products, coir fiber and coir fiber-based composite materials are utilized. There are other projects underway to create further goods from coconut fibers for use in car interior door coverings, trunk liners, and flooring. Coconut fibers have been employed in composites for non-structural parts in civil engineering as reinforcement. The performance of coconut fiber-based concrete for structural elements including beams, columns, and walls needs be studied, nevertheless. Coconut fiberboards made from coir fiber can be used in place of building materials like ceiling tiles, bricks, and cement hollow blocks. It is used for partitioning, ceilings, and internal and exterior walls. Additionally, it can be used to make furniture. Due to its thermal stability, coir fiber can be utilized to produce particle boards with low thermal conductivity (in the range of 0.054–0.1854 W/m·K), depending on the density of the board (Hirunlabh et al., 2003). Due to its high lignin and phenolic content, coconut pith is chemically reactive and can be hot-pressed into binderless particle board with significant commercial potential. Agopyan et al. (2005) investigated the effects of sisal and coconut fibers as alternatives to asbestos in roofing tiles. The experiment studied the influence of weather conditions on the tiles with a 2% total fiber volume fraction. The greatest load that coir-based tiles could support after ageing for 16 and 60 months was 235 and 248 N, respectively, compared to 237 and 159 N for sisal-based tiles. The main advantage of reinforced tiles was found to be that they at least 22% more effectively absorbed energy than unreinforced tiles. Therefore, this might short-term aid to prevent the fragile tile rupture during shipping or installation. After 28 days of hydration, Asasutjarit et al. (3005) identified the physical, mechanical, and thermal characteristics of the coconut-based lightweight cement board. Fiber length, coir pretreatment, and mixing ratio were the variables examined. It was determined that boiling and washing 6cm long fibers produced the best results when mixed with cement in a 2:1:2 weight-to-volume ratio. It was found that the produced board had less thermal conductivity than commercial boards made of flake-based composite. Researchers Paramasivam et al. (1965) looked at the viability of creating corrugated slabs reinforced with coir fiber for use in low-cost housing for poor countries. It was found that casting technology can be used to create corrugated slabs reinforced with coconut fiber. The findings demonstrated that low frequency asbestos boards and ordinary asbestos boards had equivalent thermal conductivity and sound absorption coefficients. Comparative research on cement sand mortar (1:3) slabs' resistance to impact loading was done by Agopyan et al. (2005). The chosen biofibers, coconut, sisal, jute, and hibiscus cannabinum fibers, with fiber concentrations ranging from 0.5 to 2.5% by cement weight and fiber lengths of 20, 30, and 40 mm, were used to strengthen the slab samples. According to the findings, coconut fibers with a 2% fiber content and a 40-mm fiber length among evaluated fiber-based composites provided the best impact energy absorption at 254 J. Additionally, all fibers, with the exception of coconut fiber, demonstrated fiber pullout upon failure. Li et al. used nonwoven coir mesh matting to study the fiber volume fraction and fiber surface treatment with a wetting agent for coir mesh-reinforced mortar. The findings indicated a 40% increase in maximum flexural strength, a 25-fold increase in flexural toughness, and around a 20-fold increase in flexural ductility. Mohammad examined wall panels composed of reinforced gypsum and cement with coconut fiber. The findings demonstrated that, with increasing coconut fibers but no appreciable change in moisture level, compressive strength rises. The moisture content did, however, rise over time. Slopes are firmly supported by coir erosion textiles because of their durability. With sufficient strength, coir fiber can endure degradation for up to five years. They come in a variety of shapes, including rolls, matting, and logs, which added to their suitability for stabilizing soil. Applications for coconut fiber include slope stabilization in railway cutting and embankments, reinforcement of temporary walls, protection of water-courses, unpaved roads in rural areas, providing a sub-base layer in road pavements, land reclamation and filtration in road drains, temporary seeding slopes for highways, controlling gully erosion and shallow mass waste, and many more (Sampaio and Santos, 2010).

Military applications for coir fiber-reinforced composites include ballistic armor, motorcycle helmets, and bulletproof vests. When making motorcycle helmets with epoxy resins as the matrix materials, Yuhazri and Dan used coconut fibers. Coconut fibers performed admirably as an appropriate reinforcement in epoxy resin for the production of a safety helmet, according to the mechanical characteristics results. They created a special bulletproof vest composed of coir fiber that offers all the protection of a regular vest while being lighter and more affordable than a typical bulletproof vest. They demonstrated that the vest could block 9-mm bullets at a 5-m distance. Additionally, they evaluated a high-impact hybrid composite material reinforced with coconut fibers for use in ballistic armor, and they found positive results.

Coir fiber composites are employed in automotive applications because of their strong mechanical characteristics and moderate weight, resulting in specific mechanical properties equal to those of glass fiber composites. Mercedes Benz car seat cushions are made from coir fiber-reinforced composites, which are utilized in industrial automotive. Coconut fibers are utilized in polymer composites that do not require a lot of strength and stiffness and are used in impact loading. The coir fiber composites have beneficial qualities, but they also have certain unfavorable traits, such as dimensional instability, flammability, which makes them unsuitable for high-temperature applications, and degradability with humidity, ultraviolet (UV) radiation, acids, and bases (Ben Brahim and Ben Cheikh, 3007). Numerous studies on the use of natural fiber composites in interior and exterior auto-body components have been conducted by the auto industry (Davoodi et al., 2011). Numerous automotive components made by German automakers such as Mercedes Benz use plant fiber composites, such as the seats in the

Mercedes Benz A-class model, which are made of coir fiber rubber latex composites, and the door panels in the Mercedes Benz E-class model, which are made of fax-sisal fiber mat-reinforced epoxy (Shinoj et al., 2011).

For automotive applications, Sah et al. (2017) reinforced polyvinyl chloride (PVC) using coconut shell powder. According to the investigation's findings, the composites' tensile and impact strengths were improved when compared to regular polyvinyl chloride. The lightweight, increased strength, and cost-effectiveness of composites, according to the authors, demonstrate their usefulness as a material for making car parts including seat covers, dash boards, and air intake pipes.

6.2.5 COIR FIBER-REINFORCED CEMENT-BASED COMPOSITE MATERIALS

Several coir fiber shapes, such as coir fiber rope, coir mesh, and monofilament fiber reinforcement, have been reported to be able to reinforce cement-based composite materials. The coir yarn is spun from a batch of coir fibers to create the coir rope and mesh. The friction between the twisted fibers, which is controlled by the contact area and surface roughness of the fibers, is a key factor in the mechanical performance of coir rope and mesh. The contact area between fibers is often larger the longer the fiber is. Coir fiber is a seed fiber that is typically thin and thick, measuring between 150 and 400 m in diameter and 3.5 to 15 mm in length. Because they are long and thin, stem fibers are better suited for use as yarn. For instance, flax fiber had an average diameter of 12–16 m and a maximum length of 900 mm. Coir fiber is better suited to be employed as monofilament fiber reinforcement in cement-based composite materials than other stem fibers such as flax, and this was the configuration that has been studied the most frequently during the past 20 years. Additionally, among plant-based fibers, coir fiber showed the highest toughness in tension, leading to extensive research on coir fiber as monofilament reinforcement for concrete structures (Ali et al., 2012).

6.2.5.1 PHYSICAL PROPERTIES

Coir fiber has a lesser density when compared to composite materials made of cement. The density of the concrete can be decreased by adding coir fiber to cementitious ingredients. Existing research shown that the density of the resulting concrete might be reduced by up to 12% with a coir fiber addition of less than 5% of the cement weight (i.e., the typical coir fiber content for structural application). The hydrophilic nature of coir fibers and other natural fibers allows them to absorb moisture from the cementitious matrix. Lower workability will come from a decrease in the amount of free water. The coir fibers have comparatively strong thermal and acoustic insulation qualities because of their porous structure, which has a porosity of between 21 and 31%.

Using heat flow meters, Bui et al. (2020) examined the thermal conductivity of coir fiber mat. The observed thermal conductivity ranged from 0.024 to 0.052 W/m·K, which was in line with the design value of typical thermal insulation materials. Even though CFRC has high thermal and acoustic insulation properties, it was discovered that the majority of research solely focused on one aspect. Its capacity for sound insulation was not thoroughly examined. More research should be done on the sound insulation capabilities of CFRC because coir fiber mat is good at sound absorption, especially for high frequency. The use of CFRC may be expanded if it performs similarly to other soundproofing materials. The increased use of coir fiber will move us closer to sustainability and circularity on a global scale.

6.2.5.2 MECHANICAL PROPERTIES

The inclusion of coir fiber increases the compressive strength of cementitious mortar with a coir fiber content to binder in weight of between 1 and 5%. Unlike compressive strength, adding coir fiber can increase the flexural strength of mortar even when there is a low coir fiber percentage (coir fiber content of 0.26%). According to research by Andiç-Akir et al. (Andiç-Çakir et al., 2014) the improvement of coir fiber in fracture toughness was also discovered. The fracture toughness increase was up to 62% as up to 3.4% of untreated coir fiber was added. Due to the fiber "bridge effect," adding monofilament short fibers can significantly increase the impact resistance of cementitious materials. The higher ductility of coir fiber compared to other plant-based fibers, or the plastic deformation under tensile, was primarily responsible for the coir fiber-cement mortar's higher impact resistance. As an eco-friendly material, soil-cement, a composite made of cement and soil, has been studied. This composite was frequently utilized as channel lining for highways and bridges, slope support, and reinforcement of soft soil foundations. Danso et al. added coir fiber and lime to the composite to improve the stabilization of soil–cement mortar (Danso and Manu, 2020). The findings indicated that, compared to samples with various coir fiber contents (i.e.,

0.4, 0.6, and 0.8%) and lime ratios (i.e., 0, 10, and 15%), those with 0.2% coir fiber and 5% lime by total weight had the greatest compressive strength, tensile strength, and density.

6.2.6 PRACTICAL APPLICATION OF COIR FIBERS AND COIR FIBER-REINFORCED CEMENT-BASED COMPOSITE MATERIALS

The light weight and superior insulating properties of coir fibers account for their practical use. It can be manufactured into thermal and acoustic insulation boards for roofs, floors, walls, and façades as well as ply board for interiors and furnishings. To improve the thermal insulation capabilities of brick walls, coir fiber can also be utilized as a filler. Coir fiber was used by Iwaro et al. (Iwaro and Mwasha, 2019) to fill hollow concrete blocks (150 mm ? 200 mm × 400 mm) and clay masonry blocks (100 mm ? 200 mm × 300 mm). By setting up tiny demonstrations, the insulating capabilities of coir fiber filled block as masonry walls were explored (around 1.5-m long, 1.2-m wide, and 1.5-m high with 26G corrugated, galvanized sheeting as roof). It was discovered that coir fiber filled blocks performed well in terms of thermal insulation in hot climates and might cut down on the energy needed for air conditioning. For instance, a coir fiber filled concrete block had an average internal temperature of 27.8°C without air conditioning, while an uninsulated wall had a temperature of 28.5°C. When glass fiber was utilized as the block's filler, hardly any difference was noticed. The study's average indoor temperature of 24°C could be maintained with the use of air conditioning. In comparison to uninsulated and glass fiber filled concrete blocks, the energy consumption for coir fiber filled concrete blocks was found to be 82 and 97%, respectively. The CFRC was seldom actually used as construction materials as opposed to a direct application of coir fiber. In the Philippines, the PCA-Zamboanga Research Center created a coir fiber cement board. This coir fiber cement board (CFB) had a cement content of 60–70% by weight and a coir fiber content of 30–40%. The CFB fared well in the flame test, burning slowly and emitting little smoke, despite having a low thermal conductivity of 0.9 W/mK. This research center collaborated with CFB to build a two-story home in the early 2000s. The CFB was utilized in the home's ceiling, walls, and dividers. Additionally, it was claimed that CFRC might be used as a façade coating layer for homes. Based on the findings, the authors noted that low-income housing constructions in tropical regions could benefit from CFRC as a façade coating (Goyat et al., 2022).

6.3 CONCLUSIONS AND FUTURE TRENDS

In conclusion, coir is a natural fiber with low density, low cost, high stiffness, medium strength, and high elongation. It is also sustainable and biodegradable. With various materials, particularly polymers like polyester, polypropylene, epoxy, high-density polyethylene, low-density polyethylene, linear density polyethylene, starch-based polymers, vinyl alcohol-based polymers, etc., coir is successfully used as reinforcement (as short fiber, long fiber, tangled or compressed mat, etc.). Researchers investigated coir as a successful reinforcement for cement- and rammed-earth-type construction materials in addition to the polymers. The interior of automobiles, brake pads, sound-absorbing panels, wall panels, storage tanks, shoe insoles, fire board, pots, insulation board, and biomedical items are all found to be acceptable applications for coir-based composites. It is shown in this review that it can be widely employed as a reinforcement material when combined with structural materials and polymers. The mechanical and interfacial properties of coir and the matrix are significantly enhanced by surface modification. Although it is noted that the choice of coir's surface treatment varies on the fiber type and matrix material, 4–10% NaOH treatment is frequently found to be appropriate. Additionally, it has been noticed that the compatibilizer's involvement in coir-reinforced composites is crucial. Future developments in coir-based composites could include hybrid composites, applications for dynamic loads, and dampening.

KEYWORDS

- **coir-reinforced biocomposites**
- **engineering properties**
- **natural fiber with low density**
- **low cost**
- **high stiffness**

REFERENCES

Oladele, I. O.; Adelani, S. O.; Makinde-Isola, B. A.; Omotosho, T. F.; Coconut/coir Fibers, Their Composites and Applications. *Plant Fibers Compos. Appl.* **2022,** 181–208. DOI: 10.1016/b978-0-12-824528-6.00004-7

Peças, P.; Carvalho, H.; Salman, H.; Leite, M. Natural Fibre Composites and their Applications: A Review. *J. Compos. Sci.* **2018,** *2* (4), 1–20.

Mohammed, L.; Ansari, M. N. M.; Pua, G.; Jawaid, M.; Islam, M. S. A Review on Natural Fiber Reinforced Polymer Composite and Its Applications. *Int. J. Polym. Sci.* **2015,** *2015.* DOI: 10.1155/2015/243947

Kanitkar, Y. M.; Kulkarni, A. P.; Wangikar, K. S. Characterization of Glass Hybrid Composite: A Review. *Mater. Today Proc.* **2017,** *4* (*9*), 9627–9630.

Witayakran, S.; Smitthipong, W.; Wangpradid, R.; Chollakup, R.; Clouston, P. L. *Natural Fiber Composites: Review of Recent Automotive Trends*; Elsevier Ltd., 2017.

Väisänen, T.; Das, O.; Tomppo, L. A Review on New Bio-based Constituents for Natural Fiber-polymer Composites. *J. Clean. Prod.* **2017,** *149,* 582–596.

Safri, S. N. A.; Sultan, M. T. H.; Jawaid, M.; Jayakrishna, K. Impact Behaviour of Hybrid Composites for Structural Applications: A Review. *Compos. Part B Eng.* **2018,** *133,* 112–121.

Shinoj, S.; Visvanathan, R.; Panigrahi, S.; Kochubabu, M. Oil Palm Fiber (OPF) and Its Composites: A Review. *Ind. Crops Prod.* **2011,** *33* (1), 7–22.

Mukherjee, T.; Kao, N. PLA Based Biopolymer Reinforced with Natural Fibre: A Review. *J. Polym. Environ.* **2011,** *19* (3), 714–725.

Gaurav, Gohal, H.; Kumar, V.; Jena, H. Study of Natural Fibre Composite Material and Its Hybridization Techniques. *Mater. Today Proc.* **2019,** *26,* 1368–1372.

Verma, D.; Gope, P. C.; Shandilya, A.; Gupta, A.; Maheshwari, M. K. Coir Fibre Reinforcement and Application in Polymer Composites: A Review. *J. Mater. Environ. Sci.* **2013,** *4* (2), 263–276.

Sudhakara, P.; *et al.* Fabrication of Borassus Fruit Lignocellulose Fiber/PP Composites and Comparison with Jute, Sisal and Coir Fibers. *Carbohydr. Polym.* **2013,** *98* (1), 1002–1010.

Munawar, S. S.; Umemura, K.; Kawai, S. Characterization of the Morphological, Physical, and Mechanical Properties of Seven Nonwood Plant Fiber Bundles. *J. Wood Sci.* **2007,** *53* (2), 108–113.

C. O. P. D et al., Mechanical Property Evaluation of Coconut Fibre. *BioResources* **2008,** *7* (1), 923–932.

Ramakrishna, G.; Sundararajan, T. Studies on the Durability of Natural Fibres and the Effect of Corroded Fibres on the Strength of Mortar. *Cem. Concr. Compos.* **2005,** *27* (5), 575–582.

Adeniyi, A. G.; Onifade, D. V.; Ighalo, J. O.; Adeoye, A. S. A Review of Coir Fiber Reinforced Polymer Composites. *Compos. Part B Eng.* **2019,** *176,* 107305.

Yan, L.; Chouw, N.; Huang, L.; Kasal, B. Effect of Alkali Treatment on Microstructure and Mechanical Properties of Coir Fibres, Coir Fibre Reinforced-polymer Composites and Reinforced-cementitious Composites. *Constr. Build. Mater.* **2016,** *112,* 168–182.

Wang, B.; Yan, L.; Kasal, B. A Review of Coir Fibre and Coir Fibre Reinforced Cement-based Composite Materials (2000–2021). *J. Clean. Prod.* **2022,** *338,* 130676.

Essabir, H.; Bensalah, M. O.; Rodrigue, D.; Bouhfid, R.; Qaiss, A. Structural, Mechanical and Thermal Properties of Bio-based Hybrid Composites from Waste Coir Residues: Fibers and Shell Particles. *Mech. Mater.* **2016,** *93,* 134–144.

Zhang, L.; Hu, Y. Novel Lignocellulosic Hybrid Particleboard Composites Made from Rice Straws and Coir Fibers. *Mater. Des.* **2014,** *55,* 19–26.

Rout, J.; Tripathy, S. S.; Misra, M.; Mohanty, A. K.; Nayak, S. K. The Influence of Fiber Surface Modification on the Mechanical Properties of Coir-polyester Composites. *Polym. Compos.* **2001,** *22* (4), 468–476.

Lai, C. Y.; Sapuan, S. M.; Ahmad, M.; Yahya, N.; Dahlan, K. Z. H. M. Mechanical and Electrical Properties of Coconut Coir Fiber-reinforced Polypropylene Composites. *Polym. Plast. Technol. Eng.* **2005,** *44* (4), 619–632.

Li, Z.; Wang, L.; Wang, X. Cement Composites Reinforced with Surface Modified Coir Fibers. *J. Compos. Mater.* **2007,** *41* (12), 1445–1457.

Santos, E. F.; Mauler, R. S.; Nachtigall, S. M. B. Effectiveness of Maleated- and Silanized-PP for Coir Fiber-filled Composites. *J. Reinf. Plast. Compos.* **2009,** *28* (17), 2119–2129.

Yang, Z.; Peng, H.; Wang, W.; Liu, T. Crystallization Behavior of Poly(ε-caprolactone)/Layered Double Hydroxide Nanocomposites. *J. Appl. Polym. Sci.* **2010,** *116* (5), 2658–2667.

Haque, M.; Rahman, R.; Islam, N.; Huque, M.; Hasan, M. Mechanical Properties of Polypropylene Composites Reinforced with Chemically Treated Coir and Abaca Fiber. *J. Reinf. Plast. Compos.* **2010,** *29* (15), 2253–2261.

Lomelí Ramírez, M. G.; Satyanarayana, K. G.; Iwakiri, S.; De Muniz, G. B.; Tanobe, V.; Flores-Sahagun, T. S. Study of the Properties of Biocomposites. Part I. Cassava Starch-green Coir Fibers from Brazil. *Carbohydr. Polym.* **2011,** *86* (4), 1712–1722.

Arrakhiz, F. Z.; *et al.* Mechanical Properties of High Density Polyethylene Reinforced with Chemically Modified Coir Fibers: Impact of Chemical Treatments. *Mater. Des.* **2012,** *37,* 379–383.

Yousif, B. F.; Ku, H. Suitability of Using Coir Fiber/Polymeric Composite for the Design of Liquid Storage Tanks. *Mater. Des.* **2012,** *36,* 847–853.

Diani, J.; Gall, K. Finite Strain 3D Thermoviscoelastic Constitutive Model. *Society* **2006,** 1–10.

Wambua, P.; Ivens, J.; Verpoest, I. Natural Fibres: Can They Replace Glass in Fibre Reinforced Plastics? *Compos. Sci. Technol.* **2003,** *63* (9), 1259–1264.

Bensalah, H.; Raji, M.; Abdellaoui, H.; Essabir, H.; Bouhfid, R.; Qaiss, A. L. K. Thermo-mechanical Properties of Low-Cost 'Green' Phenolic Resin Composites Reinforced with Surface Modified Coir Fiber. *Int. J. Adv. Manuf. Technol.* **2021,** *112* (7–8), 1917–1930.

Amoako, G.; Mensah-Amoah, P.; Sam, F.; Sackey, S. S. Some Mechanical Properties of Coconut Fiber Reinforced Polyethylene Composite to Control Environmental Waste in Ghana. *Energy Environ. Res.* **2018,** *8* (1), 1.

Hirunlabh, J.; Khedari, J.; Charoenvai, S. New Insulating Particleboards from Durian Peel and Coconut Coir. *Build. Environ.* **2003,** *38* (3), 435–441.

Agopyan, V.; Savastano, H.; John, V. M.; Cincotto, M. A. Developments on Vegetable Fibre-cement Based Materials in São Paulo, Brazil: An Overview. *Cem. Concr. Compos.* **2005,** *27* (5), 527–536.

Asasutjarit, C.; Hirunlabh, J.; Khedari, J.; Daguenet, M.; Quenard, D. In *Coconut Coir Cement Board*, Int. Conf. Durab. Build. Mater. Components; 2005, no. April, pp 1–9.

Paramasivam, P.; Nathan, G. K.; Das Gupta, N. C. Reviews. *High. Educ. Q.* **1965,** *19* (4), 414–423.

Sampaio, A. Z.; Santos, J. P. Journal of Civil Engineering and Construction Technology. *J. Civ. Eng. Constr. Technol.* **2010,** *2* (6), 125–137.

Ben Brahim, S.; Ben Cheikh, R. Influence of Fibre Orientation and Volume Fraction on the Tensile Properties of Unidirectional Alfa-polyester Composite. *Compos. Sci. Technol.* **2007,** *67* (1), 140–147.

Davoodi, M. M.; Sapuan, S. M.; Ahmad, D.; Aidy, A.; Khalina, A.; Jonoobi, M. Concept Selection of Car Bumper Beam with Developed Hybrid Bio-composite Material. *Mater. Des.* **2011,** *32* (10), 4857–4865.

Sah, M. H. M.; Noor, A. M.; Abbas, M. R.; Bakar, A. A. Mechanical Properties of Coconut Shell Powder reinforced PVC Composites in Automotive Applications. *J. Mech. Eng.* **2017,** *14* (2), 51–63.

Ali, M.; Liu, A.; Sou, H.; Chouw, N. Mechanical and Dynamic Properties of Coconut Fibre Reinforced Concrete. *Constr. Build. Mater.* **2012,** *30,* 814–825.

Bui, H.; Sebaibi, N.; Boutouil, M.; Levacher, D. Determination and Review of Physical and Mechanical Properties of Raw and Treated Coconut Fibers for their Recycling in Construction Materials. *Fibers* **2020,** *8* (6), 1–18.

Andiç-Çakir, Ö.; Sarikanat, M.; Tüfekçi, H. B.; Demirci, C.; Erdoğan, Ü. H. Physical and Mechanical Properties of Randomly Oriented Coir Fiber-cementitious Composites. *Compos. Part B Eng.* **2014,** *61,* 49–54.

Danso, H.; Manu, D. Influence of Coconut Fibres and Lime on the Properties of Soil-Cement Mortar. *Case Stud. Constr. Mater.* **2020,** *12,* e00316.

Iwaro, J.; Mwasha, A. Effects of Using Coconut Fiber–Insulated Masonry Walls to Achieve Energy Efficiency and Thermal Comfort in Residential Dwellings. *J. Archit. Eng.* **2019,** *25* (1), 1–12.

Goyat, V.; Ghangas, G.; Sirohi, S.; Kumar, A.; Nain, J. A Review on Mechanical Properties of Coir Based Composites. *Mater. Today Proc.* **2022,** *62,* 1738–1745.

CHAPTER 7

Porous Polymeric Composite: A Next-Generation Material for Bioactivity, Environment, and Energy

NEETU TALREJA[1], DIVYA CHAUHAN[2], and MOHAMMAD ASHFAQ[3,4]

[1]*Faculty of Science and Technology, Department of Science, Alliance University, Bengaluru, Karnataka, India*

[2]*Department of Drinking Water and Sanitation, Ministry of Jal Shakti, Pandit Deendayal Antyodaya Bhawan, New Delhi*

[3]*University Centre for Research & Development (UCRD), Chandigarh University, Gharaun, Mohali, Punjab, India*

[4]*Department of Biotechnology, Chandigarh University, Gharaun, Mohali, Punjab, India*

ABSTRACT

The porous polymeric composite materials provide numerous advantages due to their surface texture like high/selective permeability, high tensile strength/flexibility, and high surface area that makes them exceptional materials for various applications such as water treatments, filtration membranes, catalysis, sensors, and biomedical applications. Carbon-based-NMs (CB-NMs) such as graphene oxide (GO), graphene, carbon nanotubes (CNTs), carbon nanofibers (CNFs), and its hybrid materials *are* mostly applied in numerous applications. Moreover, these porous CB-NMs have been synthesized with tunable porosity by changing their synthesis temperature. Another class of porous materials, metal–organic frameworks (MOFs), porous organic solids, and covalent organic frameworks (COFs),

Application of Engineering Principles and Practices in Biotechnology.
Ann Rose Abraham, Leonardo Sepúlveda Torre, Tamara Tatrishvili, and A. K. Haghi (Eds.)

are newly emerging materials with high porosity and are widely used for numerous applications. We mainly focus on different porous polymeric composite materials and their applications. Finally, discussed the role of porosity in environmental remediation, biomedical, energy, and solar cell applications.

7.1 INTRODUCTION

Technological innovation in material science and engineering is one of the core research areas for developing society and the country. The advent of nanotechnology and nanomaterials (NMs) has expanded the scope and applicability of the materials in numerous areas, mainly sensors, environmental remediation, energy storage devices, solar cells, agriculture, and biomedicine. The extraordinary characteristics of the NMs, such as high surface area, and mechanical, electrical, and thermal ability, make them suitable candidates for numerous applications. Moreover, an intelligent combination of materials (such as NMs, polymers, and surface functional groups) is required for tuning properties or developing materials with desirable characteristics for particular applications (Bayda et al., 2019; Afreen et al., 2018; Chauhan et al., 2020; Omar et al., 2019; Afreen et al., 2020; Chauhan et al., 2021; Shahcheraghi et al., 2022). In this aspect, porous materials or materials with high porosity have the potential for numerous applications because of their structure and active sites.

The porous polymeric composite materials provide numerous advantages due to their surface texture like high/selective permeability, high tensile strength/flexibility, and high surface area that makes them exceptional materials for various applications such as water treatments, filtration membranes, catalysis, sensors, and biomedical applications. Moreover, the conjoining of porous properties or porosity in advanced technology such as three-dimensional printing (3D printing) is one of the eye-catching alternatives for developing materials with multifaceted geometries/shape like electrodes for battery, midsoles of shoes, lining of football helmet, biomimicking composite, and tissue frameworks (Ahumada et al., 2019; Mahdavi et al., 2022; Cipriani et al., 2021; Dong et al., 2021; Nikolova and Chavali, 2019; du Plessis et al., 2022). However, material scientist are uninterruptedly looking toward the development of newer porous polymeric composites that effectively use their potential ability within 3D-printing-based materials.

Recently, porous polymeric materials brought the industrial revolution due to their excellent properties, including chemical stability, mechanical strength, flexibility, lightweight, permeability, transparency, size exclusion or adsorption capacity, high specific surface area, high-temperature resistance, and low process cost. Pore diversity and morphological variation are major attracting features that are attracting attention in numerous applications primarily treatment of environmental pollution, biomedical, battery storage, sensor, oil–water separation, and agriculture (Agboola et al., 2021; Mishra et al., 2018; Wang et al., 2021; Chauhan et al., 2022; Zhang et al., 2022). Despite great demand, research is still needed to optimize controlled pore size and structure depending on the specific targeted application.

For controlling the pore size/porous texture of the composite materials various processes has been used mainly template process, leaching, and solvent evaporation. In this way, one of the most critical tasks is to create the porosity inside the structure and then apply it to various end applications. The porosity's primary factor is the templates' application and sorption during annealing. High annealing temperature can impact the formation of different pore sizes with pore volume and structure (Tan and Rodrigue, 2019; Baig et al., 2021; Farmahini et al., 2021; Kruželák et al., 2021). In this aspect, one major task is selecting the desired temperature for creating porosity.

Numerous carbon-based-NMs (CB-NMs) such as graphene oxide (GO), graphene, carbon nanotubes (CNTs), carbon nanofibers (CNFs), and their hybrid materials have been developed with their tunable porosity by changing their synthesis temperature. These porous CB-NMs and their composite are comprehensively used in numerous applications, including water treatment technology, antibiotic materials, drug delivery systems, sensors, agriculture, energy, supercapacitors, and biomedicine (Navrotskaya et al., 2020; Rathinavel et al., 2021; Shoukat and Khan, 2022). Another class of porous materials like metal–organic frameworks (MOFs), porous organic solid, and covalent organic frameworks (COFs) are newly emerging materials that have high porosity and are widely used for numerous applications, including water treatments, pharmaceuticals, biomedical, battery, supercapacitors, and solar cells applications (Samanta et al., 2019; Khan et al., 2013; Rangnekar et al., 2015). Figure 7.1 shows the different porous materials and their application. This book chapter covered synthesizing porous polymeric composite materials concerning the micro/mesoporosity that provides desirable characteristics for end applications. We also discuss the porous polymeric composite materials and their applicability in the end application.

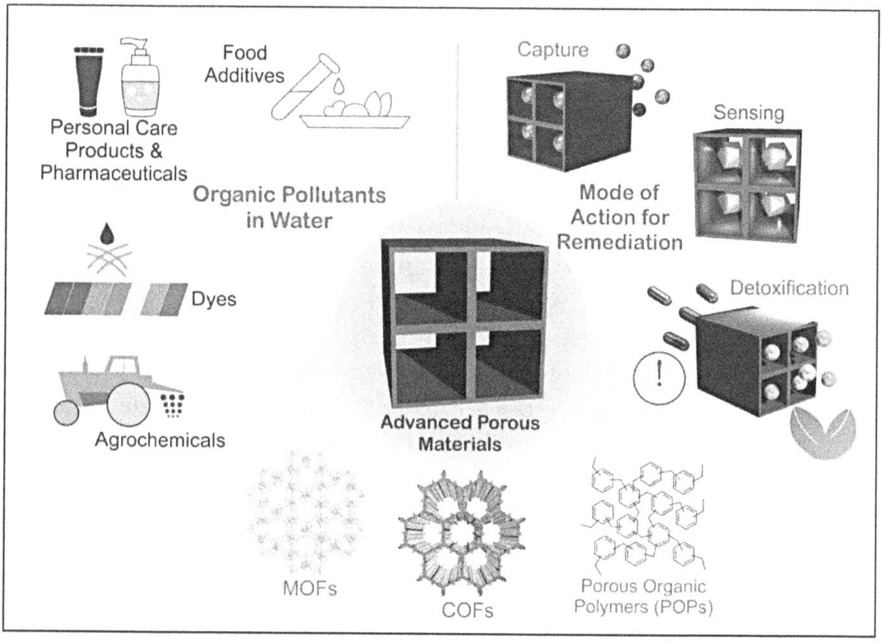

FIGURE 7.1 A schematic illustration of the different porous materials and their application. The image was taken with permission.

Source: Reprinted with permission from Samanta et al., 2019. Copyright 2019. American Chemical Society.

7.2 POROUS POLYMERIC COMPOSITE AND ITS APPLICATION

Usually, polymeric porous composite are organic/inorganic, porous texture/hierarchical porous, and amorphous/crystalline, which might be advantageous in many applications. The porous polymeric composite materials exhibit an extensive range of applications to balance our daily life due to their extraordinary properties, mainly high surface area, thermal, mechanical, low weight, and porous surface texture. Here, our primary focus is environmental remediation, biomedical, battery, supercapacitors, and solar cell applications.

7.2.1 *ENVIRONMENTAL REMEDIATION APPLICATIONS*

Environmental contamination increases with increasing population, industrialization, and urbanization, enhancing environmental contamination. Environmental contamination is a serious threat affecting the quality of human life. Several pollutants such as heavy metal ions, pharmaceutical compounds, dyes, and biological contamination can cause severe health effects on humans and animals (Adil and Thalji, 2022). Therefore, removing these contaminations is necessary from the environment to provide a safer and healthier environment.

The porous CB-NMs, metals/metal-oxide, MOFs, COFs, and porous organic solid-based composite materials might be next-generation materials that efficiently remove environmental contamination from water bodies. For example, Kumar et al. (2011) Al/Fe doped polymeric beads (Al/Fe-PB) for the sorption of fluoride (F) and arsenic (As) from water. The metals (Al/Fe) were incorporated during the polymerization process. Next, the prepared Al/Fe-PB were carbonized and activated to develop a porous texture. The data indicate the synthesized porous Al/Fe-PB materials effectively remove F and As from water with the sorption ability of ~ 100 and 40 mg/g, respectively. The sorption ability of the porous Al/Fe-PB materials is mainly due to their porosity and metal nanoparticles (NPs) (Kumar et al., 2011). Saraswat et al. (2012) synthesized porous Ni-doped polymeric beads (Ni-PB) to remove vitamin b_{12} from water. The synthesized Ni-PB materials have high porosity with interconnected pores. The data indicate that the prepared porous Ni-PB materials effectively remove vitamin B_{12} in both batch and continuous adsorption modes with a sorption ability of ~300 mg/g. The high loading/sorption ability of vitamin B_{12} is mainly due to the porosity with interconnected pores and Ni metal-NPs (Saraswat et al., 2012). Khare et al. (2013) synthesized porous CNFs on Ni and Fe-doped PB (Ni-PB-CNFs and Fe-PB-CNFs) using the chemical vapor deposition (CVD) process to remove vitamin B_{12} and As from water. The data indicate that the prepared Ni-PB-CNFs and Fe-PB-CNFs effectively remove vitamin B_{12} and As from water with the sorption ability of ~180 and 18 mg/g, respectively. The high loading ability of the prepared porous polymeric Ni-PB-CNFs and Fe-PB-CNFs is predominantly due to the materials' micro/mesoporosity and metal-NPs (Khare et al., 2013). Talreja et al. (2014) developed CNFs on Fe-PB (Fe-PB-CNFs) using suspension polymerization followed by a CVD process to remove chromium (Cr) ions. The developed Fe-PB-CNFs proficiently remove Cr from water under batch and continuous adsorption mode with the sorption capability of 41 mg/g (Talreja et al., 2014). Another study of a similar group synthesized CNFs using the CVD process, and the surface was functionalized using ethylenediamine (EDA) to prepare EDA-CNFs to remove salicylic acid from water. The data indicate that the EDA-CNFs proficiently adsorbed salicylic acid water with a high loading ability, ~682 mg/g. The high loading efficiency of the EDA-CNFs is mainly due to the porous texture and surface functional group present at the surface of CNFs (Talreja et al., 2016). Zhou et al. (2016) synthesized GO and incorporated zeolite-imidazole frameworks-8

(ZIF-8) (GO-ZIF-8) for the sorption of volatile organic carbon (VOCs). The prepared GO-ZIF-8-based composite materials effectively remove VOCs with a sorption ability of 240 mg/g (Zhou et al., 2016). Rahimi and Mohaghegh (2017) synthesized the graphene-incorporated Cu-terephthalate-based MOFs (G-Cu-P-MOFs) to remove metal ions (Pb, Cu, Zn, Mn, Cd, and Fe) from acid mine drainage. The data indicate that the prepared G-Cu-P-MOFs based composite materials effectively remove Pb, Cu, Zn, Mn, Cd, and Fe metal ions with sorption abilities of 37, 235, 89, 150, 53, and 78 mg/g, respectively. Moreover, more active sites and extraordinary surface texture significantly improved the sorption ability. Additionally, the adsorption of metals is mainly due to the interaction of metals with the surface functional group of the G-Cu-P-MOFs based composite materials (Rahimi and Mohaghegh, 2017). Zhao et al. (2017) synthesized Ni-MOFs and GO-MOFs based composite materials to remove Congo red (CR) dye. The data indicate that the prepared GO-Ni-MOFs effectively remove CR dye from water with an extraordinary loading ability of 2489 mg/g. Moreover, more active sites enhance the sorption ability of CR dye (Zhao et al., 2017). Zhao et al. (2018) synthesized graphene-oxide incorporated MOFs (GO-MOFs) to eliminate methylene blue (MB) dye. The data indicate that the prepared GO-MOFs effectively remove MB dye from water with 274 mg/g. Moreover, the high loading ability of the GO-MOFs-based composite materials, mainly acid–base, and electrostatic interaction (Zhao et al., 2018). Sun et al. synthesized MOFs and polydopamine composite (Fe-BTC-PDA) materials to remove Pb and mercury (Hg) from water. The data indicate that the Fe-BTC-PDA efficiently removes Hg and Pb contaminants from water with 1634 and 394 mg/g. Moreover, the extraordinary sorption ability of the Fe-BTC-PDA-based composite materials is mainly due to the porous surface texture of the materials (Sun et al., 2018). Kumar and Talreja (2019) synthesized Ni-doped CNFs using the CVD process and then functionalized them with rhodamine B dye (RhB) to prepare Ni-RhB-CNFs for detecting Cr and Pb ions from water. The data indicate that the developed Ni-RhB-CNFs efficiently detect Cr and Pb ions from water with a high detection limit of 203 and 132 nM, respectively. Moreover, developed Ni-RhB-CNFs colorimetric probes show sensing response within 30 s of the exposure (Kumar and Talreja, 2019). Peng et al. (2012) synthesized ZIF-NPs incorporated PAN nanofibers (ZIF-PAN-NFs) by using electrospinning and hot-press methods for the sorption of Cu. The data indicate that the ZIF-PAN-NFs effectively filtered Cu from water with ~96.5% filtration ability. Moreover, high porosity and surface of MOFs one of the determining factors for the sorption of Cu from water (Peng et al., 2020). Sasidharan et al. (2021) synthesized PMC materials for the sorption of both chemical and biological contamination from water. Figure 7.2 shows the SEM images of materials such as PU foam, graphene, Cu-PU, and PMC materials. The SEM images clearly indicate that the rough and porous texture of PMC. The adsorption data indicate that the PMC materials effectively remove Cr and Congo red (CR) dye from water with the sorption ability of 76.9 and 714 mg/g, respectively. Moreover, synthesized PMC materials effectively kill/inhibit both *Escherichia coli* and *Staphylococcus aureus.* The high loading efficiency mainly due to the surface functional group, metal nanosheets, rough surface, and porous texture (Sasidharan et al., 2021). Ashfaq et al. (2021) synthesized bimetallic (Fe/Bi)-povidone-iodine based photocatalyst materials for the sorption RhB dye and bacteria. The data indicate that the synthesized porous Fe/Bi- povidone-iodine completely degrades RhB dye and inhibits both Gram-negative and Gram-positive bacterial strains (Ashfaq et al., 2021). Table 7.1 summarized different porous materials and their environmental remediation applications. The literature data suggested that the porous polymeric composite materials or hybrid composite materials effectively remove heavy metal ions, and dye, and inhibit/kill bacterial strains. The high adsorption ability of the composite materials is mainly due to porosity, surface texture, electrostatic interaction, and acid–base interaction. Moreover, the surface functional group is also an important factor for augmenting the adsorption ability.

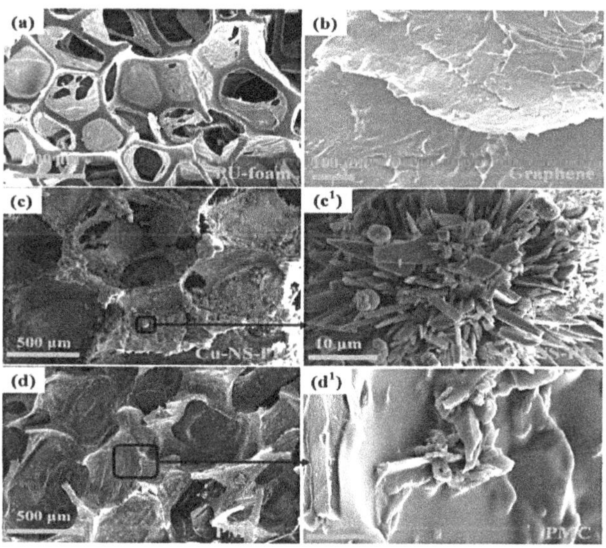

FIGURE 7.2 SEM images of the different materials (a) PU foam, (b) graphene, (c) Cu-PU, and (d) PMC composite materials. The image was taken with permission.

Source: Reprinted with permission from Sasidharan et al., 2021. https://creativecommons.org/licenses/by/4.0/

TABLE 7.1 Different Porous Materials and Their Environmental Remediation Applications.

S. No.	Porous materials	Environmental contamination	Sorption efficiency	References
1.	Al/Fe-PB	F and As	F: 100 mg/g As: 40 mg/g	(Kumar et al., 2011)
2.	Ni-PB	Vitamin B_{12}	300 mg/g	(Saraswat et al., 2012)
3.	Ni-PB-CNFs	Vitamin B_{12}	180 mg/g	(Khare et al., 2013)
4.	Fe-PB-CNFs	As	18 mg/g	(Khare et al., 2013)
5.	Fe-PB-CNFs	Cr	41 mg/g	(Talreja et al., 2014)
6.	EDA-CNFs	Salicylic acid	682 mg/g	(Talreja et al., 2016)
7.	GO-ZIF-8	VOCs	240 mg/g	(Zhou et al., 2016)
8.	GO-MOFs	CR dye	2489 mg/g	(Zhao et al., 2017)
9.	G-Cu-P-MOFs	Pb, Cu, Zn, Mn, Cd, and Fe	37, 235, 89, 150, 53, and 78 mg/g, respectively	(Rahimi and Mohaghegh, 2017)
10.	GO-MOFs	MB dye	274 mg/g	(Zhao et al., 2018)
11.	Fe-BTC-PDA	Hg and Pb	1634, and 394 mg/g	(Sun et al., 2018)
12.	Ni-RhB-CNFs	Cr and Pb	Detection limit Cr-203 nM Pb-132 nM	(Kumar and Talreja, 2019)
13.	ZIF-PAN-NFs	Cu	96.5% sorption	(Peng et al., 2020)
14.	PMC	Cr	76.9 mg/g	(Sasidharan et al., 2021)
15.	PMC	CR	714 mg/g	(Sasidharan et al., 2021)
16.	PMC	*E. coli* and *S. aureus*	Inhibiting the both Gram-negative and Gram-positive bacteria	(Sasidharan et al., 2021)
17.	Fe/Bi-povidone-iodine	RhB dye *E. coli* and *S. aureus*	100% degradation and inhibiting the both Gram-negative and Gram-positive bacteria	(Ashfaq et al., 2021)

7.2.2 BIOMEDICAL APPLICATIONS

Presently, porous polymeric composite materials significantly gain the interest of researchers due to their extraordinary characteristics like high surface area, easy functionalization, and tunable ability (mainly a combination of two/three types of materials) according to the application. Moreover, porosity and surface texture might be easily tuned by changing their size, shape, and surface functional group, thereby effectively used in biomedical applications. Numerous porous polymeric composite materials incorporated with CNTs, CNFs, COFs, and MOFs, has been comprehensively used in biomedical applications such as drug delivery system, photothermal treatment, biosensing, bioimaging, antibiotic materials, wound dressing, and hemostatic dressing materials. For example, Aw et al. (2011) polymeric micelles in the porous implant (PM-PI) for drug delivery systems. The data indicate that the prepared PM-PI effectively releases the poorly soluble drug. Moreover, release behavior might be tuned according to the pore size (Aw et al., 2011). Susanto et al. (2013) synthesized glucose oxidase enzyme immobilized onto the CNTs-porous chitosan membranes (GOXY-CC) for biosensor. The data indicate that the prepared GOXY-CC-based biosensor is effectively used in sensing applications. Moreover, CNTs increase the conductivity of the materials (Susanto et al., 2013). Ashfaq et al. (2014) synthesized polyvinyl alcohol (PVA)-cellulose acetate phthalate (CAP) encapsulated Cu-CNFs (PVA-CAP-Cu-CNFs) based composite materials for the delivery of the antibiotic. The Cu-CNFs were used as antibiotic materials, whereas PVA-CAP was used as a delivery system. Figure 7.3 shows the SEM images of the prepared PVA-CAP-Cu-CNFs and their components. The SEM images indicate that incorporating Cu-CNFs antibiotics creates internal pores. The internal porous texture of the PVA-CAP-Cu-CNFs might be advantageous for the delivery of antibiotics. Interestingly, the beauty of this PVA-CAP-Cu-CNFs based biomaterials is pH-sensitive behavior, as they release Cu-CNFs antibiotics when the solution pH is ~6 or more. Moreover, the high biocompatibility of the PVA-CAP-Cu-CNFs-based biomaterials makes them safer to use in the drug delivery system (Ashfaq et al., 2014). Another study of a similar group developed Cu/Zn-CNFs using the CVD process as antibiotic materials. The asymmetrical distribution of the metals (Cu-nanoparticles (Cu-NPs) and Zn-NPs) makes them promising antibiotic materials that inhibit both Gram-negative and Gram-positive bacteria, as CNFs hold Cu-NPs that move along with the fibers. In contrast, Zn remains to adhere on the surface of ACFs. The controlled release of Cu and robust release of Zn have initial and prolonged effects on the Cu/Zn-CNFs. Moreover, the prepared Cu/Zn-CNFs antibiotic materials did not show any toxic effects on erythrocytes (Ashfaq et al., 2016). Ashfaq et al. (2017) synthesized polymer encapsulated Cu/Zn-CNFs (PMC) biomaterials for wound dressing application. It tested against multidrug resistance (MDR) and extensively-drug resistance (XDR) bacterial strains isolates from different types of wounds. The data indicate that the PMC materials effectively inhibit/kill bacterial strains without any toxic effects. Moreover, the internal porous texture might increase the exposure and applicability (Ashfaq et al., 2017). Thakur et al. (2017) synthesized melamine foam-based porous carbon and Prussian blue-based composite materials (PCPB) for the glucose sensor. The porous carbon might be advantageous for immobilizing glucose oxide, improving the biosensor's sensitivity. The prepared PCPB-based biosensor effectively detect glucose molecules with high sensitivity of 0.03 mM (Thakur et al., 2017).

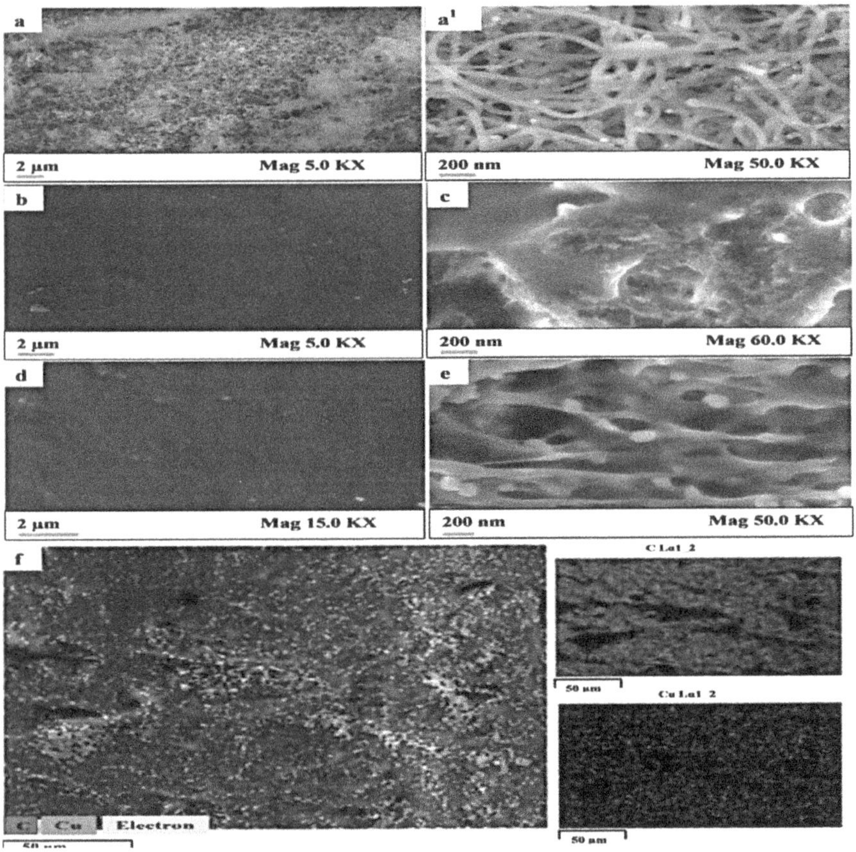

FIGURE 7.3 SEM images of (a-a') Cu-CNFs, (b-c) PVA-CAP, (d-e) PVA-CAP-Cu-CNFs, and (f) elemental mapping of PVA-CAP-Cu-CNFs.

Source: Reprinted with permission from Ashfaq et al. 2014.

Kanhed et al. (2018) synthesized microporous ZnO/AgO-hydroxyapatite-based composite (M-HAP) materials for tissue engineering. The data indicate that the porous M-HAP composite material's high hardness and flexural strength are used effectively in bone tissue regeneration (Kanhed et al., 2018). Bhadauriya et al. (2018) synthesized yeast immobilized Cu-CNFs (YI-Cu-CNFs) based biomaterials for wound dressing materials, especially for diabetic patients. The data suggested that the prepared YI-Cu-CNFs-based biomaterials effectively utilized glucose and controlled bacterial infection. Moreover, *in-vivo* experiments suggested that the YI-Cu-CNFs-based biomaterials effectively heal the wound compared to Cu-CNFs (Bhadauriya et al., 2018). Singh et al. (2019) synthesized polylactic acid and nanohydroxyapatite (PLA-HA) based porous polymeric composite using microwave curing for bone tissue engineering. The porous texture of the composite was developed through a leaching process. The developed PLA-HA-based composite materials have interconnected pores that might benefit tissue engineering applications (Kumar Singh et al., 2019). Xiao et al. (2021) synthesized calcium and PLA (Ca-PLA) based porous polymeric composite materials for tissue engineering. The data indicate that the Ca-PLA-based porous polymeric composite materials have high mineralization activity. Moreover, prepared Ca-PLA-based porous polymeric composite shows nontoxic and high biocompatibility (Xiao et al., 2021). Sharikova et al. (2022) synthesized tricalcium phosphate and reduced-GO incorporated chitosan (Ca-rGO-chitosan) based composite materials for bone tissue regeneration. The data indicate that the prepared Ca-rGO-chitosan effectively regenerates bone tissue without cellular toxicity (Sharikova et al., 2022). Akram et al. (2022) synthesized calcium phosphate nanoparticles incorporated chitosan (CCP) based biomaterials for a hemostatic bandage. The data indicate that the prepared CCP biomaterials are effectively used as hemostatic dressing materials. The CCP biomaterials have high blood clotting ability, adsorption of protein, and activation of platelets with high biocompatibility (Akram et al., 2022). Table 7.2 summarizes different polymeric composite materials and its biomedical applications. The literature suggested that the porous surface texture of the composite materials is one of the important factors of any biomedical applications. The porous texture, pore size, and interconnected pore mainly depends on the biomaterials and its synthesis process. The surface porous texture, pore size, and interconnected pores might be easily tuned by incorporating metal, nonmetals, and polymers within the composite. Moreover, electrospinning might be a next-generation process that creates porous biomaterials. Additionally, solvent casting, 3D printing, and leaching processes are the most appropriate processes to create a

TABLE 7.2 Different Porous Polymeric Composite Materials and their Biomedical Application.

S. No.	Composite materials	Biomedical applications	Remarks	References
1.	PM-PI	Drug delivery system	Effectively releases poorly soluble drugs	(Aw et al., 2011)
2.	GOXY-CC	Biosensor	Effectively used in biosensors.	(Susanto et al., 2013)
3.	PVA-CAP-Cu-CNFs	Drug delivery system	Release of Cu-CNFs antibiotics in a controlled manner.	(Ashfaq et al., 2014)
4.	Cu/Zn-CNFs	Antibiotic materials	Effectively inhibits both Gram-negative and Gram-positive bacterial strains without any cellular toxicity.	(Ashfaq et al., 2016)
5.	PMC	Wound dressing	Effectively inhibits both MDR and XDR clinical isolates.	(Ashfaq et al., 2017)
6.	PCPB	Biosensor	Effectively detects glucose with the detection limit of 0.03 mM.	(Thakur et al., 2017)
7.	M-HAP	Tissue engineering	High porosity, hardness, and flexural strength make effective materials for bone regeneration.	(Kanhed et al., 2018)
8.	YI-Cu-CNFs	Wound dressing	Efficiently utilized glucose and controlled the bacterial infection.	(Bhadauriya et al., 2018)
9.	PLA-HA	Tissue engineering	The porous texture might be beneficial for tissue engineering.	(Kumar Singh et al., 2019)
10.	Ca-PLA	Tissue engineering	High mineralization activity.	(Xiao et al., 2021)
11.	Ca-rGO-chitosan	Tissue engineering	Effectively regenerates bone tissue.	(Sharikova et al., 2022)
12.	CCP	Hemostatic bandage	Effectively clots blood within 15 s.	(Akram et al., 2022)

controlled pore. Therefore, easily fabricated porous polymeric composite is effectively used in biomedical applications.

7.2.3 ENERGY STORAGE APPLICATION

Energy storage is one of the imperative components of energy systems to provide energy, especially when required. Energy storage devices and their related area of research are one of the emerging areas of research nowadays because of their high demands in society. A supercapacitor is a device that stores energy by using surface redox reactions and ion adsorptions. Supercapacitors are one of the auspicious candidates for energy storage devices mainly due to their low maintenance, extraordinary life cycle, and high power density. The performance of the supercapacitor devices is mainly due to the characteristics of electrode materials porosity and surface functional groups. Moreover, controlling the pore size and surface texture by changing their synthesis parameters, precursor, and synthesis process that might be beneficial for the supercapacitor's performance (Presser et al., 2011; Borchardt et al., 2014; Zhang et al., 2014; Frackowiak, 2007; Swain et al., 2021; Tian et al., 2015; Sun et al., 2016; Noori et al., 2019). Numerous porous CB-NMs and polymeric composites have been used for supercapacitors application. For example, Deng et al. (2015) synthesized hierarchical porous carbon (HPC) using biomass with $KHCO_3$ for supercapacitor application. The data indicate that the prepared HPC-based materials have a high specific surface area (~1893 m^2/g) and are effectively used in supercapacitor applications with a specific capacitance of 253 F/g. Moreover, the prepared HPC-based materials have high stability up to 10,000 cycles (Deng et al., 2015). Li et al. (2017) synthesized porous graphene paper (PGP) using thermal shock for supercapacitor application. The data suggested that the prepared PGP-based materials are effectively used as supercapacitor applications with a specific capacitance of ~100 F/g. Moreover, high specific capacitance is mainly due to the high surface area and high conductivity of the PGP material (Li et al., 2017). Dong et al. (2018) rise husk-derived carbon (RHC) for supercapacitors application. The data indicate that the prepared RHC-based materials have sheet-like structures and small pores, effectively used in supercapacitor applications with 315 and 189 F/g at 0.1 and 50 A/g, respectively. Moreover, RHC texture, pores, and surface functional groups effectively improved the specific capacitance (Dong et al., 2018). Ramesh et al. (2018) synthesized tamarind seed-based carbon (TSC) using the carbonization and activation process for the supercapacitor application. Figure 7.4 shows a schematic representation of the synthesized TSC. The data indicate that the prepared TSC-based porous materials have a high surface area (1702 m^2/g) and are effectively used in supercapacitor applications with a specific capacitance of 157 F/g. Moreover, the prepared TSC-based porous materials have high stability over 1000 cycles (Ramesh et al., 2018).

Ramesh et al. (2019) synthesized nitrogen-doped graphene oxide (N-GO) incorporated SnO_2 (N-GO-SnO_2) based porous composite materials for supercapacitor application. Figure 7.5 shows the SEM images of porous

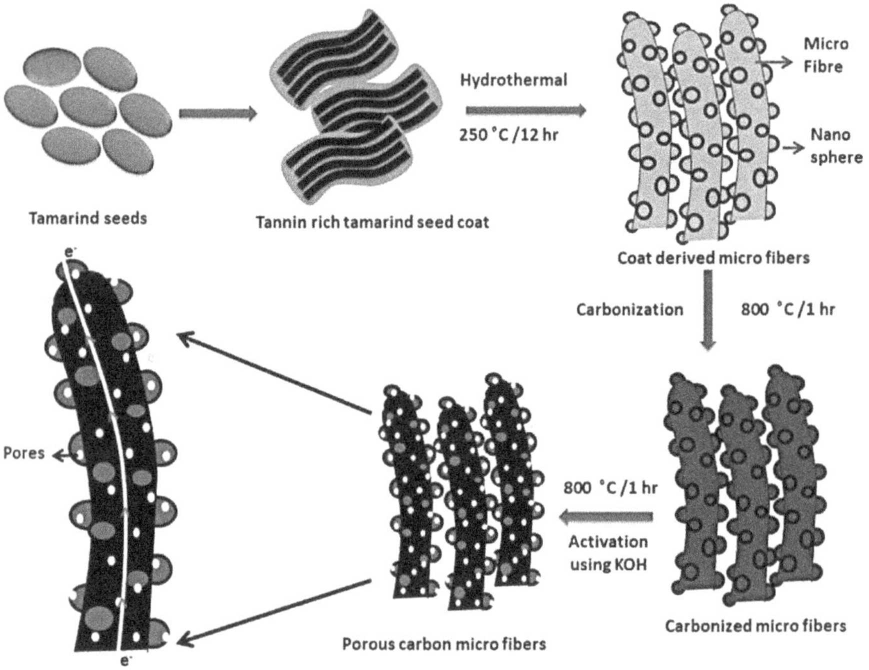

FIGURE 7.4 A schematic representation of the synthesized TSC. The image was taken with permission.

Source: Reprinted with permission from Ramesh et al., 2018. Open Access.

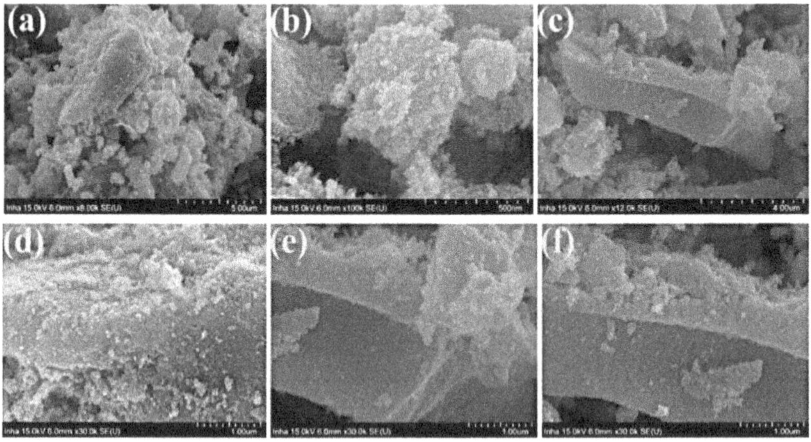

FIGURE 7.5 SEM images of porous N-GO-SnO_2 composite materials. The image was taken with permission.

Source: Reprinted with permission from Ramesh et al., 2018. Open Access.

N-GO-SnO_2-based composite materials. The SEM images show the porous and rough texture of the prepared N-GO-SnO_2-based composite materials. The data indicate that the prepared N-GO-SnO_2-based composite materials are effectively used in the supercapacitor application with ~378 F/g super capacitance. Moreover, the prepared N-GO-SnO_2-based composite materials have high stability over 5000 cycles, an attribute possibly used for supercapacitor application (Ramesh et al., 2019).

Bazan-Aguilar et al. (2020) synthesized reduced graphene oxide (RGO) and incorporated it within the commercial cotton fibers (RGO-CCFs) using the impregnation process for the supercapacitor's applications. The data indicate that the RGO-CCFs are effectively utilized in supercapacitor applications with a specific capacitance of 74.1 F/g and high cycling stability. Figure 7.6 shows the SEM images of the commercial cotton fibers (CCFs) and RGO-CCFs. The SEM images of CCFs indicate that the porous texture of CCFs, whereas incorporation of the RGO, significantly increases the RGO-CCFs materials' porosity. The high cycling stability and specific capacitance are mainly due to the porous texture and conductivity of the RGO-CCFs materials (Bazan-Aguilar et al., 2020). Talreja et al. (2020) synthesized metal incorporated phenol-formaldehyde resin-based beads and then carbonized them to prepare (Fe-CMP and Zn-CMP) using simple polymerization, carbonization, and activation process for supercapacitors application. The pore size was controlled using different metals according to the ionic radii and sonicated to create a specific pore size (Fe-CMP-S and Zn-CMP-S). The data indicate that the CMP-S is effectively used for supercapacitor application with a specific capacitance of 132 and 152 F/g of Fe-CMP-S and Zn-CMP-S, respectively. Moreover, super capacitance performance might be tuned by changing their pore size (Talreja et al., 2020). Nath et al. (2022) synthesized corn starch polymers (CSP) using the carbonization process for supercapacitors application. The data indicate that the prepared porous CSP-based materials are effectively used for the supercapacitor's application with a specific capacitance of 188 F/g (Nath et al., 2022). Table 7.3 Summarize the different porous materials and their supercapacitor application. The data indicate that porosity is one of the essential factors for supercapacitor applications. The supercapacitor performance might increase the high surface area, more active sites, high mass transfer, and shortened diffusion pathways. Therefore, porous materials can potentially store energy with high cyclic ability.

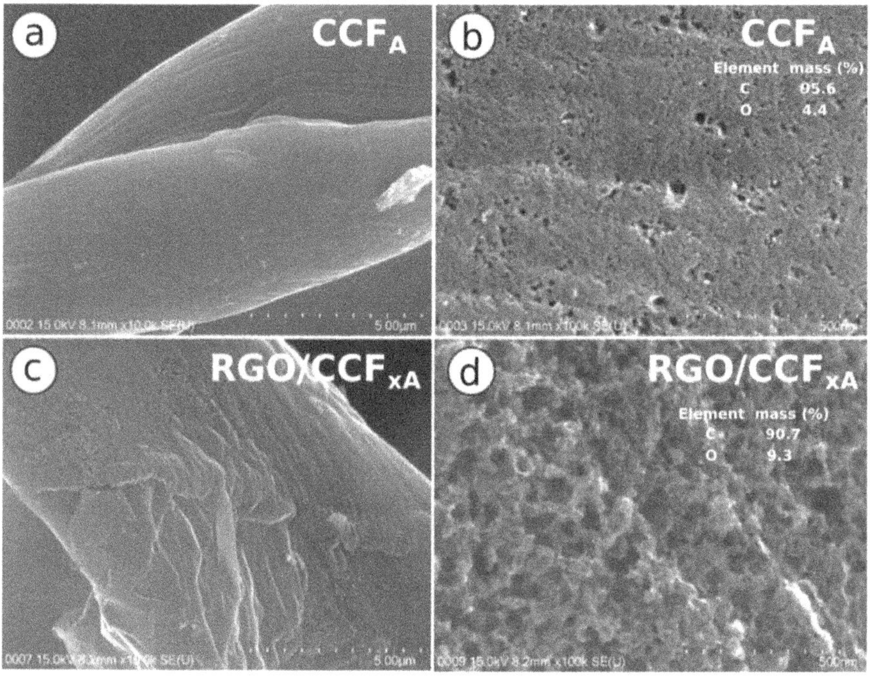

FIGURE 7.6 SEM images of CCF and RGO-CCF. The image was taken with permission.
Source: Reprinted with permission from (Bazan-Aguilar et al., 2020). Open Access.

TABLE 7.3 Different Porous Materials and Their Supercapacitor Application.

S. No.	Porous materials	Synthesis process	Specific capacitance	References
1.	HPC	Leavening	253 F/g	(Deng et al., 2015)
2.	PGP	Thermal shock	100 F/g	(Li et al., 2017)
3.	RHC	Pyrolysis	315 F/g at 0.1 A/g 189 F/g at 50 A/g	(Dong et al., 2018)
4.	TSC	Carbonization and activation	157 F/g	(Ramesh et al., 2018)
5.	N-GO-SnO_2	Thermal reduction process	~378 F/g at 4 A/g	(Ramesh et al., 2019)
6.	RGO-CCFs	Impregnation	74.1 F/g at 0.2 A/g	(Bazan-Aguilar et al., 2020)
7.	Fe-CMP-S	Template method	132 F/g	(Talreja et al., 2020)
8.	Zn-CMP-S	Template method	152 F/g	(Talreja et al., 2020)
9.	CSP	Carbonization process	~188 F/g at 5 mV/s	(Nath et al., 2022)

7.2.4 SOLAR CELL APPLICATION

The global conversion of solar light into energy has been of considerable interest to the researcher. Solar cell technologies mainly depend on the p-n junction, which allows for the use of the photovoltaic ability of semiconductor materials. Researchers continue focusing on improving the conversion efficiency of solar cells, mainly by (1) synthesis of excellent materials and (2) designing materials to improve the conversion efficiency of solar cells. Numerous porous semiconductor materials are effectively used in solar cell applications. For example, Durr et al. (2005) synthesized composite porous layer-based dye-sensitized solar cells (DSSCs) at low-temperature. The data indicate that the fabricated composite porous layer is effectively used in DSSCs with a conversion efficiency of ~7.3% (Dürr et al., 2005). Hsu et al. synthesized low-temperature TiO2-based DSSCs. The data indicate that the TiO_2-based DSSCs are less than 150°C temperature. The prepared TiO_2-based DSSCs increased the short-circuit current density and conversation efficiency by 7.4–8.8 Ma/cm^2 and 3.7–4.2%, respectively (Hsu et al., 2008). Kim and Hong synthesized flexible DSSCs using three layers based on poly(vinylidene fluoride-*co*-hexafluoropropylene) as both the lower and upper layers. In contrast, the middle layer was made of poly(ethylene terephthalate) to create a sandwich-like structure. The prepared sandwich, like flexible DSSCs, effectively converts solar light with a conversion efficiency of 8.4% (Kim and Hong, 2018). Sudhakar et al. (2020) synthesized platinum-free counter electrode-based DSSCs using nanographene incorporated PEDOT: PSS-PG composite. The data indicate that the prepared DSSCs efficiently convert solar light to energy with a conversion efficiency of 9.64% (Sudhakar et al., 2020). Sun et al. (2022) synthesized the 3D porous composite materials using porous Ni/Al. The CNTs deposited onto the surface of Ni/Al to produce a solar steam generator. The data indicate that the Ni/Al-CNTs-based solar steam generator uses around 94.4% solar adsorption and 2.41 kg/m^2/h evaporation (Sun et al., 2022). The literature suggested that the porosity/porous texture of the materials improved short-circuit current density and conversation efficiency. Moreover, the porous texture of the materials increased dye molecules' adsorption and improved the adsorption of solar irradiation, thereby high conversation efficiency. Additionally, materials design using nanotubes/nanotubes/wires incorporated within the polymeric composite might be beneficial for high conversation efficiency of the solar cells.

7.3 CONCLUSION

The porous CB-NMs and their composite are comprehensively used in numerous applications, including water treatment technology, antibiotic materials, drug delivery systems, sensors, agriculture, energy, supercapacitors, and biomedicine. Another class of porous materials, MOFs, porous organic solid, and COFs, are newly emerging materials with high porosity and are widely used for numerous applications. The porous polymeric or hybrid composite materials effectively remove heavy metal ions and dye, inhibiting/killing bacterial strains. The high sorption/removal ability of the porous polymeric composite is mainly due to porosity, surface texture, electrostatic interaction, and acid–base interaction. Moreover, functional group present at the surface of porous polymeric composite is also essential for augmenting the adsorption ability. Furthermore, the porous texture, pore size, and interconnected pore mainly depend on the biomaterials and their synthesis process. The porous surface texture, pore size, and interconnected pores might be easily tuned by incorporating metal, nonmetals, and polymers within the composite. Moreover, electrospinning might be a next-generation process that creates porous biomaterials. Additionally, solvent casting, 3D printing, and leaching process are the most appropriate processes to create a controlled pore. Therefore, quickly fabricated porous polymeric composite is effectively used in biomedical applications. It is important to mention here that the high surface area, more active sites, high mass transfer, and shortened diffusion pathways might increase the supercapacitor performance. Therefore, porous materials can potentially store energy with high cyclic ability. Incorporating multiscale porosities into one material might improve the overall performance in environment remediation, biomedical, energy, and solar cells.

KEYWORDS

- **porous materials**
- **polymers**
- **carbon**
- **metal-organic frameworks**
- **nanomaterials**

REFERENCES

Adil, H. I.; Thalji, M. R. Metal-organic Frameworks (MOFs) Based Nanofiber Architectures for the Sorption of Heavy Metal Ions. *RSC Adv.* **2022,** *12* (3), 1433–1450.

Afreen, S.; Omar, R. A.; Talreja, N.; Chauhan, D.; Ashfaq, M. Carbon-Based Nanostructured Materials for Energy and Environmental Remediation Applications. In*Approaches in Bioremediation: The New Era of Environmental Microbiology and Nanobiotechnology*; Prasad, R., Aranda, E., Eds.; Springer International Publishing: Cham, 2018.

Afreen, S.; Talreja, N.; Chauhan, D.; Ashfaq, M. Chapter 15 - Polymer/Metal/Carbon-Based Hybrid Materials for the Detection of Heavy Metal Ions. In *Multifunctional Hybrid Nanomaterials for Sustainable Agri-Food and Ecosystems*; Abd-Elsalam, K. A., Ed.; Elsevier, 2020.

Agboola, O.; Fayomi, O. S. I.; Ayodeji, A.; Ayeni, A. O.; Alagbe, E. E.; Sanni, S. E.; Okoro, E. E.; Moropeng, L.; Sadiku, R.; Kupolati, K. W.; Oni, B. A. A Review on Polymer Nanocomposities and their Effective Applications in, Membranes and Adsorbents for Water Treatment and Gas Separation. *Membranes* **2021,** *11* (2), 139.

Ahumada, M.; Jacques, E.; Calderon, C.; Martínez-Gómez, F. Porosity in Biomaterials: A Key Factor in the Development of Applied Materials in Biomedicine. In *Handbook of Ecomaterials*; Martínez, L. M. T., Kharissova, O. V., Kharisov, B. I., Eds.; Springer International Publishing: Cham, 2019.

Akram, A. M.; Omar, R. A.; Ashfaq, M. Chitosan/Calcium Phosphate-Nanoflakes-Based Biomaterial: A Potential Hemostatic Wound Dressing Material. *Polym. Bull.* **2022,** *80* (5), 1–16.

Ashfaq, M.; Khan, S.; Verma, N. Synthesis of PVA-CAP-Based Biomaterial in situ Dispersed with Cu Nanoparticles and Carbon Micro-nanofibers for Antibiotic Drug Delivery Applications. *Biochem. Eng. J.* **2014,** *90*, 79–89.

Ashfaq, M.; Talreja, N.; Chauhan, D.; Rodríguez, C. A.; Mera, A. C.; Mangalaraja, R. V. A Novel Bimetallic (Fe/Bi)-Povidone-Iodine Micro-Flowers Composite for Photocatalytic and Antibacterial Applications. *J. Photochem. Photobiol. B Biol.* **2021,** *219*, 112204.

Ashfaq, M.; Verma, N.; Khan, S. Copper/Zinc Bimetal Nanoparticles-Dispersed Carbon Nanofibers: A Novel Potential Antibiotic Material. *Mater. Sci. Eng. C* **2016,** *59*, 938–947.

Ashfaq, M.; Verma, N.; Khan, S. Highly Effective Cu/Zn-Carbon Micro/Nanofiber-Polymer Nanocomposite-Based Wound Dressing Biomaterial Against the P. aeruginosa Multi- and Comprehensively Drug-Resistant Strains. *Mater. Sci. Eng. C* **2017,** *77*, 630–641.

Aw, M. S.; Simovic, S.; Addai-Mensah, J.; Losic, D. Polymeric Micelles in Porous and Nanotubular Implants as a New System for Extended Delivery of Poorly Soluble Drugs. *J. Mater. Chem.* **2011,** *21* (20), 7082–7089.

Baig, N.; Kammakakam, I.; Falath, W. Nanomaterials: A Review of Synthesis Methods, Properties, Recent Progress, and Challenges. *Mater. Adv.* **2021,** *2* (6), 1821–1871.

Bayda, S.; Adeel, M.; Tuccinardi, T. The History of Nanoscience and Nanotechnology: From Chemical-Physical Applications to Nanomedicine. *Molecules* **2020,** *25* (1), 112

Bazan-Aguilar, A.; Ponce-Vargas, M.; Caycho, C. L.; La Rosa-Toro, A.; Baena-Moncada, A. M. Highly Porous Reduced Graphene Oxide-Coated Carbonized Cotton Fibers as Supercapacitor Electrodes. *ACS Omega* **2020,** *5* (50), 32149–32159.

Bhadauriya, P.; Mamtani, H.; Ashfaq, M.; Raghav, A.; Teotia, A. K.; Kumar, A.; Verma, N. Synthesis of Yeast-Immobilized and Copper Nanoparticle-Dispersed Carbon

Nanofiber-Based Diabetic Wound Dressing Material: Simultaneous Control of Glucose and Bacterial Infections. *ACS Appl. Bio Mater.* **2018,** *1* (2), 246–258.

Borchardt, L.; Oschatz, M.; Kaskel, S. Tailoring Porosity in Carbon Materials for Supercapacitor Applications. *Mater. Horiz.* **2014,** *1* (2), 157–168.

Chauhan, D.; Afreen, S.; Talreja, N.; Ashfaq, M. Chapter 8 - Multifunctional Copper Polymer-Based Nanocomposite for Environmental and Agricultural Applications. In *Multifunctional Hybrid Nanomaterials for Sustainable Agri-Food and Ecosystems*; Abd-Elsalam, K. A., Ed.; Elsevier, 2020.

Chauhan, D.; Singh, N.; Afreen, S.; Talreja, N.; Ashfaq, M.; Sankararamakrishnan, N.; Chaudhary, G. R. A Thermoresponsive CA-PNIPAM Based Electrospun Nanofibrous Membrane for Oil/Water Separation. *New J. Chem.* **2022,** *46*, 18984–18989.

Chauhan, D.; Talreja, N.; Ashfaq, M. Chapter 13 - Nanoadsorbents for Wastewater Remediation. In *Aquananotechnology*; Abd-Elsalam, K. A., Zahid, M., Eds.; Elsevier, 2021.

Cipriani, C. E.; Ha, T.; Martinez Defilló, O. B.; Myneni, M.; Wang, Y.; Benjamin, C. C.; Wang, J.; Pentzer, E. B.; Wei, P. Structure–Processing–Property Relationships of 3D Printed Porous Polymeric Materials. *ACS Mater. Au* **2021,** *1* (1), 69–80.

Deng, J.; Xiong, T.; Xu, F.; Li, M.; Han, C.; Gong, Y.; Wang, H.; Wang, Y. Inspired by Bread Leavening: One-Pot Synthesis of Hierarchically Porous Carbon for Supercapacitors. *Green Chem.* **2015,** *17* (7), 4053–4060.

Dong, Z.; Cui, H.; Zhang, H.; Wang, F.; Zhan, X.; Mayer, F.; Nestler, B.; Wegener, M.; Levkin, P. A. 3D Printing of Inherently Nanoporous Polymers via Polymerization-Induced Phase Separation. *Nat. Commun.* **2021,** *12* (1), 247.

Dong, S.; He, X.; Zhang, H.; Xie, X.; Yu, M.; Yu, C.; Xiao, N.; Qiu, J. Surface Modification of Biomass-Derived Hard Carbon by Grafting Porous Carbon Nanosheets for High-Performance Supercapacitors. *J. Mater. Chem. A* **2018,** *6* (33), 15954–15960.

du Plessis, A.; Razavi, S. M. J.; Benedetti, M.; Murchio, S.; Leary, M.; Watson, M.; Bhate, D.; Berto, F. Properties and Applications of Additively Manufactured Metallic Cellular Materials: A Review. *Prog. Mater. Sci.* **2022,** *125*, 100918.

Dürr, M.; Schmid, A.; Obermaier, M.; Rosselli, S.; Yasuda, A.; Nelles, G. Low-Temperature Fabrication of Dye-sensitized Solar Cells by Transfer of Composite Porous Layers. *Nat. Mater.* **2005,** *4* (8), 607–611.

Farmahini, A. H.; Krishnamurthy, S.; Friedrich, D.; Brandani, S.; Sarkisov, L. Performance-Based Screening of Porous Materials for Carbon Capture. *Chem. Rev.* **2021,** *121* (17), 10666–10741.

Frackowiak, E. Carbon Materials for Supercapacitor Application. *Phys. Chem. Chem. Phys.* **2007,** *9* (15), 1774–1785.

Hsu, C. P.; Lee, K. M.; Huang, J. T. W.; Lin, C. Y.; Lee, C. H.; Wang, L. P.; Tsai, S. Y.; Ho, K. C. EIS Analysis on Low Temperature Fabrication of TiO2 Porous Films for Dye-Sensitized Solar Cells. *Electrochim. Acta* **2008,** *53* (25), 7514–7522.

Kanhed, S.; Awasthi, S.; Midha, S.; Nair, J.; Nisar, A.; Patel, A. K.; Pandey, A.; Sharma, R.; Goel, S.; Upadhyaya, A.; Ghosh, S.; Balani, K. Microporous Hydroxyapatite Ceramic Composites as Tissue Engineering Scaffolds: An Experimental and Computational Study. *Adv. Eng. Mater.* **2018,** *20* (7), 1701062.

Khan, N. A.; Hasan, Z.; Jhung, S. H. Adsorptive Sorption of Hazardous Materials Using Metal-Organic Frameworks (MOFs): A Review. *J. Hazard. Mater.* **2013,** *244-245*, 444–456.

Khare, P.; Talreja, N.; Deva, D.; Sharma, A.; Verma, N. Carbon Nanofibers Containing Metal-Doped Porous Carbon Beads for Environmental Remediation Applications. *Chem. Eng. J.* **2013,** *229*, 72–81.

Kim, G. H.; Hong, S. C. Porous Composite Separator Membranes of Dye-Sensitized Solar Cells with Flexible Substrate for their Improved Stability. *J. Mater. Sci.* **2018,** *53* (17), 12365–12373.

Kruželák, J.; Kvasničáková, A.; Hložeková, K.; Hudec, I. Progress in Polymers and Polymer Composites Used as Efficient Materials for EMI Shielding. *Nanoscale Adv.* **2021,** *3* (1), 123–172.

, D.; Talreja, N. Nickel Nanoparticles-Doped Rhodamine Grafted Carbon Nanofibers as Colorimetric Probe: Naked Eye Detection and Highly Sensitive Measurement of Aqueous Cr3+ and Pb2+. *Korean J. Chem. Eng.* **2019,** *36* (1), 126–135.

Kumar, V.; Talreja, N.; Deva, D.; Sankararamakrishnan, N.; Sharma, A.; Verma, N. Development of Bi-metal Doped Micro- and Nano Multi-Functional Polymeric Adsorbents for the Sorption of Fluoride and Arsenic(V) from Wastewater. *Desalination* **2011,** *282*, 27–38.

Kumar Singh, M.; Zafar, S.; Talha, M. Development of Porous bio-Composites Through Microwave Curing for Bone Tissue Engineering. *Mater. Today Proc.* **2019,** *18*, 731–739.

, Q.; Guo, X.; Zhang, Y.; Zhang, W.; Ge, C.; Zhao, L.; Wang, X.; Zhang, H.; Chen, J.; Wang, Z.; Sun, L. Porous Graphene Paper for Supercapacitor Applications. *J. Mater. Sci. Technol.* **2017,** *33* (8), 793–799.

Mahdavi, H.; Smith, S. J. D.; Mulet, X.; Hill, M. R. Practical Considerations in the Design and use of Porous Liquids. *Mater. Horiz.* **2022,** *9* (6), 1577–1601.

Mishra, R. K.; Sabu, A.; Tiwari, S. K. Materials Chemistry and the Futurist Eco-friendly Applications of Nanocellulose: Status and Prospect. *J. Saudi Chem. Soc.* **2018,** *22* (8), 949–978.

Nath, G.; Singh, P. K.; Dhapola, P. S.; Dohare, S.; Noor, I. M.; Sharma, T.; Singh, A. Fabrication of Cornstarch Biopolymer-Derived Nano Porous Carbon as Electrode Material for Supercapacitor Application. *Biomass Convers. Biorefin.* **2022.**

Navrotskaya, A. G.; Aleksandrova, D. D.; Krivoshapkina, E. F.; Sillanpää, M.; Krivoshapkin, P. V. Hybrid Materials Based on Carbon Nanotubes and Nanofibers for Environmental Applications. *Front Chem.* **2020,** *8*, 546.

Nikolova, M. P.; Chavali, M. S. Recent Advances in Biomaterials for 3D Scaffolds: A Review. *Bioact. Mater.* **2019,** *4*, 271–292.

Noori, A.; El-Kady, M. F.; Rahmanifar, M. S.; Kaner, R. B.; Mousavi, M. F. Towards Establishing Standard Performance Metrics for Batteries, Supercapacitors and Beyond. *Chem. Soc. Rev.* **2019,** *48* (5), 1272–1341.

Omar, R. A.; Afreen, S.; Talreja, N.; Chauhan, D.; Ashfaq, M. Impact of Nanomaterials in Plant Systems. In *Plant Nanobionics: Volume 1, Advances in the Understanding of Nanomaterials Research and Applications*; Prasad, R., Ed.; Springer International Publishing: Cham, 2019.

Peng, L.; Zhang, X.; Sun, Y.; Xing, Y.; Li, C. Heavy Metal Elimination Based on Metal Organic Framework Highly Loaded on Flexible Nanofibers. *Environ. Res.* **2020,** *188*, 109742.

Presser, V.; Heon, M.; Gogotsi, Y. Carbide-Derived Carbons – From Porous Networks to Nanotubes and Graphene. *Adv. Funct. Mater.* **2011,** *21* (5), 810–833.

Rahimi, E.; Mohaghegh, N. New Hybrid Nanocomposite of Copper Terephthalate MOF-Graphene Oxide: Synthesis, Characterization and Application as Adsorbents for

Toxic Metal Ion Sorption from Sungun Acid Mine Drainage. *Environ. Sci. Pollut. Res.* **2017,** *24* (28), 22353–22360.

Ramesh, T.; Rajalakshmi, N.; Dhathathreyan, K. S.; Reddy, L. R. G. Hierarchical Porous Carbon Microfibers Derived from Tamarind Seed Coat for High-Energy Supercapacitor Application. *ACS Omega* **2018,** *3* (10), 12832–12840.

Ramesh, S.; Yadav, H. M.; Lee, Y. J.; Hong, G. W.; Kathalingam, A.; Sivasamy, A.; Kim, H. S.; Kim, H. S.; Kim, J. H. Porous Materials of Nitrogen Doped Graphene Oxide@SnO2 Electrode for Capable Supercapacitor Application. *Sci. Rep.* **2019,** *9* (1), 12622.

Rangnekar, N.; Mittal, N.; Elyassi, B.; Caro, J.; Tsapatsis, M. Zeolite Membranes – A Review and Comparison with MOFs. *Chem. Soc. Rev.* **2015,** *44* (20), 7128–7154.

Rathinavel, S.; Priyadharshini, K.; Panda, D. A Review on Carbon Nanotube: An Overview of Synthesis, Properties, Functionalization, Characterization, and the Application. *Mater. Sci. Eng. B* **2021,** *268*, 115095.

Samanta, P.; Desai, A. V.; Let, S.; Ghosh, S. K. Advanced Porous Materials for Sensing, Capture and Detoxification of Organic Pollutants toward Water Remediation. *ACS Sustain. Chem. Eng.* **2019,** *7* (8), 7456–7478.

Saraswat, R.; Talreja, N.; Deva, D.; Sankararamakrishnan, N.; Sharma, A.; Verma, N. Development of Novel in situ Nickel-Doped, Phenolic Resin-Based Micro–Nano-Activated Carbon Adsorbents for the Sorption of Vitamin B-12. *Chem. Eng. J.* **2012,** *197*, 250–260.

Sasidharan, V.; Sachan, D.; Chauhan, D.; Talreja, N.; Ashfaq, M. Three-Dimensional (3D) Polymer—Metal–Carbon Framework for Efficient Sorption of Chemical and Biological Contaminants. *Sci. Rep.* **2021,** *11* (1), 7708.

Shahcheraghi, N.; Golchin, H.; Sadri, Z.; Tabari, Y.; Borhanifar, F.; Makani, S. Nano-Biotechnology, An Applicable Approach for Sustainable Future. *3 Biotech* **2022,** *12* (3), 65.

Sharikova, N. A.; Antipova, K. G.; Lukanina, K. I.; Stolyarova, D. Y.; Vdovichenko, A. Y.; Malakhov, S. N.; Krasheninnikov, S. V.; Kulikova, O. R.; Khramtsova, E. A.; Chvalun, S. N.; Grigoriev, T. E. Chitosan-Based Porous Composites for Bone Tissue Engineering. *Macromol. Symp.* **2022,** *404* (1), 2100398.

Shoukat, R.; Khan, M. I. Carbon Nanotubes/Nanofibers (CNTs/CNFs): A Review on State of the Art Synthesis Methods. *Microsyst. Technol.* **2022,** *28* (4), 885–901.

Sudhakar, V.; Singh, A. K.; Chini, M. K. Nanoporous Reduced Graphene Oxide and Polymer Composites as Efficient Counter Electrodes in Dye-Sensitized Solar Cells. *ACS Appl. Electron. Mater.* **2020,** *2* (3), 626–634.

Sun, K.; Cui, H.; Xu, R.; Wang, L.; Li, M.; Yang, Z.; Zhao, M.; Wei, N. Constructing of 3D Porous Composite Materials of NiAl/CNTs for Highly Efficient Solar Steam Generation. *Solar Energy Mater. Solar Cells* **2022,** *240*, 111722.

Sun, M. H.; Huang, S. Z.; Chen, L. H.; Li, Y.; Yang, X. Y.; Yuan, Z. Y.; Su, B. L. Applications of Hierarchically Structured Porous Materials from Energy Storage and Conversion, Catalysis, Photocatalysis, Adsorption, Separation, and Sensing to Biomedicine. *Chem. Soc. Rev.* **2016,** *45* (12), 3479–3563.

Sun, D. T.; Peng, L.; Reeder, W. S.; Moosavi, S. M.; Tiana, D.; Britt, D. K.; Oveisi, E.; Queen, W. L. Rapid, Selective Heavy Metal Sorption from Water by a Metal–Organic Framework/Polydopamine Composite. *ACS Central Sci.* **2018,** *4* (3), 349–356.

Susanto, H.; Samsudin, A. M.; Rokhati, N.; Widiasa, I. N. Immobilization of Glucose Oxidase on Chitosan-Based Porous Composite Membranes and their Potential use in Biosensors. *Enzyme Microb. Technol.* **2013,** *52* (6), 386–392.

Swain, N.; Saravanakumar, B.; Kundu, M.; Schmidt-Mende, L.; Ramadoss, A. Recent Trends in Template Assisted 3D Porous Materials for Electrochemical Supercapacitors. *J. Mater. Chem. A* **2021,** *9* (45)**,** 25286–25324.

Talreja, N.; Jung, S.; Yen, L. T. H.; Kim, T. Phenol-formaldehyde-resin-based Activated Carbons with Controlled Pore Size Distribution for High-Performance Supercapacitors. *Chem. Eng. J.* **2020,** *379*, 122332.

Talreja, N.; Kumar, D.; Verma, N. Sorption of Hexavalent Chromium from Water using Fe-grown Carbon Nanofibers Containing Porous Carbon Microbeads. *J. Water Process Eng.* **2014,** *3*, 34–45.

Talreja, N.; Verma, N.; Kumar, D. Carbon Bead-Supported Ethylene Diamine-Functionalized Carbon Nanofibers: An Efficient Adsorbent for Salicylic Acid. *CLEAN Soil Air Water* **2016,** *44* (11)**,** 1461–1470.

Tan, X.; Rodrigue, D. A Review on Porous Polymeric Membrane Preparation. Part I: Production Techniques with Polysulfone and Poly (Vinylidene Fluoride). *Polymers (Basel)* **2019,** *11* (7)**,** 1160.

Thakur, B.; Guo, X.; Chang, J.; Kron, M.; Chen, J. Porous Carbon and Prussian Blue Composite: A Highly Sensitive Electrochemical Platform for Glucose Biosensing. *Sens. Bio-Sens. Res.* **2017,** *14*, 47–53.

Tian, W.; Gao, Q.; Tan, Y.; Yang, K.; Zhu, L.; Yang, C.; Zhang, H. Bio-Inspired Beehive-Like Hierarchical Nanoporous Carbon Derived from Bamboo-Based Industrial by-Product as a High Performance Supercapacitor Electrode Material. *J. Mater. Chem. A* **2015,** *3* (10)**,** 5656–5664.

Wang, Z.; Chen, H.; Wang, Y.; Chen, J.; Arnould, M. A.; Hu, B.; Popovs, I.; Mahurin, S. M.; Dai, S. Polymer-Grafted Porous Silica Nanoparticles with Enhanced CO2 Permeability and Mechanical Performance. *ACS Appl. Mater. Interf.* **2021,** *13* (23)**,** 27411–27418.

Xiao, Y.; Yang, Y.; Li, J.; Ma, Y.; Wang, H.; Wang, L.; Huang, Y.; Zhang, P.; Zou, Q.; Lai, X. Porous Composite Calcium Citrate/Polylactic Acid Materials with High Mineralization Activity and Biodegradability for Bone Repair Tissue Engineering. *Int. J. Polym. Mater. Polym. Biomater.* **2021,** *70* (7)**,** 507–520.

Zhang, Y.; Zhang, T.; Huang, Z.; Yang, J. A New Class of Electronic Devices Based on Flexible Porous Substrates. *Adv. Sci.* **2022,** *9* (7)**,** 2105084.

Zhang, X.; Zhang, H.; Li, C.; Wang, K.; Sun, X.; Ma, Y. Recent Advances in Porous Graphene Materials for Supercapacitor Applications. *RSC Adv.* **2014,** *4* (86)**,** 45862–45884.

Zhao, S.; Chen, D.; Wei, F.; Chen, N.; Liang, Z.; Luo, Y. Sorption of Congo Red Dye from Aqueous Solution with Nickel-Based Metal-Organic Framework/Graphene Oxide Composites Prepared by Ultrasonic Wave-Assisted Ball Milling. *Ultrason. Sonochem.* **2017,** *39*, 845–852.

Zhao, S.; Chen, D.; Wei, F.; Chen, N.; Liang, Z.; Luo, Y. Synthesis of Graphene Oxide/Metal–Organic Frameworks Hybrid Materials for Enhanced Sorption of Methylene Blue in Acidic and Alkaline Solutions. *J. Chem. Technol. Biotechnol.* **2018,** *93* (3)**,** 698–709.

Zhou, Y.; Zhou, L.; Zhang, X.; Chen, Y. Preparation of Zeolitic Imidazolate Framework-8 /Graphene Oxide Composites with Enhanced VOCs Adsorption Capacity. *Micropor. Mesopor. Mater.* **2016,** *225*, 488–493.

CHAPTER 8

Recent Advances in Biodegradable Polymer-Based Nanocomposites for Energy and Environmental Applications

A. SÁENZ-GALINDO[1], R. RAMOS-GONZÁLEZ[2], R. ARREDONDO-VALDÉS[1], J. D. GARCÍA-GARCÍA[1], L. SEPÚLVEDA-TORRE[1], E. MARTÍNEZ-MORENO[1], and M. DÁVILA-MEDINA[1]

[1]*Facultad de Ciencias Químicas, Universidad Autonoma de Coahuila, Saltillo, Coahuila, México*

[2]*Universidad Autonoma de Coahuila, Saltillo, Coahuila, México*

ABSTRACT

The depletion of energy and the worsening of environmental problems associated with the disposal of plastic waste has become an environmental crisis worldwide, causing severe damage to our ecological and aquatic environment. This has motivated innovations in the plastics industry to develop polymers obtained from renewable bio-based resources. The principal goal is to provide low-cost materials with and biodegradable characteristics and adequate mechanical and chemical properties. One of the alternatives is biopolymers made from biomass or organic waste that is obtained using natural sources as they are sufficiently available and cheap. Another option is to improve the final product, mix it with supplementary polymers, and assemble additives in the matrix. The mixtures can be synthetic or natural materials. In creating high-performance advanced polymeric nanocomposites, various nano-sized fillers are used as reinforcing materials. A promising additive is nanofillers for obtaining nanocomposite-type materials. Bio-based hybrid nanocomposites enhance the synergy of natural fibers in bio-based

Application of Engineering Principles and Practices in Biotechnology.
Ann Rose Abraham, Leonardo Sepúlveda Torre, Tamara Tatrishvili, and A. K. Haghi (Eds.)

polymers while improving performance and maintaining environmental appeal. Compared to traditional composites, polymeric nanocomposites provide the possibility to examine new performance and applications apart from classical polymers. Nanoparticles frequently effects the mechanical properties of polymers in very low volume fractions because of the nearly short distance linking nanoparticles, molecular compatibility, and interfacial interaction among polymer and particles chains.

8.1 INTRODUCTION

Plastics have been used for diverse purposes throughout history, and several researchers have studied them. The global production of plastics has reached almost 350 million tons, and three-quarters have become waste. Their unique physiochemical properties such as strength, lightness, durability, and resistance to degradation and their wide range of applications make their industrial-scale production economical and sustainable (Kalia et al., 2021). They are used in almost all industries, especially packaging, which accounts for more than 50% of total consumption. The lifetime of plastics depends on the purpose for which they are used. Plastics used for bottling and baling have short lifetime and cause serious environmental problems because they are non-degradable plastic, and their incineration leads to gas emissions (López-Cuellar et al., 2011).

This severe problem in the environment is now an international issue. Plastic contamination has reached the food chain, threatening human health. When a plastic package is found in the ecosystem, it causes a disruption that will impact directly or indirectly and has long-term effects. Chemical compounds present in plastics have been observed in rivers, marine waters, agriculture soils, and some dead animals. These compounds are bisphenol A and phthalates, plastic additives used for coating, colorant compounds such as cadmium, lead, selenium, and chromium, and some flame retardants such as bromine (Waring et al., 2018).

The earnestness of the problem has increased until the first insight into plastics ingestion by fish, that is, in the Gulf of California in Mexico. In total, 1384 particles of plastic debris were recovered from the gastrointestinal tracts of 552 specimens belonging to 13 species (Salazar-Pérez et al., 2021). Similar observations in the Amazon River estuary, the North Sea and Baltic Sea, and Western Arabian Gulf have been reported (Rummel et al., 2016; Pegado et al., 2018; Baalkhuyur et al., 2020). These affirmations conclude that marine water is contaminated, and the fauna and diversity are at high risk.

The challenge for humanity is the development of materials to replace plastic products. In recent years, there has been a growing effort to develop environmentally friendly biodegradable polymers, an alternative to avoid the pollution problems caused by commercial plastics. The main objective is to find low-cost and biodegradable materials with good mechanical and chemical properties. Several movements involve prohibiting the sale of plastic bags and imposing fees or levies on customers or retailers. However, the reality is the need for an eco-friendly solution (Moshood et al., 2022).

Biodegradability is the process in which the environmental conditions such as weather, soil conditions, anaerobic conditions, or microorganisms degrade materials completely in a timely, safe, and efficient way. Biodegradation consists of two main processes—fragmentation and mineralization. The material is firstly fragmented into small pieces, and the mineralization can benefit the environment in which this process is carried out. Both methods are necessary for being considered biodegradable materials (Havstad, 2020). The biodegradability process can be divided into groups of natural biodegradable polymers: biomass products, polymers produced by microorganisms, and polymers synthesized from renewable materials (Moshood et al., 2022). However, it is necessary to highlight that bio-feedstocks do not necessarily mean that the finished product will be biodegradable (Havstad, 2020). This property depends on the raw material source and the environmental conditions.

One of the alternatives is biopolymers made from biomass or organic waste, which come from natural sources because they are abundantly available and cheap. Another option is to improve the final product, mixing it with other polymers, and incorporating additives in the matrix.

While conventional petrol synthetic plastics represent a considerable pollution problem, bio-based plastics have received tremendous attention. Their high molecular weight, biodegradability, non-toxicity, thermoplasticity, biocompatibility, and production from renewable carbon sources made them a potential alternative instead of conventional plastics (Flores-Sánchez et al., 2020). Polyhydroxyalkanoates (PHAs) are one among the various biopolymers metabolically produced by bacterial organisms. PHAs are biodegradable but are produced in minuscule quantities by prokaryotes and certain eukaryotes; however, PHAs and polylactides are considered eco-friendly plastic resources (Kalia et al., 2021).

Nanotechnology can often overcome these challenges by encapsulating the active compounds within food-grade nanoparticles, which are then introduced into the packaging materials. Different nanocarriers can potentially be used to incorporate active agents into biopolymer-based packaging materials. This purpose uses agro-industrial wastes, natural compounds, and proteins. The size, morphology, and final use are characteristics to be considered in the process; thus, nanotechnology represents a wide area of research to find eco-friendly solutions (Khezerlou et al., 2021). Other sources and alternatives for replacing conventional plastics will be discussed further.

Therefore, the objective of this chapter is to analyze the trending advances in biopolymers and their biodegradability process; and the discussion of the current alternative substitution of biomaterials and the application in which they have been used.

8.2 BIODEGRADABLE POLYMER

The biodegradable raw material was first introduced in the 1980s and is used in several industries such as container residuals, agricultural science, medical specialty, and other industrial areas. There has been an increase in intensity and interest in biodegradable polymers. Two groups of biodegradable polymers can be distinguished: synthetic and natural polymers (Vroman and Tighzert, 2009). Biodegradable polymers add the amount to the businesses that would assist in achieving sustainable development and subsequently emphasize a green economy decreasing the burden of greenhouse gases in the ecosystem and valorizing waste biomass (Rai et al., 2021). Natural polymers are accessible in substantial amounts from renewable suppliers, while synthetic polymers are supplied from nonrenewable petroleum sources (Nagalakshmaiah et al., 2019). Biodegradation occurs through enzymes' activity and chemical deterioration correlated with organisms; the process follows two steps. The first one consists of the polymers fragmentation into lower molecular mass groups through abiotic results, that is, photodegradation, oxidation, hydrolysis, or biotic effects, that is, microorganisms' degradation. The second step begins with microorganisms' bio-assimilation of the polymer sections and their mineralization. Biodegradability depends on the origin of the polymer, its chemical structure, and the degrading environmental circumstances (Mishra, 2015).

8.2.1 NATURALS

Natural polymers are effective in multipurpose applications, including regulated drug delivery, gene distribution, regenerative medicine, and other biomedical functions. Natural polymers are macromolecular compounds that appear naturally within a variety of organisms. The living microorganisms synthesize the biopolymers consisting of repeating units connected by covalently bonded units. Natural polymers are found in microorganisms such as plants, bacteria, fungi, and algae (Balaji et al., 2018). These polymers are identified to generate fewer toxic effects when matched with synthetic polymers. They are obtained from plants, animals, and microbial supplies, which are again categorized based on their chemistry into polysaccharides, protein, polyester, and polyamide-based polymers (Doppalapudi et al., 2015). Biodegradable natural polymers classification is represented in Table 8.1.

TABLE 8.1 Categorization of Natural Polymers Biodegradable.

Origin	Chemistry composition	Examples	References
Plant origin	Polysaccharides, proteins, and polyesters.	Polymers are formed by many glucose and fructose units, cyclodextrins, cellulose, starch, inulin, pectin, glucomannan, guar gum, arabinogalactan, xhantan, dextran, and carrageenan. some proteins are casein, wheat gluten, and soy. On the other hand, polyesters can be polylactic acid and polyhydroxyalkanoates.	Doppalapudi et al., 2015; Parveen et al., 2019; Encalada et al., 2019.
Animal origin	Polysaccharides, proteins, and resin.	Chitosan, chitin, hyaluronan, chondroitin sulfate, collagen, gelatin, albumin, fibrin, silk fibroin, and shellac.	Doppalapudi et al., 2015; Rajeswari et al., 2017; Balaji et al., 2018.
Microbial origin	Polysaccharides, polyesters, polyamides, and polyanhydrides.	Alginate dextran, polyhydroxyalkanoate, poly gamma glutamate, polyphosphate, polylactic acid, hyaluronate, pullulan.	Balaji et al., 2018; Doppalapudi et al., 2015; Parveen et al., 2019.

Natural polymers demonstrate their vast possibility for multifaceted purposes. Also, they open many attractive opportunities for more development of new approaches and the development of current applications (Song et al., 2018).

8.2.2 SYNTHETIC

Few polymers are derived from natural renewable sources. Hence, they can also be processed under the classification of biopolymers (Balaji et al.,

2018). Biodegradable synthetic polymers are produced materials that are extremely practical in the biomedical sector as their properties can be modified to tissue engineering purposes. Synthetic polymers explain mechanical and physic-chemical properties equivalent to biological tissues. They can be formed under controlled conditions and thus exhibit expected and consistent physical and mechanical properties such as:

- elastic modulus,
- tensile modulus,
- tensile strength, and
- degradation rate (Song et al., 2018).

A further benefit of synthetic polymers is the control of material impurities.

Furthermore, synthetic polymers are degraded by hydrolysis, and the degradation rate does not differ from host to host (Kundu et al., 2013). Biodegradable synthetic polymers are derived from corn starch and cassava roots; they undergo chemical and enzymatic polymerization for large-scale production (Balaji et al., 2018). The most significantly active synthetic polymers are poly(glycolic acid) (PGA), poly(lactic acid) (PLA), and their copolymers poly(lactide-co-glycolide), polyanhydride, poly(propylene fumarate), polycaprolactone (PCL), polyethylene glycol (PEG), and polyurethane Kundu et al. (2013). Polymers are manufactured by chemical methods; esters, anhydrides, diacids, and amides are some chemical compositions of these polymers. The weak hydrolyzable links forming the backbones of synthetic biopolymers are the prime source of biodegradability (Balaji et al., 2018). They chemically or enzymatically break down into monomer units, among which few are biologically acceptable by the human body, making their importance significant in various biomedical applications.

Biodegradable polymers have acknowledged considerable observation in the last decades due to their possible applications in the fields associated with environmental friendly and the conservation of physical health (Vroman and Tighzert, 2009).

However, infrequent groups of the introduced biopolymers are of market importance. The most important reason is their price level, which is not yet rational. The imminent of each biopolymer is determined not only by its competitiveness but also by society's capacity to pay for it. The future expectation for development in the field of biopolymers materials is hopeful. Some modern technologies have been used to add value to biodegradable polymers (Kumar et al., 2017). They incorporate active packaging techniques and green fiber reinforcements. Lately, several reports have been published concerning nano clay with biodegradable polymers, especially with starch and aliphatic polyesters. In addition, nano-bio-composites or bio-nano composites are investigated (Basavegowda and Baek, 2021). It is thus clear that the progress of the natural and synthetic biodegradable polymers has developed in response to a progressively more explicit definition of needs for materials with exceptional qualities. It is expected that the wide variety of polymer systems with diverse and unique characteristics will allow progressively successful requests to many problems in medicine, food, agriculture, and other industrial areas.

8.3 NANOCOMPOSITES BIODEGRADABLE POLYMER

8.3.1 OBTAINING

The biodegradable polymers natural or synthetic origin play a crucial role in the life of human beings, because represent a viable alternative for the care and conservation of the environment. When are mixed with nanoparticles or nanostructure form nanocomposites, a nanocomposite is a material that is made up of at least two phases and one phases is on nanoscale, 10^{-9}m, in most cases it is usually the discontinuous phase, reinforcement or additive, which is found in lesser proportion, for the continuous phases exist numerous raw materials for the obtaining nanocomposites biodegradable polymers, this type of nanocomposites, present multiple applications in different areas, such as medicine, pharmacy, food, textiles, biotechnology, electronics, agriculture, etc. Likewise, the continuous phases can be natural or synthetic; Figure 8.1 presents example of different polymer biodegradable origin natural and synthetic (Fig. 8.1).

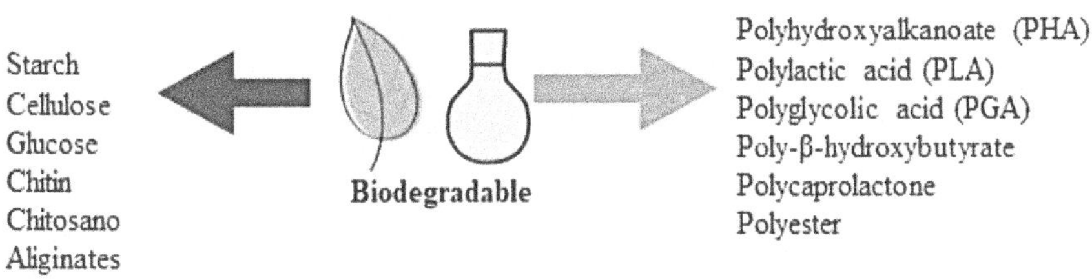

FIGURE 8.1 Example of polymer biodegradables origin natural and synthetics.

Until now there are different routes or methods to obtain this type of nanocomposites biodegradable polymers. The methods more common are: polymerization in situ, dissolution, and fusion each present advantages and disadvantages.

1. Polymerization in situ. In this method, the polymerization is carried out, in presence of the nanoparticles or nanostructure are mixed with the monomer, when the polymer chains grow, the nanoparticles or nanostructure will be dispersed homogeneously in the matrix to form the nanocomposite.
2. Melt mixed. In this method, the discontinuous phase, made up of nanoparticle or nanostructure, must be added when the polymeric material is melted without reaching degradation and in this way carry out adequate mixing. In order to carry out the homogeneous dispersion, an equipment is required that provides adequate shear stresses.
3. Mixed in solution. The nanoparticles or nanostructure are incorporated into a polymer solution. When mixing and removing the solvent, the discontinuous phase will be intercalated between the polymer chains.

Other method actually studied by biosynthesis uses microorganisms or plants, sol-gel, controlled polymerizations, among others. It is important to highlight that the three methods can be assisted by alternate energies such as ultrasound, microwave, and plasma.

Various studies reported about obtaining nanocomposites biodegradable polymers; Marmol et al. (2011) reported a study on chitin and chitosan, which showed how these types of natural polymeric materials are environmentally friendly. The chitosan is one of the most abundant polysaccharides on earth, is used in various applications and uses, such as in food, packaging, covers, in the area of agriculture and in different water treatments, is an ideal polymer natural for obtaining nanocomposites biodegradable polymers. Most of the route used to obtain type of material is by dissolving chitosan in acid solutions, employing acetic acid in most cases (Marmol et al., 2011).

Recently, Janmohammad et al. (2023) reported a detailed study about cellulose-based composite scaffolds with important applications in bone tissue engineering and localized drug delivery, highlighting that cellulose and its derivatives biodegradable natural polymers, in addition to being biocompatibility, available through renewable resources, and low cost of preparation and processing, shows unique characteristics for this type pf materials, are special in bone tissue engineering, show different work route, where biosynthesis using microorganisms for the production of bacterial cellulose (BC)—organic composites and nanocomposites; BC is usually produced by microorganisms such as *Gluconacetobacter xylinus, Gluconacetobacter, Agrobacterium tumefaciens, Sarcina ventriculi* (Janmohammad et al., 2023). A special characteristic of this type of natural organic cellulose is that it is considered highly crystalline; it has been reported that it contains more that 60% crystallinity in its chemical structure, this type of BC is incorporate with polymeric nanofibers to obtain nanocomposites with applications in tissue engineering showing promising results in this area (Jozala et al., 2016). The oxidized nanocellulose is produced by an oxidation reaction where TEMPO (2,2,6,6-tetra-methyl-piperidin-1-oxy) is used; the reactions stars by making BC reaction with TEMPO, oxidation stars, using controlled conditions, the oxidized BC is subsequently obtained and is subjected to an aqueous reaction of HAp (hydroxyapatite) in a highly dispersed solution to obtain the BC-TEMPO nanocellulose composite with HAp presenting interesting applications in tissue engineering (Park et al., 2015).

Another synthetic polymer highly studied as a biodegradable polymer is polycaprolactone; it is a natural polymer, various composites based on carbon nanostructure have been reported, such as carbon nanotubes (CTN), single-walled carbon nanotubes (SWCNT), multi-walled carbon nanotubes (MWCNT), double-walled nanotubes (DWCNT), graphene, nanofibers, such as nanoparticles polymerics, metallics, inorganics, etc., an improvement in different properties was demonstrated when using this type of nanostructure based on carbon.

Janigova et al. (2015) reported a study about obtaining biodegradable polymer/clay nanocomposites and/or composites based on poly(ε-polycaprolactone) (PCL) used by conventional melt mixing. Using three type of clays, organomodified Cloisite 15A, and Cloisite 10A with different ammonium cations located in the silicate gallery and unmodified Cloisite with Na cations were used for composites preparation; the presence of intercalated and exfoliated structures was observed for the composites PCL/Cloisite 15A and PCL/Cloisite 10A, show that nanocomposite structure was formed. The different changes of viscoelastic properties to more solid-like behavior, especially in the low frequency range were explained by formation of silicate network structure, which can be detected by modified Cole-Cole plots, the results obtained contribute to the view that biodegradable matrix-based nanocomposites can be prepared with substantially modified properties, still fulfilling the status of biodegradability according to the current standards (Janigoya et al., 2015).

Armentano et al. (2018), reported the obtaining of different biodegradable composites and nanocomposites, the importance of uses and applications in different areas, such as agriculture, materials, medicine, etc., likewise, it reports a summary of the different methods of obtaining, highlighting different reinforcing phases and natural and synthetic additives, such as silver nanoparticles, carbon nanostructures, cellulose nanocrystals, and lignin. A series of methods are also reported where it stands out, different strategies have been considered to develop and obtention of nanocomposites based on biodegradable natural or synthetic polymers, and can mainly be divided into solvent-based and melt-mixing methods. The process technology is an important step in the final nanocomposite development since it can affect the dispersion grade of the nanofillers in the polymers and hence the functional properties and the micro or nanostructure of films or 3D structures. A factor important is homogeneous dispersion of the nanofillers within a continuous polymeric matrix is a key step to benefiting from their outstanding chemical or physical properties (Armentano et al., 2018).

The main criteria for the selection of the appropriate process technology for obtention and design biodegradable nanocomposite polymeric manufacture include the desired product geometry, the performance needed, and the cost. The different processing techniques in general do not yield a method of obtention of biodegradable nanocomposite polymeric, which is a solvents-based process.

The solvent casting is one of the simplest methods to develop biodegradable nanocomposite polymeric; the main points in the method are:

- Selection of the solvent: The solvent is important in this methodology to permit a complete dissolution of the selected polymer and, at the same time, provide a good dispersion of the nanostructures in the polymer matrix; it used different energy forms as ultrasonic to disperse the nanostructure.
- The proportional concentration among polymer and solvent (as it can effect the viscosity of the solution as well as the evaporation rate); the viscosity in polymer is important for incorporation of different additive, influencing in chemical and physical properties.
- The external conditions of process (pressure, time, light exposure, temperature, and humidity) during the solvent evaporation, as they can effect the properties of the surface morphology along with nanocomposites (Armentano et al., 2018).

The major parameter to be considered is the complete evaporation of the solvent prior to using the final nanocomposite, as it can be quite toxic and also can affect the properties; this process of evaporation can be carried out at room temperature or by using heat. In both things, there are disadvantages and advantages depending on the cost of the process. In academic research laboratories and also in industrial sectors, the use of halogenated solvents like such as chloroform is in general bypass; consequently, the chance of applying a water-soluble polymer is a major approach. However, the solvent-based process restricts the number of polymer matrices that could be considered and this process is neither industrial nor economical.

Melt mixing: Melt-compounding methods, such as extrusion or injection moulding, are commonly used to process thermoplastic polymers in industrial and laboratory, and it is economical and is considered "green" (solvent-free), and industrially and economically viable. The production of the final biodegradable nanocomposite polymeric is optimized in relation to temperature, pressure, moulding time, process time, amount, etc. However, during these processes, high temperatures will be used, so thermal degradation of the polymers should be avoided, here, it is important to know the degradation temperatures of biodegradable nanocomposite polymeric, for example in the case of chitosan: 50–70 °C, PLA: 377 °C, and lignin 300–500 °C. This is a "green" method—environmentally benign—due to the absence of organic solvents, and is viable at the industrial level. Compared to other methods, this is the most viable (Armentano et al., 2018).

The obtained biodegradable nanocomposites polymers is an area of great opportunity to study. There are different factors to consider in obtaining biodegradables polymer nanocomposites, such as, availability of raw materials, process costs, pollution generated, applications, among others.

8.3.2 CHEMICAL AND PHYSICAL PROPERTIES OF BIODEGRADABLE POLYMER-BASED NANOCOMPOSITES

The need to obtain novel engineered materials with enhanced properties and characteristics has been the impulse to research and develop these specialized materials. Moreover, due to the need to reduce the environmental impact and to obtain materials with specialized properties for specific applications, such as in medicine and food technology, the specialists have appealed to materials of natural origin or with reduced environmental impact. The use of biodegradable polymers has been an alternative to these purposes.

According to their source, polymers can be classified as natural or synthetic. And, within this classification, polymers can be degradable or not. An interesting property of natural and some synthetic polymers is that they can be biodegradable. However, polymers could be improved by incorporating nanostructured fillers that bring other properties to this organic material than the bulk polymer.

Polymers are present in people's daily lives and are used for many different applications due to their low density, low cost, lightweight, chemical stability, and outstanding processability (Spinelli et al., 2022). Besides, biopolymers are natural materials obtained from animals, plants, and microorganisms. These biomaterials are elastic, flexible, and fibrous. The most widely used biopolymers are proteins and polysaccharides (Gobi et al., 2021). Biopolymers are of great interest because, due to their biological nature, it is possible to mitigate the use of polymeric materials derived from petroleum and the environmental problems they cause. In addition, nanomaterials are intensified by developing nanocomposites, which are solid materials that result when two or more different materials with different physical and chemical properties are combined to create new materials with improved properties (Basavegowda and Baek, 2021). On the other hand, polymer-based nanocomposites are a unique class of multiphase nanostructured entities formed by a continuous polymeric phase and at least one phase (polymeric, metallic, or ceramic) in the nanoscale dimension (Raza et al., 2021). Polymer-based nanocomposites exhibit unique chemical and physical properties that make them attractive materials for broad applications. Polymer-based nanocomposites can be produced by dispersing nanometric materials (nanofillers) in polymeric or continuous matrices. This reinforcement produces a matrix with unique and improved physical, chemical, and mechanical properties. Combining these materials makes it possible to create a synergistic effect with extraordinary properties not present in the individual components (Basavegowda and Baek, 2021).

Biopolymer-based films are used as an alternatively environment-friendly food packaging. Nevertheless, these materials lack mechanical and physicochemical properties compared with synthetic polymers. To improve these shortcomings, an alternative to enhance their properties is to reinforce the biopolymers with nanomaterials. Also, some nanofillers add other exciting properties, such as antioxidant and antimicrobial activities to the biodegradable polymer-based nanocomposites (Basumatary et al., 2022). Kritchenkov et al. (2021) developed a novel biopolymer-based nanocomposite for applications in food coatings. A chitosan matrix is loaded with nanoparticles of methylcellulose/PEG/chitosan functionalized with anthocyanidin and gallotannin. The nanobiocomposite film exhibit enhanced mechanical and gas barrier properties. Also, the nanocomposite presents antimicrobial, antioxidant, and UV-protective activities. As mentioned, biopolymers do not show appropriate properties for their application in food preservation. The incorporation of graphene derivatives permits obtaining nanocomposites that guarantee some interesting properties. Biodegradable polymer-based nanocomposites synthesized with graphene or graphene oxide enhanced their mechanical properties and thermal stability. Also, it has been reported that incorporating these nanofillers produces nanocomposites with better hydrophobic properties (Barra et al., 2020; Rossa et al., 2022).

On the other hand, biopolymers are commonly used in medical applications due to their biological activity, biodegradability, and biocompatibility. These properties can be enhanced by incorporating nanostructured fillers into the polymeric matrix (Feldman, 2019). Biodegradable nanocomposites have attracted attention in medical applications. Pappa et al. (2018), synthesized poly(ethylene oxide) and sodium montmorillonite clay nanocomposites. They used the composite as a drug carrier for sustained release. The clay nanofiller acts as a transport vehicle for the active molecules, thus increasing the drug stability and efficiently delivering it. Moreover, biodegradable polymer nanocomposites have been applied for ligament-tendon tissue engineering; for this application, the biological activity of the polymer is essential because the biodegradation of the nanocomposite is desirable. Furthermore, incorporating the nanofillers raises the mechanical properties of the polymer (Silva et al., 2020).

Biodegradable polymer-based nanocomposites are of interest in the field of electronics, for example, natural polymers filled with metal oxide nanoparticles (MONPs) have been developed for applications as electronic devices, optical circuits, and sensors due to the electrical and optical properties of the nanocomposites formed by natural polymers and diverse MONPs. Ezzat et al. (2021) carried out theoretical studies of diverse biopolymers such as sodium alginate, cellulose, and chitosan as polymeric matrices of zinc oxide (ZnO), copper oxide (CuO), and graphene oxide nanoparticles for its possible optoelectronic applications. They found that the inclusion of the nanofillers into the biopolymers increases the physical, chemical, and thermal stability. Also, Ezzat et al. (2020) studied the thermal stability and the electronic properties of alginate, cellulose, and chitosan biopolymers enhanced with metal oxide nanoparticles for their possible application as humidity sensors.

8.3.3 APPLICATIONS

Environmental issues have given rise to significant academic and industrial research works directed toward developing sustainable materials based on raw materials derived from green resources, as well as biodegradable and biopolymer materials. Biopolymers have attracted interest in mitigating the influence and application of petroleum-derived polymeric materials and related environmental concerns. Nanotechnology presents new opportunities to improve the performance of polymeric materials with better mechanical, thermal, and electrical properties (Liu, et al., 2019; Armentano et al., 2018; Basavegowda and Baek, 2021; Glaskova et al., 2021).

Biodegradable polymers are often considered the future materials, addressing growing environmental concerns. The advancement of biorefineries and sustainable technologies has produced several polymers with excellent properties comparable to commercial plastics. Water resistance, high dimensional stability, processability, and excellent physicochemical properties limit the reviewed materials to biodegradable polyesters and modified starch and cellulose compositions, both known for their abundance and relatively low price (Vroman and Tighzert, 2009).

The conduct of the nanostructure and also the inclusion of nanoparticles to polymers have influenced remarkable improvements in structural and functional properties in a series of polymeric systems as a material response to the continuous requirements of modern industrial sectors. The accessibility of new nanoparticles with excellent properties (carbon nanotubes, graphenes, nanocellulose, metals, and ceramics) has led to exciting new possibilities for a continued expansion of polymer markets—silver nanoparticles, single-walled carbon nanotubes, carbon nanofibers, nanohydroxyapatite, cellulose nanocrystals, and nanolignin (Peponi et al., 2014).

Nanocomposites can also display modern design opportunity, offering outstanding improvement in creating practical materials with required properties for certain types of applications. Using natural resources and being friendly to the environment have also provided new application opportunities. There are many applications of nanocomposites and a growing number of commercial products available in the market, for example, auto parts, packaging, construction materials, biotechnology, medical devices, building materials, computer cases, and automobile interiors. In addition, the balanced mechanical properties, functionalities, and biocompatibility of bionanocomposites are helpful for designing and fabricating new materials for biomedical applications, drug delivery, biosensors and electronic shielding, and tissue engineering (Rivadeneira et al., 2021).

Another area of importance for nanocomposites biodegradable polymer is the packaging industry. Improving food quality and shelf life while reducing plastic waste has spurred the development of biodegradable polymers as advanced, smart packaging. These systems include biopolymers from agricultural resources, such as polysaccharides and proteins, from biotechnology (e.g., poly (lactic acid), poly(hydroxyalkanoates), or biopolymers from petrochemical sources, e.g., PCL) (Armentano et al., 2013; Rivadeneira et al., 2021)

In science and engineering, studies on carbon nanotubes have widely turned them into possible materials due to their fascinating properties, such as high thermal and chemical stability, well-defined adsorption sites, and easy bonding of functional groups currently establishment. The growth of nanoparticles has shown an unequivocal interaction with contamination in water and gases. These properties generate potential for the stimulation of innovative and improved environmental utilization of scientific diameters in the nanometer range. Along the same lines, there is currently an establishment that the growth of nanoparticles has shown an unequivocal interaction with contamination in water and gases; These types of properties have the potential to stimulate the innovative and improved environmental use of scientific knowledge (Agboola et al., 2021; Masciangioli and Zhang, 2003).

Biodegradable electronic products can be an effective solution for waste management since they can degrade or dissolve in the surrounding environment without pollution, it has great potential to reduce the environmental footprint of devices and enable therapeutic and health monitoring technologies. Complex biodegradable electronics require biodegradable substrates, insulators, conductors, and semiconductors, all of which make up the building blocks of devices. This makes electronic components environmentally and disposal safe while reducing the cost of recycling operations and the health risks associated with harmful emissions. Additionally, biodegradable materials are often biocompatible, allowing electronics to be used in implantable biomedical applications. Biocompatibility will enable materials to contact skin tissues directly without generating adverse effects. There is a wide range of applications including fiber lasers, supercapacitors, field emission devices, and photovoltaics, where the combination of tunable optoelectronic properties as well as structural and chemical stability, high surface area, and low mass density nanofillers with polymer processability offer a new class of materials (Feig et al., 2018; Liu et al., 2019).

Research on active packaging for food has been directed toward biodegradable and ecological polymers to develop alternatives to nonrenewable polymers derived from petroleum. Starch is a widely available biopolymer in several natural sources such as corn, wheat, and potatoes, among others, and can be obtained from different crop residues and industrial processes. Taking into account the weak packing properties of this type of biopolymers (few mechanical, barrier, and thermal resistance properties, among others), the development of clay nanocomposites biopolymers has shown a significant improvement in the properties of barrier, rheological, mechanical, and thermal resistance compared to pure biopolymers, that is, starch/montmorillonite nanocomposites, chitosan/hydroxyapatite/magnetite nanocomposites natural rubber/modified montmorillonite (Campos-Requena et al., 2017; Sookyung et al., 2016; Heidari et al., 2016).

Wide technological applications have been found, including electromagnetic interference shielding/microwave absorption, high-density information storage, bimodal imaging agent, environmental remediation, and pharmaceuticals. For developing the aforementioned cutting-edge materials science and nanotechnology, highly efficient electrochemical energy storage materials, and highly kinetic recyclable nanoadsorbents for wastewater remediation, it requires a detailed understanding of the chemical structures of these wastewaters. Magnetic nanostructures. To understand remediation mechanisms and chemical stability during interactions with waste species and the charged discharge process, the chemical environments of magnetic components, such as iron species, are of vital importance (Abdulkadir et al., 2016).

8.4 ADVANTAGES OF USE OF NANOCOMPOSITES BIODEGRADABLE POLYMER

Nanocomposites have attracted much attention in academic research and industry due to their unique properties compared to conventional composites, even with low filler content; nanofillers have reinforcing solid effects, and studies have also shown their positive impact on barrier properties. The advantages of composite materials over conventional materials increase their higher specific strength, higher water absorption quality, and low fire resistance, stiffness, and fatigue characteristics. Polymer composites materials are used as a replacement for conventional materials in various applications. It can meet diverse design requirements, and because of its good mechanical and physical properties, composite materials meet the requirements of a particular application (Peponi et al., 2014). Growing environmental concerns have led to research on the potential use of renewable resources for specific applications, such as biomedical and packaging.

As mentioned, materials such as polymers are of great importance in different areas such as packaging and storage, in the energy, security, transport, electrical, chemical areas, among others, as well as for research purposes, since polymeric nanocomposites can mean a solution for different needs of daily life (Darwish et al., 2022). According to the United Nations Environment Program (UNEP), from the 1950s to the present, about 8.3 billion tons of plastic have been produced, of which 60% has ended up as a pollutant; in addition, the production of these plastics employ the use of non-biodegradable and, in some cases, toxic additives (Rivadeneira-Velasco et al., 2021). Given the footprint of the use of nonrenewable materials in the production of polymers and the growing concern for the environment, the main advantage offered by using biodegradable nanocomposites is the low environmental impact due to their degradation. The biodegradation of these materials is mainly caused by fungi, bacteria, and algae in the environment, so the degradation mechanism of a biodegradable polymer is given by the metabolism of microorganisms. A combination of heat, light, and microbial presence result in physical and chemical changes in polymers leading to material disintegration. It is worth mentioning that the polymeric material has to be in contact with the environment (soil), so burial would favor degradation (Glaskova-Kuzmina et al., 2021).

The search for materials of renewable and ecological origin to reduce the use of petroleum derivatives has led to the production of biomaterials of plant origin; such materials are produced from organic waste or biomass, coming from natural sources, being a cheap and abundant raw material, which represents an advantage. Polymers such as cellulose, chitosan, or starch are found in abundance, however, despite being successful in a variety of applications, they cannot completely replace the functions of fossil plastics, so the main research is based on the embedding of nanofillers in polymeric matrices improving their properties (Glaskova-Kuzmina et al., 2021; Liu et al., 2019; Rivadeneira-Velasco et al., 2021).

It has been reported that adding nanocomposites to a polymeric matrix can influence its degradation rate, causing the material to be biodegradable. Currently, the use of biodegradable nanocomposites to manufacture biopolymers represents an advantage compared to conventional materials; the addition of nanocomposites to a polymeric matrix results in the synergy between both components and can present properties that individually each material is not capable of demonstrate, that is, it improves the physicochemical properties, the mechanical and barrier properties, the stability to humidity or affinity to water, the durability, the weight, and the flexibility of the materials according to the objective of the biomaterial, among other characteristics. Likewise, it should be emphasized that composite biomaterials can have a long useful life, which favors their use in different areas; in addition to their functional properties, some provide additional characteristics to polymers (antimicrobial properties, "intelligent," etc.) (Armentano et al., 2018; Basavegowda and Baek, 2021; Keya et al., 2019).

In the biomedical area, the use of biomaterials represents a significant advantage over other materials. They have the ability to adjust to the body due to the chemical structure of the material and its morphology, as well as its dissolution scale, which can be modified by changing the properties of the polymer such as molecular weight, chemical composition, the crystalline structure through erosion or polymerization mechanisms that thus change their hydrophobic and hydrophilic nature. Protein-based biopolymers such as collagen, chitosan, or gelatin, or polysaccharides such as alginate, cellulose, dextran, or starch have been used for the manufacture of medical devices due to their biodegradability and biocompatibility, in addition to their inherent bioactivity due to their similarities with the macromolecules of the human body, being used as transitory components for implants. On the other hand, synthetic biopolymers provide greater control regarding the physicochemical properties of device materials since these are manufactured under controlled and reproducible conditions (Hosseini et al., 2021).

KEYWORDS

- **nanocomposites**
- **renewable**
- **biodegradable**
- **plastics, nanocomposites**

REFERENCES

Abdulkadir, A.; Sarker, T.; He, Q.; Guo, Z.; Wei, S. Mössbauer Spectroscopy of Polymer Nanocomposites. In *Spectroscopy of Polymer Nanocomposites*; Elsevier: Amsterdam, The Netherlands, 2016; pp 393–409.

Agboola, O.; Fayomi, O. S. I.; Ayodeji, A.; Ayeni, A. O.; Alagbe, E. E.; Sanni, S. E.; Okoro, E. E.; Moropeng, L.; Sadiku, R.; Kupolati, K. W.; et al. A Review on Polymer Nanocomposites and Their Effective Applications in Membranes and Adsorbents for Water Treatment and Gas Separation. *Membranes* **2021,** *11*, 139.
https:// doi.org/10.3390/membranes11020139.

Armentano, I.; Puglia, D.; Luzi, F.; Arciola, C. R.; Morena, F.; Martino, S.; Torre, L. Nanocomposites Based on Biodegradable Polymers. *Materials* **2018,** *11* (5). https://doi.org/10.3390/MA11050795.

Baalkhuyur, F. M.; Mohammad A. Q.; Premlal P.; Duarte C. M. Microplastics in Fishes of Commercial and Ecological Importance from the Western Arabian Gulf. *Marine Pollut. Bull.* **2020,** 110920. https://doi.org/10.1016/j.marpolbul.2020.110920.

Balaji, A. B.; Pakalapati, H.; Khalid, M.; Walvekar, R.; Siddiqui, H. Natural and Synthetic Biocompatible and Biodegradable Polymers. In *Biodegradable and Biocompatible Polymer Composites*, 2018; pp 3–32. https://doi.org/10.1016/b978-0-08-100970-3.00001-8.

Barra, A.; Santos, J. D. C.; Silva, M. R. F.; Nunes, C.; Ruiz-Hitzky, E.; Gonçalves, I.; Yildirim, S.; Ferreira, P.; Marques, P. A. A. P. Graphene Derivatives in Biopolymer-Based Composites for Food Packaging Applications. *Nanomaterials* **2020,** *10* (10), 2077.
https://doi.org/10.3390/nano10102077.

Basavegowda, N.; Baek, K. H. Advances in Functional Biopolymer-Based Nanocomposites for Active Food Packaging Applications. *Polymers* **2021,** *13* (23), 4198. https://doi.org/10.3390/POLYM13234198.

Basumatary, I. B.; Mukherjee, A.; Katiyar, V.; Kumar, S. Biopolymer-Based Nanocomposite Films and Coatings: Recent Advances in Shelf-Life Improvement of Fruits and Vegetables. *Crit. Rev. Food Sci. Nutr.* **2022,** *62* (7), 1912–1935.
https://doi.org/10.1080/10408398.2020.1848789.

Campos-Requena, V. H.; Rivas, B. L.; Pérez, M. A.; Figueroa, C.; Figueroa, N. E.; Sanfuentes, E. A. Thermoplastic Starch/Clay Nanocomposites Loaded with Essential Oil Constituents as Packaging for Strawberries In vivo Antimicrobial Synergy Over *Botrytis cinere*a. *Postharvest Biol. Technol.* **2017,** *129*, 29–36.

Darwish, M. S. A.; Mostafa, M. H.; Al-Harbi, L. M. Polymeric Nanocomposites for Environmental and Industrial Applications. *Int. J. Mol. Sci.* **2022,** *23* (3), 1023. https://doi.org/10.3390/IJMS23031023.

Doppalapudi, S.; Katiyar, S.; Domb, A. J.; Khan, W. Biodegradable Natural Polymers. In *Advanced Polymers in Medicine*; Puoci, F., Eds.; Springer: Cham, 2015. https://doi.org/10.1007/978-3-319-12478-0_2.

Encalada, K.; Bélen-Aldás, M.; Proaño, E.; Valle, V. An Overview of Starch-Based Biopolymers and their Biodegradability. *Ciencia e Ingenieria* **2018,** *39* (3), 245–258. https://www.redalyc.org/journal/5075/507557607005/html/.

Ezzat, H. A.; Hegazy, M. A.; Nada, N. A.; Osman, O.; Ibrahim, M. A. Application of Natural Polymers Enhanced with ZnO and CuO as Humidity Sensor. *NRIAG J. Astron. Geophys.* **2020,** *9* (1), 586–597.
https://doi.org/10.1080/20909977.2020.1821573.

Ezzat, H. A.; Hegazy, M. A.; Nada, N. A.; Osman, O.; Ibrahim, M. A. Development of Natural Polymer/Metal Oxide Nanocomposite Reinforced with Graphene Oxide for Optoelectronic Applications. *NRIAG J. Astron. Geophys.* **2021,** *10* (1), 10–22. https://doi.org/10.1080/20909977.2020.1846246.

Feig, V. R.; Tran, H.; Bao, Z. Biodegradable Polymeric Materials in Degradable Electronic Devices. *ACS Cent Sci.* **2018**, *4* (3), 337–348. DOI: 10.1021/acscentsci.7b00595.

Feldman, D. Polymers and Polymer Nanocomposites for Cancer Therapy. *Appl. Sci.* **2019,** *9* (18), 3899. https://doi.org/10.3390/app9183899.

Flores-Sánchez, A.; et al. Biosynthesis of Polyhydroxyalkanoates from Vegetable Oil under the Co-Expression of FadE and PhaJ Genes in Cupriavidus Necator. *Int. J. Biol. Macromol.***2020,** *164*, 1600–1607.
https://doi.org/10.1016/j.ijbiomac.2020.07.275.

Glaskova-Kuzmina, T.; Starkova, O.; Gaidukovs, S.; Platnieks, O.; Gaidukova, G. Durability of Biodegradable Polymer Nanocomposites. *Polymers* **2021,** *13* (19), 3375.
https://doi.org/10.3390/POLYM13193375.

Gobi, R.; Ravichandiran, P.; Babu, R. S.; Yoo, D. J. Biopolymer and Synthetic Polymer-Based Nanocomposites in Wound Dressing Applications: A Review. *Polymers* **2021,** *13* (12), 1962. https://doi.org/10.3390/polym13121962.

Havstad, M. R. Biodegradable Plastics. In *Plastic Waste and Recycling*, 2020; pp 97–129..
DOI: 10.1016/b978-0-12-817880-5.00005-0.

Heidari, F.; Razavi, M.; Bahrololoom, M. E.; Bazargan-Lari, R.; Vashaee, D.; Kotturi, H.; Tayebi, L. Mechanical Properties of Natural Chitosan/Hydroxyapatite/ Magnetite Nanocomposites for Tissue Engineering Applications. *Mater. Sci. Eng.* **2016,** *65*, 338–344. https://doi: 10.1016/j.msec.2016.04.039.

Hosseini, E. S.; Dervin, S.; Ganguly, P.; Dahiya, R. Biodegradable Materials for Sustainable Health MonitoringDevices. *ACS Appl. Bio Mater.* **2021,** *4* (1), 163.
https://doi.org/10.1021/ACSABM.0C01139.

Janigova, I.; Lednicky, F.; Jochec Moskova, D.; Chodak, I. Nanocomposites with Biodegradable Polycaprolactone Matrix. *Macromol. Symp.* **2011,** *301*, 1–8. DOI: 10.1002/ masy.201150301.

Janmohammadi, M.; Nazemi, Z.; Orash Mahmoud, A. O.; Seyfoori, A.; John, J.; Sadegh Nourbakhsh, M. S.; Mohsen Akbari, M. Cellulose-Based Composite Scaffolds for Bone Tissue Engineering and Localized Drug Delivery. *Bioact. Mater.* **2023,** *20*, 137–163. Jozala, A. F.; de Lencastre-Novaes, L. C.; Lopes, A. M.; Santos-Ebinuma, V. C.; Mazzola, P. G.; Pessoa-Jr, A.; Grotto, D.; Gerenutti, M.; Chaud, M. V. Bacterial Nanocellulose Production and Application: a 10-Year Overview. *Appl. Microbiol. Biotec.* **2016,** *100* (5), 2063–2072. DOI: 10.1007/s00253-015-7243-4.

Kalia, V. C.; Sanjay K. S.; Ramasamy S.; Jung K. L. Polyhydroxyalkanoates: Trends and Advances Toward Biotechnological Applications. *Bioresour. Technol.* **2020,** *326*, 124737. https://doi.org/10.1016/j.biortech.2021.124737.

Keya, K. N.; Kona, N. A.; Koly, F. A.; Maraz, K. M.; Islam, M. N.; Khan, R. A. Natural Fiber Reinforced Polymer Composites: History, Types, Advantages and Applications. *Mater. Eng. Res.* **2019,** *1* (2), 69–85. https://doi.org/10.25082/MER.2019.02.006.

Khezerlou, A.; et al. Application of Nanotechnology to Improve the Performance of Biodegradable Biopolymer-Based Packaging Materials. *Polymers* **2021,** *13* (24), 1–21.

Kritchenkov, A. S.; Egorov, A. R.; Volkova, O. V.; Artemjev, A. A.; Kurliuk, A. V.; Anh Le, T.; Hieu Truong, H.; Le-Nhat-Thuy, G.; Van Tran Thi, T.; Van Tuyen, N.; Khrustalev, V. N. Novel Biopolymer-Based Nanocomposite Food Coatings that Exhibit Active and Smart Properties due to a Single Type of Nanoparticles. *Food Chem.* **2021,** *343*, 128676. https:// doi.org/10.1016/j.foodchem.2020.128676.

Kumar, R.; Singh, N.; Singh, R. An Introduction of Biodegradable Polymers, Modes of Biodegradation and Designing of Biodegradable Polymers. *Res. J. Pharm. Tech.* **2017,** *10* (2), 625–640. https://doi.org/10.5958/0974-360X.2017.00121.4.

Kundu, J.; Pati, F.; Hun Jeong, Y.; Cho, D. W. Biomaterials for Biofabrication of 3D Tissue Scaffolds. In *Biofabrication*, 2013; pp 23–46. https://doi.org/10.1016/b978-1-4557-2852-7.00002-0.

Liu, H.; Jian, R.; Chen, H.; Tian, X.; Sun, C.; Zhu, J.; Yang, Z.; Sun, J.; Wang, C. Application of Biodegradable and Biocompatible Nanocomposites in Electronics: Current Status and Future Directions. *Nanomaterials* **2019,** *9* (7).
https://doi.org/10.3390/NANO9070950.

López-Cuellar, M. R.; Alba-Flores, J.; Gracida Rodríguez, J. N.; Pérez-Guevara, F. Production of Polyhydroxyalkanoates (PHAs) with Canola Oil as Carbon Source. *Int. J. Biol. Macromol.* **2011,** *48* (1), 74–80.

Masciangioli, T.; Zhang, W. X. Environmental Technologies at the Nanoscale. *Environ. Sci. Technol.* **2003,** *37*, 102A–108A.

Mishra, M. Ed.; In *Handbook of Encapsulation and Controlled Release*, 1st Ed.; CRC Press, 2015. https://doi.org/10.1201/b19038.

Moshood, T. D.; et al. Biodegradable Plastic Applications towards Sustainability: A Recent Innovations in the Green Product. *Cleaner Eng. Technol.* **2022,** *6*, 100404. https://doi.org/10.1016/j.clet.2022.100404.

Nagalakshmaiah, M.; Afrin, S.; Malladi, R. P.; Elkoun, S.; Robert, M.; Ansari, M. A.; Svedberg, A.; Karim, Z. Biocomposites. In *Green Composites for Automotive Applications*, 2019; pp 197–215. https://doi.org/10.1016/b978-0-08-102177-4.00009-4.

Pappa, C.; Nanaki, S.; Giliopoulos, D.; Triantafyllidis, K.; Kostoglou, M.; Avgeropoulos, A.; Bikiaris, D. Nanostructured Composites of Sodium Montmorillonite Clay and PEO Used in Dissolution Improvement of Aprepitant Drug by Melt Mixing. *Appl. Sci.* **2018,** *8* (5), 786. https://doi.org/10.3390/app8050786.

Park, M.; Lee, D.; Shin, S.; Hyun, J. Effect of Negatively Charged Cellulose Nanofibers on the Dispersion of Hydroxyapatite Nanoparticles for Scaffolds in Bone Tissue Engineering. *Colloids Surf. B Biointerfaces* **2015,** *130*, 222–228. https://doi.org/ 10.1016/j.colsurfb.2015.04.014.

Parveen, I.; Mahmud, Md. I.; Khan, R. A. Biodegradable Natural Polymers for Biomedical Applications. Academic Research Publishing Group, 2019; vol *5* (3), pp 67–80.
https://doi.org/10.32861/sr.53.67.80.

Pegado, T. de S. E. S.; et al.: First Evidence of Microplastic Ingestion by Fishes from the Amazon River Estuary. *Mar. Pollut. Bull.* **2018,** *133*, 814–21. https://doi.org/10.1016/j.marpolbul.2018.06.035.

Peponi, L.; Puglia, D.; Torre, L.; Valentini, L.; Kenny, J. M. Processing of Nanostructured Polymers and Advanced Polymeric Based Nanocomposites. *Mater. Sci. Eng.* **2014,** *85*, 1–46.

Rai, P.; Mehrotra, S.; Priya, S.; Gnansounou, E.; Sharma, S. K. Recent Advances in the Sustainable Design and Applications of Biodegradable Polymers. *Bioresour. Technol.* **2021,** *325*, 124739. https://doi.org/10.1016/j.biortech.2021.1247.

Rajeswari1, A.; Prasanthi1, T.; Sudha1, N.; Swain, R. P.; Panda, S.; Goka, V. Natural Polymers: A Recent Review. *World J. Pharm. Pharm. Sci.* **2021,** *6* (8), 472–494. https://doi.org/10.20959/wjpps20178-9762 .

Raza, S.; Ansari, A.; Siddiqui, N. N.; Ibrahim, F.; Abro, M. I.; Aman, A. Biosynthesis of Silver Nanoparticles for the Fabrication of Non Cytotoxic and Antibacterial Metallic Polymer Based Nanocomposite System. *Sci. Rep.* **2021,** *11* (1), 10500.
https://doi.org/10.1038/s41598-021-90016-w.

Rivadeneira-Velasco, K. E.; Utreras-Silva, C. A.; Díaz-Barrios, A.; Sommer-Márquez, A. E.; Tafur, J. P.; Michell, R. M. Green Nanocomposites Based on Thermoplastic Starch: A Review. *Polymers* **2021,** *13* (19). https://doi.org/10.3390/POLYM13193227.

Rossa, V.; Ferreira, L. E. M.; Vasconcelos, S. da C.; Shimabukuro, E. T. T.; Madriaga, V. G. da C.; Paula Carvalho, A.; Pergher, S. B. C.; da Silva, F. de C., Francisco Ferreira, V.; Junior, C. A. C.; de Melo Lima, T. Nanocomposites Based on the Graphene Family for Food Packaging: Historical Perspective, Preparation Methods, and Properties. *RSC Adv.* **2022,** *12* (22), 14084–14111. https://doi.org/10.1039/D2RA00912A.

Rummel, C. D.; et al. Plastic Ingestion by Pelagic and Demersal Fish from the North Sea and Baltic Sea. *Marine Pollut. Bull.* **2016,** *102* (1), 134–141.
http://dx.doi.org/10.1016/j.marpolbul.2015.11.043.

Salazar-Pérez, C.; Amezcua, F.; Rosales-Valencia, A.; Rosales-Valencia, L.; Green, L.; Pollorena-Melendrez, J. E.; Sarmiento-Martínez, M. A.; Tomita Ramírez, I.; Gil-Manrique, B. D.; Hernandez-Lozano, M. Y.; Muro-Torres, V. M.; Green-Ruiz, C.; Piñon-Colin, T. D. J.; Wakida, F. T.; Barletta, M. First Insight into Plastics Ingestion by Fish in the Gulf of California, Mexico. *Marine Pollut. Bull.* **2021,** *171*, 112705. DOI: 10.1016/j.marpolbul.2021.112705.

Silva, M.; Ferreira, F. N.; Alves, N. M.; Paiva, M. C. Biodegradable Polymer Nanocomposites for Ligament/Tendon Tissue Engineering. *J. Nanobiotechnol.* **2020,** *18* (1),23. https://doi.org/10.1186/s12951-019-0556-1.

Song, R.; Murphy, M.; Li, C.; Ting, K.; Soo, C.; Zheng, Z. Current Development of Biodegradable Polymeric Materials for Biomedical Applications. *Drug Des. Devel. Ther.* **2018,** *24* (12), 3117–3145. https://doi.org/10.2147/DDDT.S165440 .

Sookyung, U.; Nakason, C.; Venneman, N.; Thaijaroend, W. Influence Concentration of Modifying Agent on Properties of Natural Rubber/Organoclay Nanocomposites. *Polym. Test* **2016,** *54*, 223–232.

Spinelli, G.; Guarini, R.; Kotsilkova, R.; Batakliev, T.; Ivanov, E.; Romano, V. Experimental and Simulation Studies of Temperature Effect on Thermophysical Properties of Graphene-Based Polylactic Acid. *Materials* **2022,** *15* (3), 986.
https://doi.org/10.3390/ma15030986.

Vroman, I.; Tighzert, L. Biodegradable Polymers. *Materials* **2009,** *2* (2), 307–344. https://doi.org/10.3390/ma2020307.

Waring, R. H.; Harris, R. M.; Mitchell, S. C. Plastic Contamination of the Food Chain: A Threat to Human Health?. *Maturitas* **2018,** *115*, 64–68. https://doi.org/10.1016/j.maturitas.2018.06.010.

Zulay Mármol, Z.; Páez, G.; Rincón, M.; Araujo, K.; Aiello, C.; Chandler, C.; Gutiérrez, E. Quitina y Quitosano polímeros amigables.: Una revisión de sus aplicaciones. *Revista Tecnocientífica URU* **2011,** *1*, 53–58.

PART 4

CASE STUDIES

CHAPTER 9

Biotechnology Applications in Invertebrate Biological Control Agents: An Environmentally Friendly Approach

REBECA CASIQUE-VALDÉS[1], SERGIO RENÉ SÁNCHEZ-PEÑA[2], and LEONARDO SEPÚLVEDA-TORRE[3]

[1]*Instituto de Ciencias y Humanidades, Lic.Salvador González Lobo, Universidad Autónoma de Coahuila, México*

[2]*Dpto. Parasitología Agrícola, Universidad Autónoma Agraria Antonio Narro, México*

[3] *Dpto. Biotecnología, Facultad de Ciencias Químicas, Universidad Autónoma de Coahuila, México*

ABSTRACT

The agri-food industry has always faced many adversities; one of the biggest challenges is to increase food production for a world population that is experiencing exponential growth. Insect pests and plant diseases cause severe damage and losses of agricultural and horticultural crops every year, that result in excessive use of pesticides and fertilizers, reduced food supplies, poorer quality, and higher prices. There is an existent concern to reduce the actual chemical consumption used in agriculture; therefore, it is necessary to develop new alternatives to insect-pest control due to its resistance to current insecticides. Biotechnology is positioned as a tool that uses multidisciplinary knowledge, to provide solutions capable of meeting the demands of efficient agri-food production that are environmentally friendly. These techniques will be less dependable on mechanical or chemical innovations and will

Application of Engineering Principles and Practices in Biotechnology.
Ann Rose Abraham, Leonardo Sepúlveda Torre, Tamara Tatrishvili, and A. K. Haghi (Eds.)

be based on an in-depth application of reliable data as well as molecular and cellular technology. Recombinant technology provides potential new methods to modify entomopathogens in order to manage pests. The biological agents that play an important role in pest-control and diseases are viruses, bacteria, fungi, and nematodes. The biotechnology has contributed to the development of biocontrol agents from identification to formulation. When biocontrol agents are used to control insects, they produce metabolites such as hydrolytic enzymes and secondary metabolites, compounds that can be used as bioinsecticides or fungicides, and can be produced by fermentative processes. This opens new areas of agrobiotechnological development, in accordance with the new strategies in the agricultural research worldwide. This chapter reviews the contribution of biotechnology in the development of biocontrol agents.

9.1 INTRODUCTION

There are more than 700 species of entomopathogenic fungi (EPF) distributed in 100 genera (Jaber and Ownley, 2018) on the phyla Oomycota, Chytridiomycota, Microsporidia, Entomophtoromycota, Basidiomycota, and Ascomycota (Araújo and Hughes, 2016; Shukla and Afzal, 2021); these fungi include various genera that can infect and kill insects efficiently; moreover, EPF have considerable host specificity and can be produced quickly in bulk quantity (Islam et al., 2021). Despite its use as biological control agents, only some of these have been thoroughly studied and used commercially (Toledo-Hernández et al., 2019); however, the action of these microorganisms against pests are influenced on environmental conditions of temperature, relative humidity, solar radiation, and wind (Beris, 2021), and are usually marketed in spore-based formulation that must be prepared under certain conditions for their effectiveness (De Costa, 2020). An alternative to these formulations is to incorporate metabolites that EPF produce, they consist in chemically diverse secondary metabolites that cause severe adverse reactions in other organisms, eliminate the competition of nutrients, and facilitate the establishment of the pathogen (Chen and Wu, 2021). The main parameters that explains the validity of the infection process include lytic enzymes, secondary metabolites, and adhesins (Litwin et al., 2020); some fungi produce mycotoxins, such as cyclic peptides and macromolecular proteins which can cause paralysis or disrupt physiological processes including the immune responses of the insect (Kazek et al., 2021). The ecological importance of EPF secondary metabolites, rely on toxins production (Mannino et al., 2021), some of these are destruxins, beauverincins, and efrapeptins that are described chemically along with the process of pathogenesis by Kidanu and Hagos (2020). The isolation of these toxins generates a source of natural pesticides with low toxicity in humans, high insecticide action, and do not need special requirements for their use (Rios-Moreno et al., 2016). It is noteworthy that the production of a specific metabolite can be significantly altered by optimizing culture conditions, such as nutrients, temperature, and pH (St Leger et al., 1996). Furthermore to their use in pest control, baculoviruses showed a functional and effective eukaryotic vector for the production of great amount of recombinant proteins (Martínez-Solis et al., 2019), as the expression of recombiant toxins in an insect-specific baculovirus or a fungus (Deng et al., 2019); from the time of the first recombinant protein was revealed in 1983 using the baculovirus expression system (BEVS) (Grose et al., 2021), various methods have been advanced for the generation of recombinant viruses and to augment the stability, yield, and posttranslational conversion of recombinant proteins. The baculovirus expression system is a workhorse for recombinant protein expression for over 35 years, the system has been designed and modified many times for fast and clear expression and scale-up of the recombinant proteins (Mishra, 2020). In this chapter, we summarize the secondary metabolites, toxins, and enzymes that EPF produce and some promising avenues for biotechnological applications of EPF and entompathogenic viruses.

9.1.1 METABOLITES FROM ENTOMOPATHOGENS

EPF synthesize metabolites that are toxic against insects and are generally synthesized when the fungus has penetrated the exoskeleton and has reached the hemocoel as part of the virulence factors during pathogenesis (Brivio and Mastore, 2020). Many of these fungal toxins are low molecular weight secondary metabolites with commercial potential as insect control agents (Subbanna et al., 2020). Secondary metabolites can be divided into cyclic depsipeptides (cyclic tetradepsipeptides and cyclic hexadepsipeptides), peptides (octadepsipeptides, dipeptides, and depsipeptides), amino acid derivatives, polyketides, peptide hybrids, and terpenoids (Wang et al., 2018). Destruxins are cyclic hexadepsipeptides isolated mostly from *Metarhizium* sp. More than 40 kinds of destruxins have been reported, with biological properties such as cytotoxic, antimicrobial, antiproliferative, antiviral, and immunosuppressive properties (Litwin et al., 2020). *Beauveria bassiana* (Ascomycota: Hypocreales) produces an overabundance of toxic secondary metabolites as beauvericin (BEA) that either facilitate fungal invasion or act as immunosuppressive compounds (Olleik et al., 2019); also, it biosynthesizes and accumulates different depsipeptides beauvenniatins (BEAEs) or enniatins (ENNs) (Urbaniak et al., 2019; Weng et al., 2019). In a study conducted by Urbaniak et al. (2020), where *Beauveria, Cordyceps, Isaria,* and phytopathogenic *Fusarium* genera were evaluated, the most efficient producers of BEA were *Fusarium* strains, such as *F. proliferatum* and *F. concentricum*. These toxins have divergent chemical natures, such as polyketides and nonribosomal peptides (Pedrini, 2022); also synthesize bassianolide (cyclooligomeric nonribosomal peptides), a variety of beauverolides (cyclic peptides), oosporein (dibenzoquinone), bassiatin (diketomorpholine), and tenellin (2-pyridone) (Zhang et al. 2020).

Most of the studies on the entomophagous fungi are on *M. anisopliae* and *B.bassiana* and less on equally important species of commercial importance such as *V. lecanii*, *I. fumosorosea*, *Tolypocladium* spp. and *Hirsutella* spp. (Yadav et al., 2019). Secondary metabolites such as destruxins of *Metarhizium*, beauvericins of *Beauveria*, hirsutellides of *Hirsutella*, isarolides of *Isaria*, cordyols of *Cordyceps*, vertihemipterins of *Verticillium*, directly and indirectly disable the defense mechanism of insect hosts and accelerate the EPF infection process (Vongvanich et al., 2002; Unagul et al., 2005). The chemical nature of secondary metabolites from entomopathogenic fungi ranges from simple non-peptide pigments like oosporine to highly complex piperazine derivatives, like vertihemiptellides (Paschapur et al., 2021).

On the other hand, other used organisms in biological control are entomopathogenic nematodes (EPN); they belong to the genus *Steinernema* and *Heterorhabditis*, one of the most important biocontrol agents against insect pests (Boszormeny et al., 2009; Sharma et al., 2022). The free-living form of EPNs is protected from the environment by an external cuticle, only the third larvae stage (encapsulated) called infective juveniles (IJs), are unable to feed and can survive outside a host for several months (Gaugler and Campbell, 1993); IJs are harmful to insects, while all other developmental stages are only found inside infected hosts (Dillman and Sternberg, 2012); more detailed discussion of symbiosis could be found in Lewis et al. (2006), Stock and Blair (2008), and Sharma et al. (2022). The infective juvenile (IJ) is a bacterial-vectoring stage that seeks out insects to infect and kill (Sharma et al., 2022). The nematode and its pathogenic bacteria cargo, *Xenorhabdus* and *Photorhabdus*, gram-negative bacteria belonging to the family

Enterobacteriaceae, live in symbiosis with the nematodes *Heterorhabditis* and *Steinernema*, respectively (Kumar et al., 2014). The IJs enter the hemoecel of the insect and release the symbiotic bacteria, then multiply in the hemolymph causing insect death within 48–72 h (Ibrahim et al., 2019). The bacteria are known to produce a toxic cocktail of secondary metabolites that not only are lethal to the insect hosts, but also prevent opportunistic bacteria and fungi from utilizing the nutrient-rich cadaver, sequestering the resources for themselves and their nematode partners (Dillman and Sternberg, 2012). *Xenorhabdus* spp. have been reported to produce a variety of antibacterial peptides, depsipeptides such as xenematides, xenomacins, szentiamide, and xenobactin, lipodepsipeptides, xenocoumacins, fabclavines, pristinamycin, xenortides, rhabdopeptides, bicornitun, PAX peptides, cabanillasin, nemaucin, dithiolopyrrolone derivatives, indole-containing compounds, benzylideneacetone, rhabdicin, bacteriocins, and a few unnamed peptides (Booysen and Dicks, 2020; Shan et al., 2020). Joyce et al. (2011) studied three compounds from *Photorhabdus* genus, 3,5-dihydroxy-4-isopropylstilbene, the β-lactam antibiotic carbapenem, and an anthraquinone pigment. Clarke (2016) has carried out an intensive search for metabolites produced by *Photorhabdus* including stilbene and rhabduscin as prophenoloxidase inhibitors, pyrone, anthraquinone, glidobactin, and cepafungin as proteasome inhibitors, among others.

Toxicity in the secondary metabolites from invertebrate entomopathogens showed over the insect cellular lines, opening the probability of spreading new bioinsecticides (Sánchez-Perez, 2014). Peptides, dipeptides, and depsipeptides are the best known metabolites that EPF produce (Yadav et al., 2019), they have a wide range of harmful effects on insects that include membrane depolarization due to the opening of Ca^{2+} channels, causing tetanic paralysis and death (Samuels et al., 1988), affect part of the immune response such as encapsulation and phagocytosis (Wrońska and Boguś, 2019); reduce the expression of antimicrobial peptides that have an important role in the humoral immune response of insects (Pedrini, 2022); induce structural changes in epithelial cells that cause membrane disruption and oxidative stress in cells (Ma et al., 2021). Another type of metabolites are the alkaloids, although the β-carboline alkaloids harman and norharman are considered as plant metabolites, they can also be secreted by fungi such as the entomopathogen *Conidiobolus coronatus* (Wrońska and Boguś, 2019), such alkaloids have the capability to bind to serotonin receptors, a noticeable immune regulatory molecule in both invertebrates and vertebrates. The Entomophthorales (Zoopagomycota) comprise all known species with active host transmission conduct where the fungus continue or advancing "normal" host endeavor during sporulation, enabling fast and extensive diffusion initial to host death (Hajek et al., 2018). Hypocrealean entomopathogens have helped disengaged infection processes and host responses, mainly for the "zombie ant fungus" *Ophiocordyceps unilateralis* (Fredericksen et al., 2017). This pathogen is believed to adjust host conduct via fungus-derived neurogenic metabolites and enterotoxins, hence considering a chemical basis for this observable phenotype. Boyce et al. (2019) have shown compounds as cathinone, an amphetamine formely known from plants, and psilocybin, a tryptamine formerly known from basidiomycete mushrooms in *Massospora* genera. Boyce et al. (2019) shown the detection, using global and targeted metabolomics supported by metagenomics and proteomics, of the plant amphetamine, cathinone, in *Massospora cicadina* infected periodical cicadas, and tryptamine and psilocybin in *M. platypediae* and *M. levispora* infected annual cicadas. The neurogenic activities of these alkaloids consider a hypothetical structure for a chemically activate extended phenotype of *Massospora* that alters cicada behavior by augmented capacity and elimination feeding before death. Kazek et al. (2021) observed that *C. coronatus* releases dodecanol into its culture approach which not only does appear to be an productive potential insecticide, it is also known to be safe towards vertebrates, and presently was considered for use as a food additive.

The genus *Metarhizium* have the potential to make lysergic acid-derived ergot alkaloids, isolates of *M. brunneum* and *M. anisopliae* gathered the lysergic acid amides lysergic acid α-hydroxyethyl amide, ergine, and ergonovine on sucrose-yeast extract agar, isolates of *M. brunneum, M. flavoviride, M. robertsii, M. acridum*, and *M. anisopliae* produced high concentrations of ergot alkaloids in infected larvae of the model insect *Galleria mellonella* (Leadmon et al., 2020). Ergot alkaloids are a various family of fungus-specialized metabolites, in addition to simple clavine ergot alkaloids and additional complex lysergic acid derivatives. Lysergic acid-derived ergot alkaloids have been very dominant in medicine and agriculture. It should be noted that the derivatives of lysergic acid are considered to synthesize a range of pharmaceuticals applied to treat migraines, Parkinson's disease, dementia, and hyper-prolactinemia (Steen et al., 2021).

9.1.2 ENTOMOPATHOGENIC METABOLITES PRODUCTION

Mycelial culture on potato dextrose agar of EPF has been utilized (Woo et al., 2020) and then its cultivation in dextrose broth for obtaining mycelial biomass was proposed by Anggiani et al. (2020), they dried the mycelia and mixed it with chloroform to obtain the crude extract for determination in HPLC, they quantified in this methodology quinidine. For volatile organic compounds, Bojke et al. (2018) harvested mycelium from the Petri dishes, 0.50 g of mycelia was placed into a headspace solid-phase microextraction (HS-SPME) vial (4 mL); volatile organic compounds were extracted by HS-SPME employing a 50/30 μm, divinylbenzene/carboxen/polydimethylsiloxane fiber, the analyses were performed using the HS-SPME/GC single bond MS technique identifying 63 volatile compounds: aldehydes, ketones, alcohols, esters, acids, terpenes, and others.

The production of beauvericin (BEA) by *Fusarium oxysporum* in liquid medium was compared to a solid medium on inert support by Vásquez-Bonilla et al. (2022), they found that the production of BEA under solid medium was higher relative to liquid medium after seven days of incubation, using polyurethane foam as a solid support as a new culture system for obtaining secondary metabolites, on the other hand, Roswanjaya et al. (2022) proposed the biphasic system in which the fungus was first grown under submerged conditions and then was allowed to conidiate in solid-state conditions, they indicated that potato dextrose broth was the optimum culture medium to produce blastophore and BEA. The toxic effect of depsipeptides on different species of insects has opened up a great opportunity for their production as an insecticide by liquid fermentation (Liu et al., 2000), finding that their production strongly depends on the availability of nitrogen (Wang, 2009).

Some novel techniques such as genetic engineering will be required to increase the efficiency of various entomopathogens for increasing the virulence, for example, some *Metarhizium* spp. strains are pathogenic to adult mosquitoes but with slow killing and low persistence; to remedy these deficiencies, it has been engineered a strain of *Metarhizium pingshaense* (Mp-Hybrid) to express the U.S. Environmental Protection Agency (EPA)–approved calcium activated potassium (KCa) and voltage-gated calcium (CaV) blocker w/k-hexatoxin-Hv1a (Hybrid) under the control of a hemolymph-specific promoter; in laboratory studies, Mp-Hybrid killed mosquitoes faster and at lower spore doses than the wild-type strain (Bilgo et al., 2018). Transcription parameters considered in different processes during fungal growth and pathogenesis via regulating a series of genes and are main competitor for fungal development via genetic engineering. For example, overexpression of MaSom1, a key transcription factor gene in the cAMP/PKA direction, enhance the biocontrol traits of *Metarhizium acridum* in multiple respects. When compared with the wild type of *M. acridum* strain, the MaSom1-overexpression showed improved tolerances to UV-B and heat shock, with greater mean of 50% inhibition times by 66.9% and 155%, respectively (Du et al. 2022). Boyce et al. (2019) applied global and targeted liquid chromatography–mass spectrometry (LC-MS)-based metabolomics to freshly collected and stored parasitized cicadas to identify candidate small molecules potentially contributing to a hypersexual behavioral phenotype of 3 *Massospora* species. Sbaraini et al. (2021) analyzed an unusual carnitine acyltransferase domain-containing highly reducing polyketide synthase found in the genome of *M. anisopliae*, they employed heterologous expression in *Aspergillus nidulans*, to obtain polyketides.

Various methods have been employed to increase the production of secondary metabolites produced by *Xenorhabdus* spp. These include non-ribosomal peptide synthesis (NRPS), or a combination of polyketide synthesis (PKS), ribosomal peptide synthesis (RPS), and NRPS (NRPS/PKS) (Booysen et al., 2021). Booysen and Dicks (2020) elucidated an extensive review on antimicrobial compound synthesis by *Xenorhabdu*s spp.

The metabolic pathways responsible for the production of both stilbene and AQ have been described by Clarke (2016), it has been proposed the action of enzymes to produce these metabolites called polyketide synthases (PKS) and non-ribosomal peptide synthases (NRPS) (Hutchinson, 2003). A major component of this secondary metabolism is a stilbene molecule, called ST. The first step in ST biosynthesis is the non-oxidative deamination of phenylalanine resulting in the production of cinnamic acid catalyzed by phenylalanine-ammonium lyase, an enzyme encoded by the stlA gene (Lango-Scholey et al., 2013). Bode (2009) has listed diversity of loci that encodes for PKS, NRPS, and PKS-NRPS on the *Photorhabdus* genome, despite the high diversity of loci that makes peptide molecules, only three have been characterized for make a carbapenem antibiotic, an anthraquinone pigment, and the ST antibiotic (Wilkinson et al., 2009).

9.1.3 LYTIC ENZYMES OF ENTOMOPATHOGENIC FUNGI

EPF synthesize a different class of enzymes to proliferate in the hemolymph following cuticle penetration that will allow them to utilize carbohydrates (Lovett and St. Leger, 2018). The pathogenicity of this group of fungi depends majorly on the ability of their enzymatic machinery to degrade insects' integument and on the secretion of bioactive volatile organic compounds and antibiotics (Dhawan and Joshi, 2017). Different type of enzymes that produce EPF include proteases, chitinases, lipases, and lipoxygenases

(Sharma and Sharma, 2021). Table 9.1 indicates some of the lytic enzymes that entomopathogenic fungi produces.

TABLE 9.1 Entomopathogenic Fungi Reported Enzymes.

Entomopathogenic fungi	Enzyme	Reference
A. aleyrodis, B. bassiana, M. anisopliae, H. thompsonii, I. fumosorosea, N. rileyi, O.sinensis, V. lecanii	Chitinases	St Leger et al., 1986a; St Leger et al., 1986b; Kang et al., 1999; Fang et al., 2005; Agrawal et al., 2015; Mondal et al., 2016
B. bassiana, B. brongniartii, I. fumosorosea, M. anisopliae, M. robertsii, V. lecanii,	N-acetyl-β-glucosaminidase	St Leger et al., 1986b; Lopusiewicz et al., 2020
A. aleyrodis, B. bassiana, M. anisopliae, N. rileyi, Vertidllium lecanii,	Chymoelastases	St. Leger et al., 1988; St. Leger et al., 1987; Bidochka and Meltzer, 2000
B. bassiana, I. fumosorosea, M. anisopliae, M. flavoviride, N. rileyi, V. lecanii	Lipases	Silva et al., 2005; Fernandes et al., 2012; Supakdamrongkul et al., 2010; Gómez et al., 2017; Hasan et al., 2013; Parveen, 2021
B. bassiana , I. fumosorosea, M.anisopliae, V. fungicola, V. lecanii,	Subtilisin-like (Pr1) and trypsin-like (Pr2) activity	Castellanos-Moguel et al., 2007; Dias et al., 2008; Zibaee and Bandani, 2009; St Leger et al., 1997; Sheng et al., 2006
B. bassiana, B. brongniartii, I. fumsorosea, L. giganteum, M. anisopliae, N. rileyi, V. lecanii, T. niveum	Proteases	Mondal et al., 2016
M. anisopliae	Glucose phosphate isomerase, triosephosphate isomerase	St. Leger, 1992
B. bassiana, I. fumsorosea, M. anisopliae	Trehalose-hydrolysing enzyme	Hallsworth et al., 1994; Xia et al., 2002
B. bassiana, M. flavoviride, Paecilomyces sp., *V. lecanii,*	Amylase	Hasan et al., 2013; Fernandes et al., 2012; Amobonye et al., 2020; Parveen, 2021
B. bassiana, Paecilomyces sp.	Pectinase and caseinase	Fernandes et al., 2012
B. bassiana, M. anisopliae, M. robertsii	β-galactosidases	
B. bassiana ,Paecilomyces sp.	Cellulase activity	Fernandes et al., 2012; Amobonye et al., 2020

The pathogenicity of this group of fungi depends majorly on the ability of their enzymatic machinery to degrade insects' integument and also on the secretion of bioactive volatile organic compounds and antibiotics (Amobonye et al., 2020), the proteases and peptidases help in the degradation of the insect cuticle because insect cuticle is composed of chitin and protein. The fungi *B. bassiana, B. brongniartii, Lagenidium giganteum, Nomuraea rileyi, M. anisopliae, and V. lecanii* have been identified with protein degrading enzymes (Sheng et al., 2006). Chitinases play important roles in the cleavage of N-acetylglucosamine (Table 9.1), they help to break down the insect cuticle into monomers; also, lipases production is a critical part of the cuticle degrading reserve and the pathways involved in triglyceride metabolism and phospholipid homeostasis have revealed to contribute to host invasion (Keyhani, 2018). The pathogenic mechanism of these fungi begins with the adhesion of the conidia in an insect's exoskeleton surface, formation of an appressorium or a mucilaginous structure that remains adhered to a germinal tubule and penetration by mechanical pressure and enzymatic activity (Barranco-Florido et al., 2013); as a result, many studies have been dedicated to the potential of various entomopathogenic fungi for the production of important enzymes and other important metabolites (Amobonye et al., 2020).

EPF infect their insect hosts mainly by penetrating through the cuticle necessitating an ability to confront and overcome surface lipids and other molecules that often include antimicrobial compounds (Keyhani, 2018). In order to guarantee an effective infection, EPF produce a variety of degrading enzymes that help to infringe the insect cuticle, and then, secrete toxic secondary metabolites that facilitate fungal invasion of the hemolymph (Pedrini, 2018) (Fig. 9.1).

9.1.4 ENTOMOPATHOGENIC FUNGI ENZYMES PRODUCTION

Several entomopathogenic fungi when grown in liquid cultures containing locust cuticle as sole carbon source, produce a variety of hydrolytic enzymes with activity against the major components of insect cuticle, namely, protein, chitin, and lipid (St Lcgcr ct al., 1986a). It has been reported that most effective inducers of chitinase and chitosanase were N-acetylglucosamine and chitosan respectively (St Leger et al., 1986c).

It has been predicted that *Beauveria bassiana* genome encode 10,366 protein genes which include proteases genes (23 trypsins, 43 subtilisins, 21

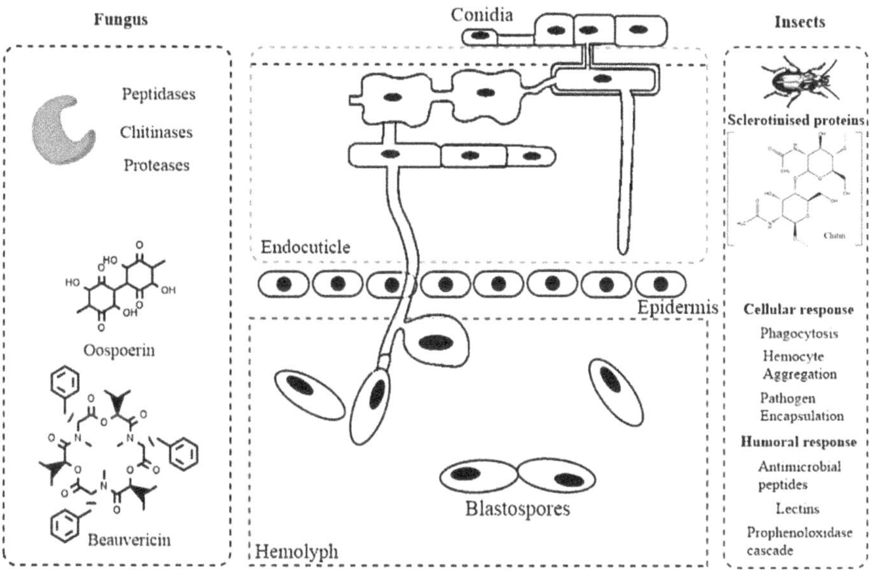

FIGURE 9.1 Overview of infecting process by entomopathogenic fungi.

aspartic proteases, 52 carboxypeptidases, 47 cysteine peptidases, 20 threonine peptidases, and 98 metallopeptidases), 145 carbohydrate active enzymes such as chitinases, cellulases, hemicellulases, ketolases, etc. (Amobonye et al., 2020).

Various kinds of insect plagues have been controlled extensively by extracellular lipases produced by *M. anisopliae*; the different lipid sources that best induced lipase production in *M. Anisopliae* were rice oil, soybean oil, olive oil, sunflower oil, sesame oil, and hydrogenated soybean fat (Silva et al., 2005). A significant review on biotechnological application of lipases has been done by Keyhani et al. (2018). Supakdamrongkul et al. (2010) studied *Metarhizium rileyi* strain as productor of lipase, they yield 1.69% of lipase using ammonium sulfate precipitation; the purified lipase hydrolyzed synthetic and natural triglycerides and also enhanced toxicity toward *Spodoptera litura* larvae. Besides from proteases, lipases, and chitinases, EPF also produce acid trehalase, it hydrolyzes trehalose, the main disaccharide of insect hemolymph (Jin et al., 2015). Saleem et al. (2019) tested three EPF for their abilities to produce extracellular protease enzyme, they inoculated casein broth with mycelial discs of tested fungi and incubated at 28 °C for seven days. Then the mycelium was harvested by filtration and the supernatants were assayed for proteolytic activity, according to the method of casein agar cup plate clearing zone assay, the results showed that the maximum activity of protease, was recorded after six days of incubation periods at 28 °C, in a medium initially adjusted to pH 6. In a assay conducted by Lovera et al. (2020), a soluble recombinant chitinase from a gene from the Colombian *B. bassiana* isolate using an *Escherichia coli* expression system was achieved; the recombinant protein (rChit37) was produced in both soluble and insoluble fractions of an *E. coli* culture. Both fractions expressing endo- (90 mU/μL) and exochitinase (170 mU/μL) enzymatic activity, with optimum conditions for enzyme activity of 45 °C and pH 5.0. In another study, the BbepnL-1 gene encoding the endothiapepsin-like protein as a model to investigate the function of the aspartic proteinase in *B. bassiana* was expressed in *Pichia pastoris* used vector pPIC9K, and the epidermis of the silkworm was used as a substrate to detect the ability of the recombinant protein to release the cuticle proteins (Gu et al., 2020); as well, Liu et al. (2020), cloned and expressed a chitosanase gene (BbCSN-1) from *Beauveria bassiana* in *P. pastoris*. They found that the amount of BbCSN-1 in the fermentation broth of *P. pastoris* gradually increased after induction with methanol reaching 398 μg/mL on the sixth day with optimum activity at pH 5 and 30 °C. By the other hand, Nguyen et al. (2018) cloned, sequenced, and overexpressed an endochitinase gene without signal peptide (mchit1) from *Lecanicillium lecanii* strain in *Pichia pastoris*.

9.1.5 RECOMBINANT ENTOMOPATHOGENIC BACULOVIRUSES

Entomopathogenic viruses (EVs) are important agents of biological control with features such as a narrow host range, non-toxicity to vertebrates, and eco-friendliness (Karabörklü et al., 2018). Use of these EPVs in sustainable pest management has many advantages as these viruses are highly specific toward their host range and will not infect nontarget organisms. Baculoviruses, a prominently group of EPVs, are highly specific in nature and they can be used in either augmentative or inoculative releases (Raj et al., 2022). Baculoviruses, mainly the nucleo-polyhedral viruses, are the most commonly used for development as microbial bio-insecticides largely for the control of lepidopteran insects pests on crops, however, not much success has been achieved due to a relatively slow speed of kill, less persistence in the field, and a narrow spectrum of activity (Tyagi, 2021); recently, genes of recombinant baculoviruses have been manipulated using insertions and deletions for increasing the killing speed of the agents and reduce feeding capacity of the host (Karabörklü et al., 2018) as well as lower insect resistance and lower spraying requirements (Azizoglu and Karabörklü, 2021).

The typical characteristic of insect baculoviruses is that the virus particle has two different structural forms, namely budded virus (BV) and occlusion-derived virus (ODV). BVs and ODVs are responsible for cell and oral infections, respectively, and they are widely used as high-efficiency expression vectors (Zheng et al., 2022). Baculovirus genomes are composed of a single covalently closed circular supercoiled dsDNA molecule with a size range of 80–180 kilobase pairs (Kbp) encoding for 80 of 200 potential genes. So far, only 85 different baculovirus species genomes have been sequenced. During the baculovirus life cycle, two virion phenotypes can be produced at chronologically distinct stages. The ODV are occluded in a protein matrix formed by the assembling of the highly expressed late-phase viral proteins units (polyhedrin in NPVs or granulin in GVs), into occlusion bodies (OB) (Sosa-Gómez et al., 2020). EPVs have been used as eukaryotic protein expression vectors in biotechnology (van Oers et al., 2015) for medical research and biotechnology of protein using the baculovirus expression vector system (BEVS), which is used to express thousands of recombinant targets genes due to its high level of gene expression driven by the polyhedrin promoter in virus-infected insect cells by replacing the polyhedrin gene with the foreign gene of interest (Fig. 9.2) (Karabörklü et al., 2018; Kim, 2022).

9.1.6 ARTHROPOD TOXINS INTO ENTOMOPTHOGNIEC FUNGI

A wide range of genes encoding insect-specific toxins isolated from spiders and scorpions have been introduced into the genomes of *Metarhizium* spp (Pava-Ripoll et al., 2008) or *Beauveria* spp. These toxins generally produce rapid paralysis by targeting one or more major ion channels (Wang and St Leger, 2007).

Karabörklü et al. (2018) conducted an extensive search on biotechnological approaches to pest insect control as the expression of neurotoxin genes from scorpions, mites, spiders, sea anemone, and ants who have been inserted into baculoviruses and assessed against pest insects, Harrison and Hoover (2012) modified *Metarhizium robertsii* by integrating genes that encode for the cuticle-degrading protease Pr1A and the scorpion neurotoxin BjαIT, which works in the insect haemocoel, by activating the insect immune responses against fungal infections, Timofeev et al. (2019) used a beta/delta agatoxin-1 from the *Agelena orientalis* spider venom as a potentially

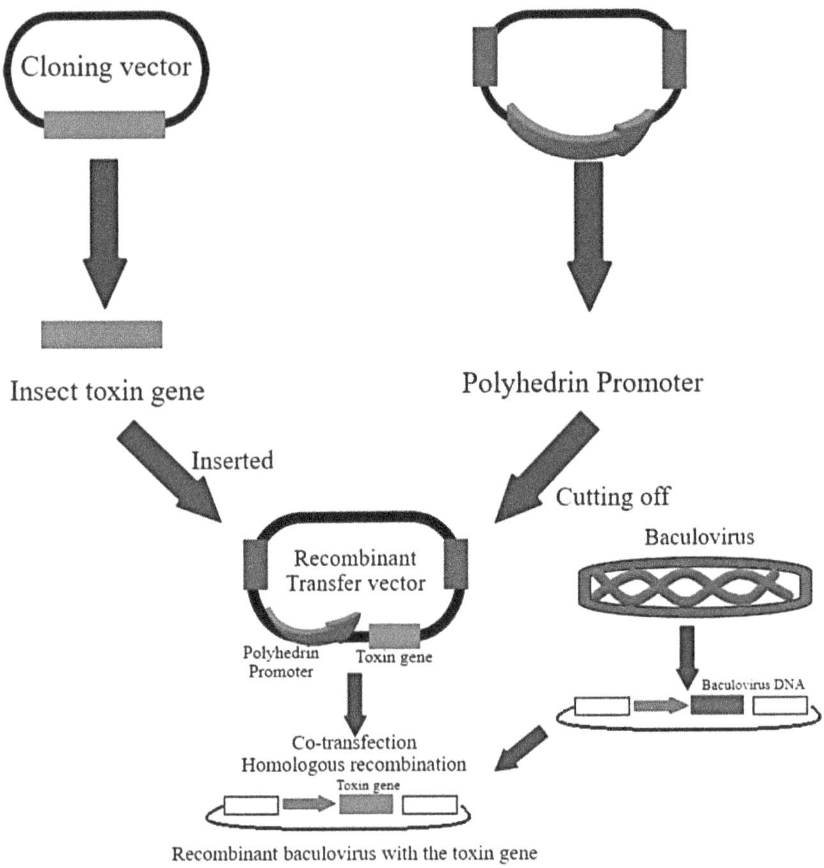

FIGURE 9.2 Summary of recombinant baculovirus production. (1) Construction of the transfer vector; (2) linearized baculovirus DNA; (3) co-transfection of recombinant transfer vector with the baculovirus DNA into the insect cells; (4) recombinant baculovirus carrying the toxin gene.

insecticidal recombinant product for the transformation of *Lecanicillium muscarium*; using the transformation of *L. muscarium* and the heterologous expression of a recombinant protein fused with Mcl1 signal peptide of *M. anisopliae*; they were able to obtain a strain that intensively expressed and secreted the inserted sequence. It has been documented the expression of heterologous proteins from scorpion *Leiurus quinquestriatus* excitatory toxin β-BUTX Lqq1a, defense protein from snowdrop plant *Galanthus nivalis* agglutinin (GNA), and *Bacillus thuringiensis* insecticidal toxins (Cyt1Aa and Cry1Ac) to empower *M. anisopliae* and *B. bassiana* pathogenicity towards insect pests (Dhanasingh, 2019).

The virulence of *M. acridum* has been enhanced by expressing the LqhIT2, an insect-specific neurotoxin from the venom of scorpion *Leiurus quinquestriatus* and Bj$\alpha\alpha$IT from the scorpion *Buthotus judaicus* (Peng and Xia, 2015). Li and Xia (2018) cloned the insect neurotoxin BjαIT gene into the pET32 expression vector and the resulting thioredoxin (Trx)-BjαIT fusion protein in *Escherichia coli.*

9.2 CONCLUSION

Entomopathogenic fungi play a crucial role in controlling insect populations in biological control; however, these pathogens need a special condition to proliferate and invade the host. Genetically modified entomopathogenic fungi might provide a relatively safe and cost-effective method of biological insect control for crops affected by certain pests. Some synthetic genes have been inserted into entomopathogen genome like neurotoxic peptides, proteases and chitinases that degrade the insect cuticle. The principal approach of genetic engineering is the expression of recombinant proteins using biological expression systems including baculovirus transfer vector containing the gene for the protein of interest, a donor plasmid, an *E. coli* host strain containing a cloned baculoviral genome, and *Pichia pastoris* expression as the most popular and standard tools to produce recombinant protein in molecular biology.

KEYWORDS

- **baculoviruses**
- **entomopathogenic fungi**
- **enzymes**
- **secondary metabolites**
- **toxins**

REFERENCES

Agrawal, Y.; Khatri, I.; Subramanian, S.; Shenoy, B. D Genome Sequence, Comparative Analysis, and Evolutionary Insights into Chitinases of Entomopathogenic Fungus *Hirsutella thompsonii*. *Genome Biol. Evol.* **2015,** *7,* 916–930.

Amobonye, A.; Bhagwat, P.; Pandey, A.; Singh, S.; Pillai, S. Biotechnological Potential of *Beauveria bassiana* as a Source of Novel Biocatalysts and Metabolites. *Crit. Rev. Biotechnol.* **2020,** *40,* 1019–1034.

Anggiani, J. P.; Listiyowati, S.; Rahayu, G. Entomopathogenic Fungi *Beauveria* sp. and *Aspergillus sclerotiorum* can Produce Secondary Metabolite Quinidine. *IOP Conf. Ser. Earth. Environ Sci.* **2020,** *457,* 1–7.

Araújo, J. P.; Hughes, D. P. Diversity of Entomopathogenic Fungi: Which Groups Conquered the Insect Body? *Adv. Genet.* **2016,** *94,* 1–39.

Azizoglu, U.; Karabörklü, S. Role of Recombinant DNA Technology to Improve the Efficacy of Microbial Insecticides. In *Microbes for Sustainable Insect Pest Management*; Springer: Cham, Copenhagen, Denmark, 2021; pp 159–182.

Barranco-Florido, E.; García-Hernández, L. A.; Rodríguez-Navarro, S.; Flores-Macías, A.; Ramos-López, M. A. Regulation of Gene Expression in Entomopathogenic Fungi in Three Different Environmental Conditions: A Review. *Afr. J. Biotechnol.* **2013,** *12,* 989–995.

Beris, E. Evaluation and Environmental Testing of Entomopathogenic Fungi for their Effectiveness as Bio-control Agents of Major Vineyard Pests. *Plant Protect.* **2021,** *5,* 13–23.

Bidochka, M. J.; Meltzer, M. J. Genetic Polymorphisms in Three Subtilisin-Like Protease Isoforms (Pr1A, Pr1B, and Pr1C) from *Metarhizium* Strains. *Can. J. Microbiol.* **2000,** *46,* 1138–1144.

Bilgo, E.; Lovett, B.; Bayili, K.; Millogo, A. S.; Saré, I.; Dabiré, R. K.; Diabate, A. Transgenic *Metarhizium pingshaense* Synergistically Ameliorates Pyrethroid-Resistance in Wild-Caught, Malaria-Vector Mosquitoes. *PloS One* **2018,** *13,* e0203529.

Bode, H. B. Entomopathogenic Bacteria as a Source of Secondary Metabolites. *Curr. Opin. Chem. Biol.* **2009,** *13,* 224–230.

Bojke, A.; Tkaczuk, C.; Stepnowski, P.; Gołębiowski, M. Comparison of Volatile Compounds Released by Entomopathogenic Fungi. *Microbiol. Res.* **2018,** *214,* 129–136.

Booysen, E.; Dicks, L. M. T. Does the Future of Antibiotics Lie in Secondary Metabolites Produced by *Xenorhabdus* spp.? A Review. Probiotics Antimicrob. Proteins **2020,** *12,* 1310–1320.

Booysen, E.; Rautenbach, M.; Stander, M. A.; Dicks, L. M. Profiling the Production of Antimicrobial Secondary Metabolites by *Xenorhabdus khoisanae* J194 Under Different Culturing Conditions. *Front. Chem.* **2021,** *9,* 626653.

Boszormeny, E.; Rsek, T. E.; Fodor, A.; Fodor, A. M.; Szldes, F. L.; Hevesi, M.; Hogan, J. S.; Katona, Z.; Klein, M. G.; Kormány, A.; Pekár, S.; Szentirmai, A.; Sztaricskai, F.; Taylor, R. A. J. Isolation and Activity of *Xenorhabdus* Antimicrobial Compounds Against the Plant Pathogens *Erwinia amylovora* and *Phytophthora nicotianae*. *J. Appl. Microbiol.* **2009,** *107,* 746–759.

Boyce, G. R.; Gluck-Thaler, E.; Slot, J. C.; Stajich, J. E.; Davis, W. J.; James, T. Y.; Cooley, J. R.; Panaccione, D. G.; Eilenberg, J.; De Fine Licht, H. H.; Macias, A. M.; Berger, M. C.; Wickert, K. L.; Stauder, C. M.; Spahr, E. J.; Maust, M. D.; Metheny, A. M.; Simon, C.; Kritsky, G.; Hodge, K. T.; Humber, R. A.; Guillion, T.; Short, D. P. G.; Kijimoto, T.; Mozgai, D.; Arguedas, N.; Kasson, M. T. Psychoactive Plant-and Mushroom-Associated Alkaloids from Two Behavior Modifying Cicada Pathogens. *Fungal Ecol.* **2019,** *41,* 147–164.

Brivio, M. F.; Mastore, M. When Appearance Misleads: The Role of the Entomopathogen Surface in the Relationship with its Host. *Insects* **2020,** *11,* 387.

Castellanos-Moguel, J.; González-Barajas, M.; Mier, T.; del Rocío Reyes-Montes, M.; Aranda, E.; Toriello, C. Virulence Testing and Extracellular Subtilisin-Like (Pr1) and Trypsin-like

(Pr2) Activity During Propagule Production of *Paecilomyces fumosoroseus* Isolates from Whiteflies (Homoptera: Aleyrodidae). *Rev. Iberoam Micol.* **2007**, *24*, 62.

Chen, W.; Hu, Q. Secondary Metabolites of *Purpureocillium lilacinum. Molecules* **2021,** *27*, 18.

Clarke, D. J. The Regulation of Secondary Metabolism in *Photorhabdus*. In *The Molecular Biology of Photorhabdus Bacteria*; Springer: Copenhagen, Denmark, 2016; pp 81–102.

De Costa, D. M. Microbial Pesticides Towards Eco-friendly Agriculture: Present Status and Future Prospects in Sri Lanka. In *Agricultural Research for Sustainable Food Systems in Sri Lanka*; Springer: Singapore, 2020; pp 159–186.

Deng, S. Q.; Chen, J. T.; Li, W. W.; Chen, M.; Peng, H. J. Application of the Scorpion Neurotoxin AaIT Against Insect Pests. *Int. J. Mol. Sci.* **2019,** *20*, 3467.

Dhanasingh, M.; Studies on Engineering Entomopathogenic Fungi *Metarhizium anisopliae* and *Beauveria bassiana* to Express Heterologous Insect-Specific Toxins. Doctoral Thesis, Indian Institute of Technology Guwahati, Department of Biotechnology, New Delhi, India, 2019.

Dhawan, M.; Joshi, N. Enzymatic Comparison and Mortality of *Beauveria bassiana* against Cabbage Caterpillar *Pieris brassicae* LINN. *Braz. J. Microbiol.* **2017,** *48*, 22–529.

Dias, B. A.; Neves, P. M. O. J.; Furlaneto-Maia, L.; Furlaneto, M. C. Cuticle-Degrading Proteases Produced by the Entomopathogenic Fungus *Beauveria bassiana* in the Presence of Coffee Berry Borer Cuticle. *Braz. J. Microbiol.* **2008,** *39*, 301–306.

Dillman, A. R.; Sternberg, P. W. Entomopathogenic Nematodes. *Curr. Biol.* **2012,** *22*, R430–R431.

Du, Y.; Xia, Y.; Jin, K. Enhancing the Biocontrol Potential of the Entomopathogenic Fungus in Multiple Respects via the Overexpression of a Transcription Factor Gene MaSom1. *J. Fungi* **2022,** *8*, 105.

Fang, W.; Leng, B.; Xiao, Y.; Jin, K.; Ma, J.; Fan, Y.; Pei, Y. Cloning of *Beauveria bassiana* Chitinase Gene Bbchit1 and its Application to Improve Fungal Strain Virulence. *Appl. Environ. Microbiol.* **2005**, *71*, 363–370.

Fernandes, E. G.; Valerio, H. M.; Feltrin, T.; Van der Sand, S. T. Variability in the Production of Extracellular Enzymes by Entomopathogenic Fungi Grown on Different Substrates. *Braz. J. Microbiol.* **2012,** *43*, 827–833.

Fredericksen, M. A.; Zhang, Y.; Hazen, M. L.; Loreto, R. G.; Mangold, C. A.; Chen, D. Z.; Hughes, D. P.; Three-dimensional Visualization and a Deep-Learning Model Reveal Complex Fungal Parasite Networks in Behaviorally Manipulated Ants. *Proc. Natl. Acad. Sci.* **2017,** *114*, 12590–12595.

Gaugler, R.; Campbell, J. F. Nictation Behaviour and its Ecological Implications in the Host Search Strategies of Entomopathogenic Nematodes (Heterorhabditidae and Steinernematidae). *Behaviour* **1993,** *126*, 155–169.

Gómez, C.; Amaya, I.; Cruz-Quiroz, R. D. L.; Rodríguez-Herrera, R.; Aguilar, C. N. T*enebrio monitor* Biomass as Inducer of Lipases Proteases Produced by *Peacilomyces fumosoroseus*. *Mex. J. Biotechnol.* **2017,** *2*, 142–150.

Grose, C.; Putman, Z.; Esposito, D. A Review of Alternative Promoters for Optimal Recombinant Protein Expression in Baculovirus-Infected Insect Cells. *Protein Expr. Purif.* **2021,** *186*, 105924.

Gu, C. X.; Zhang, B. L.; Bai, W. W.; Liu, J.; Zhou, W.; Ling, Z. Q.; Wan, Y. J. Characterization of the Endothiapepsin-Like Protein in the Entomopathogenic Fungus *Beauveria bassiana* and its Virulence Effect on the Silkworm, *Bombyx mori*. *J. Invertebr. Pathol.* **2020,** *169*, 107277.

Hajek, A. E.; Steinkraus, D. C.; Castrillo, L. A. Sleeping Beauties: Horizontal Transmission Via Resting Spores of Species in the Entomophthoromycotina. *Insects* **2018,** *9*, 102.

Hallsworth, J. E.; Magan, N. Effect of Carbohydrate Type and Concentration on Polyhydroxy Alcohol and Trehalose Content of Conidia of Three Entomopathogenic Fungi. *Microbiology* **1994,** *140*, 2705–2713.

Harrison, R. L.; Hoover, K. Baculoviruses and Other Occluded Insect Viruses. In *Insect Pathology*; London Academic Press: Cambridge, Massachusetts, 2012; pp 73–131.

Hasan, S.; Ahmad, A.; Purwar, A.; Khan, N.; Kundan, R.; Gupta, G. Production of Extracellular Enzymes in the Entomopathogenic Fungus *Verticillium lecanii*. *Bioinformation* **2013,** *9*, 238.

Hutchinson, C. R. Polyketide and Non-Ribosomal Peptide Synthases: Falling Together by Coming Apart. *Proc. Natl. Acad. Sci. USA* **2003,** *100*, 3010–3012.

Ibrahim, S. A. M.; Salem, H. H. A; Taha, M. A. Dual Application of Entomopathogenic Nematodes and Fungi on Immune and Antioxidant Enzymes of the Greater Wax Moth, *Galleria mellonella* L. *Egypt J. Biol. Pest Control* **2019,** *29*, 20.

Islam, W.; Adnan, M.; Shabbir, A.; Naveed, H.; Abubakar, Y. S.; Qasim, M.: Ali, H. Insect-Fungal-Interactions: A Detailed Review on Entomopathogenic Fungi Pathogenicity to Combat Insect Pests. *Microb. Pathog.* **2021,** *159*, 105122.

Jaber, L. R.; Ownley, B. H. Can we use Entomopathogenic Fungi as Endophytes for Dual Biological Control of Insect Pests and Plant Pathogens?. *Biol. Control* **2018,** *116*, 36–45.

Jin, K.; Peng, G.; Liu, Y.; Xia, Y. The Acid Trehalase, ATM1, Contributes to the In Vivo Growth and Virulence of the Entomopathogenic Fungus, *Metarhizium acridum*. *Fungal Genet. Biol.* **2015,** *77*, 61–67.

Joyce, S. A.; Lango, L.; Clarke, D. J. The Regulation of Secondary Metabolism and Mutualism in the Insect Pathogenic Bacterium *Photorhabdus luminescens*. In *Advances in Applied Microbiology*; Academic Press: United States, 2011; vol 76, pp 1–25.

Kang, S. C.; Park, S.; Lee, D. G. Purification and Characterization of a Novel Chitinase from the Entomopathogenic Fungus, *Metarhizium anisopliae*. *J. Invertebr. Pathol.* **1999,** *73*, 276–281.

Karabörklü, S.; Azizoglu, U.; Azizoglu, Z. B. Recombinant Entomopathogenic Agents: A Review of Biotechnological Approaches to Pest Insect Control. *World J. Microbiol. Biotechnol.* **2018,** *34*, 1–12.

Kazek, M.; Kaczmarek, A.; Wrońska, A. K; Boguś M. I.; Dodecanol, Metabolite of Entomopathogenic Fungus *Conidiobolus coronatus*, Affects Fatty Acid Composition and Cellular Immunity of *Galleria mellonella* and *Calliphora vicina*. *Sci. Rep.* **2021,** *11*, 15963.

Keyhani N. O. Lipid Biology in Fungal Stress and Virulence: Entomopathogenic Fungi. *Fungal Biol.* **2018,** *122*, 420–429.

Kidanu, S.; Hagos, L. Research and Application of Entomopathogenic Fungi as Pest Management Option: A Review. *J. Environ. Earth Sci.* **2020,** *10*, 31–39.

Kim, H. J. Comparative Study on the Expression and Characteristics of Lipase Genes from Entomopathogenic Fungi. Master Diss., Department of Agricultural Biotechnology, Seoul National University, Korea, 2022.

Kumar, S. N.; Nambisan, B.; Sundaresan, A.; Mohandas, C.; Anto, R. J. Isolation and Identification of Antimicrobial Secondary Metabolites from *Bacillus cereus* Associated with a Rhabditid Entomopathogenic Nematode. *Ann. Microbiol.* **2014,** *64*, 209–218.

Lango-Scholey, L.; Brachmann, A. O.; Bode, H. B.; Clarke, D. J. The expression of stlA in *Photorhabdus luminescens* is Controlled by Nutrient Limitation. *Plos One* **2013,** *8*, e82152.

Leadmon, C. E.; Sampson, J. K.; Maust, M. D.; Macias, A. M.; Rehner, S. A.; Kasson, M. T.; Panaccione, D. G. Several *Metarhizium* Species Produce Ergot Alkaloids in a Condition-Specific Manner. *Appl. Environ. Microbiol.* **2020,** *86*, e00373–20.

Lewis, E. E.; Campbell, J.; Griffin, C.; Kaya, H.; Peters, A. Behavioral Ecology of Entomopathogenic Nematodes. *Biol. Control* **2006,** *38*, 66–79.

Li, H.; Xia, Y. Recombinant Production of the Insecticidal Scorpion Toxin BjαIT in *Escherichia coli*. *Protein Expr. Purif.* **2018,** *142*, 62–67.

Litwin, A.; Nowak, M.; Różalska, S. Entomopathogenic Fungi: Unconventional Applications. *Rev. Environ. Sci. Biotechnol.* **2020,** *19*, 23–42.

Liu, B. L.; Chen, J. W.; Tzeng, Y. M. Production of Cyclodepsipeptides Destruxin A and B from *Metarhizium anisopliae*. *Biotechnol. Prog.* **2000,** *16*, 993–999.

Liu, Y.; Li, Y.; Tong, S.; Yuan, M.; Wang, X.; Wang, J.; Fan, Y. Expression of a *Beauveria bassiana* chitosanase (BbCSN-1) in *Pichia pastoris* and Enzymatic Analysis of the Recombinant Protein. *Protein Expr. Purif.* **2020,** *166*, 105519.

Lopusiewicz, L.; Mazurkiewicz-Zapalowicz, K.; Tkaczuk, C.; Bartkowiak, A. The Influence of Cobalt Ions on Growth and Enzymatic Activity of Entomopathogenic Fungi Used in Biological Plant Protection. *J. Plant Prot. Res.* **2020,** *60*, 58–67.

Lovera, A.; Belaich, M.; Villamizar, L.; Patarroyo, M. A.; Barrera, G. Enhanced Virulence of *Beauveria bassiana* Against *Diatraea saccharalis* Using a Soluble Recombinant Enzyme with Endo-and Exochitinase Activity. *Biol. Control* **2020,** *144*, 104211.

Lovett, B.; St. Leger, R. J. Genetically Engineering Better Fungal Biopesticides. *Pest Manag. Sci.* **2018,** *74*, 781–789.

Ma, X.; Ge, Q.; Taha, R. H.; Chen, K.; Yuan, Y. *Beauveria bassiana* ribotoxin (BbRib) Induces Silkworm Cell Apoptosis Via Activating Ros Stress Response. *Processes* **2021,** *9*, 1470.

Mannino, M. C.; Davyt-Colo, B.; Pedrini, N. Toxic Secondary Metabolites and Virulence Factors Expression by Entomopathogenic Fungi during Insect Infection and Potential Impact as a Tool for Pest Management. In *Microbes for Sustainable Insect Pest Management*; Springer: Cham, Copenhagen, Denmark, 2021; pp 121–134.

Martínez-Solís, M.; Herrero, S.; Targovnik, A. M. Engineering of the Baculovirus Expression System for Optimized Protein Production. *Appl. Microbiol. Biotechnol.* **2019,** *103*, 113–123.

Mishra, V. A. Comprehensive Guide to the Commercial Baculovirus Expression Vector Systems for Recombinant Protein Production. *Protein Pept. Lett.* **2020,** *27*, 529–537.

Mondal, S.; Baksi, S.; Koris, A.; Vatai, G. Journey of Enzymes in Entomopathogenic Fungi. *Pac. Sci. Rev. Nat. Sci. Eng.* **2016,** *18*, 85–99.

Nguyen, H. Q.; Vu, V. H.; Le, P. D.; Chu, H. M. High-Level Expression, Purification and Properties of an Endochitinase Gene Without Signal Peptide from *Lecanicillium lecanii* 43H in *Pichia pastoris*. *Mol. Biol. Rep.* **2018,** *45*, 1067–1075.

Olleik, H.; Nicoletti, C.; Lafond, M.; Courvoisier-Dezord, E.; Xue, P.; Hijazi, A.; Maresca, M. Comparative Structure–Activity Analysis of the Antimicrobial Activity, Cytotoxicity, and Mechanism of Action of the Fungal Cyclohexadepsipeptides Enniatins and Beauvericin. *Toxins* **2019,** *11*, 514.

Parveen, S. S. Biochemical Characterization of Entomopathogenic Fungal Isolates. *J. Entomol. Res.* **2021,** *45*, 53–54.

Paschapur, A.; Subbanna, A. R. N. S.; Singh, A. K.; Jeevan, B.; Stanley, J.; Rajashekhar, H.; Mishra, K. K. Unraveling the Importance of Metabolites from Entomopathogenic Fungi in

Insect Pest Management. In *Microbes for Sustainable Insect Pest Management*; Springer: Cham, Copenhagen, Denmark, 2021; pp 89–120.

Pava-Ripoll, M.; Posada, F. J.; Momen, B.; Wang, C.; St. Leger, R. Increased Pathogenicity Against Coffee Berry Borer, *Hypothenemus hampei* (Coleoptera: Curculionidae) by *Metarhizium anisopliae* Expressing the Scorpion Toxin (AaIT) Gene. *J. Invertebr. Pathol.* **2008,** *99*, 220–226.

Pedrini, N. Molecular Interactions Between Entomopathogenic Fungi (Hypocreales) and their Insect Host: Perspectives from Stressful Cuticle and Hemolymph Battlefields and the Potential of Dual RNA Sequencing for Future Studies. *Fungal Biol.* **2018,** *122*, 538–545.

Pedrini, N. The Entomopathogenic Fungus *Beauveria bassiana* Shows its Toxic Side Within Insects: Expression of Genes Encoding Secondary Metabolites During Pathogenesis. *J. Fungi* **2022,** *8*, 488.

Peng, G.; Xia, Y. Integration of an Insecticidal Scorpion Toxin (Bjα IT) Gene into *Metarhizium acridum* Enhances Fungal Virulence Towards *Locusta migratoria manilensis. Pest Manag. Sci.* **2015,** *71*, 58–64.

Raj, M. N.; Samal, I.; Paschapur, A.; Subbanna, A. R. N. S. Entomopathogenic Viruses and their Potential Role in Sustainable Pest Management. In *New and Future Developments in Microbial Biotechnology and Bioengineering*; Elsevier Inc.: Amsterdam, The Netherlands, 2022; pp 47–72.

Rios-Moreno, A.; Garrido-Jurado, I.; Resquín-Romero, G.; Arroyo-Manzanares, N.; Arce, L.; Quesada-Moraga, E. Destruxin A Production by *Metarhizium brunneum* Strains During Transient Endophytic Colonisation of *Solanum tuberosum. Biocontrol Sci. Technol.* **2016,** *26*, 1574–1585.

Saleem, A. R.; Ibrahim, R. A. Assessment of the Virulence and Proteolytic Activity of Three Native Entomopathogenic Fungi Against the Larvae of *Oryctes agamemnon* (Burmeister) (Coleoptera: Scarabaeidae). *Egypt J. Biol. Pest Control* **2019,** *29*, 21.

Samuels, R. I.; Charnley, A. K.; Reynolds, S. E. The Role of Destruxins in the Pathogenicity of 3 Strains of *Metarhizium anisopliae* for the Tobacco Hornworm Manduca sexta. *Mycopathologia* **1988,** *104*, 51–58.

Sánchez-Pérez, L.; Barranco-Florido, J.; Rodríguez-Navarro, S.; Cervantes-Mayagoitia, J.; Ramos-López, M. Enzymes of Entomopathogenic Fungi, Advances and Insights. *Adv. Enz. Res.* **2014,** *2*, 65–76.

Sbaraini, N.; Hu, J.; Roux, I.; Phan, C. S.; Motta, H.; Rezaee, H.; Staats, C. C. Polyketides Produced by the Entomopathogenic Fungus *Metarhizium anisopliae* Induce *Candida albicans* Growth. *Fungal Genet. Biol.* **2021,** *152*, 103568.

Shan, S.; Ma, H.; Li, Y.; Huang, C.; Gu, X.; Jiang, Z.; Ruan, W. Metabolites from Symbiotic Bacteria of Entomopathogenic Nematodes have Antimicrobial Effects Against *Pythium myriotylum. Eur. J. Plant Pathol.* **2020,** *158*, 35–44.

Sharma, H.; Rana, A.; Bhat, A. H.; Chaubey, A. K. Entomopathogenic Nematodes: Their Characterization, Bio-Control Properties and New Perspectives. In *Nematodes-Recent Advances, Management and New Perspectives*; IntechOpen: London, United Kingdom, 2022; pp 187–210.

Sharma, R.; Sharma, P. Fungal Entomopathogens: A Systematic Review. *Egypt J. Biol. Pest Control* **2021,** *31*, 1–13.

Sheng, J.; An, K.; Deng, C.; Li, W.; Bao, X.; Qiu, D. Cloning a Cuticle-Degrading Serine Protease Gene with Biologic Control Function from *Beauveria brongniartii* and its Expression in *Escherichia coli. Curr. Microbiol.* **2006,** *53*, 124–128.

Shukla, A. C.; Afzal, K. Entomopathogenic Fungi. In *Microbial Approaches for Insect Pest Management*; Springer: Singapore, 2021; pp 315–336.

Silva, W.; Mitidieri, S.; Schrank, A.; Vainstein, M. H. Production and Extraction of an Extracellular Lipase from the Entomopathogenic Fungus *Metarhizium anisopliae*. *Process Biochem.* **2005,** *40*, 321–326.

Sosa-Gómez, D. R.; Morgado, F. S.; Corrêa, R. F. T.; Silva, L. A.; Ardisson-Araújo, D. M. P.; Rodrigues, B. M. P.; Ribeiro, B. M. Entomopathogenic Viruses in the Neotropics: Current Status and Recently Discovered Species. *Neotrop. Entomol.* **2020,** *49*, 315–331.

St Leger, R. J.; Charnley, A. K.; Cooper, R. M. Cuticle Degrading Enzymes of Entomopathogenic Fungi. Synthesis in Culture on Cuticle. *J. Invertebr. Pathol.* **1986c,** *47*, 167–177.

St Leger, R. J.; Cooper, R. M.; Charnley, A. K. Cuticle-Degrading Enzymes of Entomopathogenic Fungi: Regulation of Production of Chitinolytic Enzymes. *Microbiology* **1986a,** *132*, 1509–1517.

St Leger, R. S.; Cooper, R. M.; Charnley, A. K. Cuticle-Degrading Enzymes of Entomopathogenic Fungi: Cuticle Degradation *in vitro* by Enzymes from Entomopathogens. *J. Invertebr. Pathol.* **1986b,** *47*, 167–177.

St Leger, R. S.; Cooper, R. M.; Charnley, A. K. Distribution of Chymoelastases and Trypsin-Like Enzymes in Five Species of Entomopathogenic Deuteromycetes. *Arch. Biochem. Bioph.* **1987,** *258*, 123–131.

St. Leger, R. J.; Durrands, P. K.; Cooper, R. M.; Charnley, A. K. Regulation of Production of Proteolytic Enzymes by the Entomopathogenic Fungus *Metarhizium anisopliae*. *Arch. Microbiol.* **1988,** *150*, 413–416.

St Leger, R. S.; May, B.; Allee, L. L.; Frank, D. C.; Staples, R. C.; Roberts, D. W. Genetic Differences in Allozymes and in Formation of Infection Structures Among Isolates of the Entomopathogenic Fungus *Metarhizium anisopliae*. *J. Invertebr. Pathol.* **1992,** *60*, 89–101.

St Leger, R. J.; Joshi, L.; Bidochka, M. J.; Roberts, D. W. Characterization of Chitinases from *Metarhizium anisopliae, M. falvoviride* and *Beauveria bassiana*, and Ultrastructural Localization of Chitinase Production During Invasion of Insect Cuticle. *Appl. Environ. Microbiol.* **1996,** *62*, 907–912.

St Leger, R. J.; Joshi, L.; Roberts, D. W. Adaptation of Proteases and Carbohydrases of Saprophytic, Phytopathogenic and Entomopathogenic Fungi to the Requirements of Their Ecological Niches. *Microbiology* **1997,** *143*, 1983–1992.

Steen, C. R.; Sampson, J. K.; Panaccione, D. G. A Baeyer-Villiger Monooxygenase Gene Involved in the Synthesis of Lysergic Acid Amides Affects the Interaction of the Fungus *Metarhizium brunneum* with Insects. *Appl. Environ. Microbiol.* **2021,** *87*, e00748-21.

Stock, S. P.; Blair, H. G. Entomopathogenic Nematodes and their Bacterial Symbionts: The Inside Out of a Mutualistic Association. *Symbiosis* **2008,** *46*, 67–75.

Subbanna, A. R. N. S.; Stanley, J.; Rajasekhara, H.; Mishra, K. K.; Pattanayak, A.; Bhowmick, R. Perspectives of Microbial Metabolites as Pesticides in Agricultural Pest Management. In *Co-evolution of Secondary Metabolites*; Springer: Cham, Copenhagen, Denmark, 2020; pp 925–952.

Supakdamrongkul, P.; Bhumiratana, A.; Wiwat, C. Characterization of an Extracellular Lipase from the Biocontrol Fungus, *Nomuraea rileyi* MJ, and its Toxicity Toward *Spodoptera litura*. *J. Invertebr. Pathol.* **2010,** *105*, 228–235.

Timofeev, S.; Mitina, G.; Rogozhin, E.; Dolgikh, V. Expression of Spider Toxin in Entomopathogenic Fungus *Lecanicillium muscarium* and Selection of the Strain Showing Efficient Secretion of the Recombinant Protein. *FEMS Microbiol. Lett.* **2019,** *366*, fnz181.

Toledo-Hernández, R. A.; Toledo, J.; Valle-Mora, J.; Holguín-Meléndez, F.; Liedo, P.; Huerta-Palacios, G. Pathogenicity and Virulence of *Purpureocillium lilacinum* (Hypocreales: Ophiocordycipitaceae) on Mexican Fruit Fly Adults. *Fla Entomol.* **2019,** *102*, 309–314.

Tyagi, S. Application of Biotechnology in Plant Protection. *Bioingene PSJ* **2021,** *1*, 1–8.

Unagul, P.; Wongsa, P.; Kittakoop, P.; Intamas, S.; Srikitikulchai, P.; Tanticharoen, M. Production of Red Pigments by the Insect Pathogenic Fungus *Cordyceps unilateralis* BCC 1869. *J. Ind. Microbiol. Biotechnol.* **2005,** *32*, 135–140.

Urbaniak, M.; Stepien, L.; Uhlig, S. Evidence for Naturally Produced Beauvericins Containing N-Methyl-Tyrosine in Hypocreales Fungi. *Toxins* **2019,** *11*, 82.

Urbaniak, M.; Waśkiewicz, A.; Trzebny, A.; Koczyk, G.; Stępień, Ł. Cyclodepsipeptide Biosynthesis in Hypocreales Fungi and Sequence Divergence of the Non-ribosomal Peptide Synthase Genes. *Pathogens* **2020,** *9*, 552.

van Oers, M. M.; Pijlman, G. P.; Vlak, J. M. Thirty Years of Baculovirusinsect Cell Protein Expression: From Dark Horse to Mainstream Technology. *J. Gen. Virol.* **2015,** *96*, 6–23.

Vásquez-Bonilla, J. N.; Barranco-Florido, J. E.; Ponce-Alquicira, E.; Rincón-Guevara, M. A.; Loera, O. Improvement of Beauvericin Production by *Fusarium oxysporum* AB2 Under Solid-State Fermentation Using an Optimised Liquid Medium and Co-cultures. *Mycotoxin Res.* **2022.** https://doi.org/10.1007/s12550-022-00458-y.

Vongvanich, N.; Kittakoop, P.; Isaka, M.; Trakulnaleamsai, S.; Vimuttipong, S.; Tanticharoen, M.; Thebtaranonth, Y. Hirsutellide A, a New Antimycobacterial Cyclohexadepsipeptide from the Entomopathogenic fungus *Hirsutella kobayasii. J. Nat. Prod.* **2002,** *65*, 1346–1348.

Wang, H. Destruxin Production of *Metarhizium anisopliae* Under Carbon and Nitrogen Exhaustion. *J. Basic Microbiol.* **2009,** *49*, 404–411.

Wang, X.; Gong, X.; Li, P.; Lai, D.; Zhou, L. Structural Diversity and Biological Activities of Cyclic Depsipeptides from Fungi. *Molecules* **2018,** *23*, 169.

Wang, C.; St. Leger, R. J. A Scorpion Neurotoxin Increases the Potency of a Fungal Insecticide. *Nat. Biotechnol.* **2007,** *25*, 1455–1456.

Weng, Q.; Zhang, X.; Chen, W.; Hu, Q. Secondary Metabolites and the Risks of *Isaria fumosorosea* and *Isaria farinosa. Molecules* **2019,** *24*, 664.

Wilkinson, P.; Waterfield, N. R.; Crossman, L.; Corton, C.; et al. Comparative Genomics of the Emerging Human Pathogen Photorhabdus Asymbiotica with the Insect Pathogen *Photorhabdus luminescens*. BMC Genomics. **2009,** *10*, 302.

Woo, R. M.; Park, M. G.; Choi, J. Y.; Park, D. H.; Kim, J. Y.; Wang, M.; Je, Y. H. Insecticidal and Insect Growth Regulatory Activities of Secondary Metabolites from Entomopathogenic Fungi, *Lecanicillium attenuatum. J. Appl. Entomol.* **2020,** *144*, 655–663.

Wrońska, A. K.; Boguś, M. I. Harman and Norharman, Metabolites of the Entomopathogenic Fungus *Conidiobolus coronatus* (Entomophthorales), Affect the Serotonin Levels and Phagocytic Activity of Hemocytes, Insect Immunocompetent Cells, in *Galleria mellonella* (Lepidoptera). *Cell Biosci.* **2019,** *9*, 1–17.

Xia, Y.; Clarkson, J. M.; Charnley, A. K. Trehalose-Hydrolysing Enzymes of *Metarhizium anisopliae* and their Role in Pathogenesis of the Tobacco Hornworm, *Manduca sexta. J. Invertebr. Pathol.* **2002,** *80*, 139–147.

Yadav, R. N.; Rashid, M.; Zaidi, N. W.; Kumar, R.; Singh, H. B. Secondary Metabolites of *Metarhizium* spp. and *Verticillium* spp. and their Agricultural Applications. In *Secondary Metabolites of Plant Growth Promoting Rhizomicroorganisms*; Springer: Singapore, 2019; pp 27–58.

Zhang, L.; Fasoyin, O. E.; Molnár, I.; Xu, Y. Secondary Metabolites from Hypocrealean Entomopathogenic Fungi: Novel Bioactive Compounds. *Nat. Prod. Rep.* **2020,** *37*, 1181–1206.

Zheng, H.; Pan, Y.; Wang, X.; Tian, W.; Yao, L.; Sun, J. Impact of Molecular Modification on the Efficiency of Recombinant Baculovirus Vector Invasion to Mammalian Cells and its Immunogenicity in Mice. *Viruses* **2022,** *14*, 140.

Zibaee, A.; Bandani, A. R. Purification and Characterization of the Cuticle-Degrading Protease Produced by the Entomopathogenic Fungus, *Beauveria bassiana* in the Presence of Sunn pest, *Eurygaster integriceps* (Hemiptera: Scutelleridae) Cuticle. *Biocontrol Sci Technol.* **2009,** *19*, 797–808

CHAPTER 10

Fluid Dynamics Modeling to Assess the Impact of Urban Geometry on Urban Microclimate

GEORGE THOMAS and NIKITHA MARY MONSON

Department of Physics, Catholicate College, Pathanamthitta, Kerala, India

ABSTRACT

More than half of the world's population lives in urban areas and is vulnerable to climate change. The enhancement of the urban heat island (UHI) is a major concern nowadays. The paradigm shift in the definition of UHI from the elevation in the temperature between urban, and rural areas to the thermal differentiation between local climate zones (LCZ) brings forth the potential to incorporate various modeling tools and simulations in urban microclimate studies. Although the microclimate models have been extensively studied in the context of modifying urban microclimate, they have been less explored and validated in the humid tropical, monsoon-dominated climate. The aim of this study is to investigate the responsiveness of a three-dimensional (3D) microclimate model, ENVI-met, to evaluate the impact of urban geometry on the urban thermal environment in the urban region of Kochi, a tropical coastal city on the southwest coast of India. Filed measurements were carried out at two LCZ zones in the study area. Two sets of simulations were also carried out using the area input file attributes of the compact midrise zone (CMR) and the openset midrise zone (OMR) in LCZ classification. The results of the simulation reveal that the models adequately captured the diurnal variations of temperature in the CMR and OMR zones during

Application of Engineering Principles and Practices in Biotechnology.
Ann Rose Abraham, Leonardo Sepúlveda Torre, Tamara Tatrishvili, and A. K. Haghi (Eds.)

simulation and observation. The findings simulation also emphasizes that urban geometry has a significant impact on the modification of UHI intensity.

10.1 INTRODUCTION

Urban regions have undergone unprecedented changes in the last few decades. About half of the total population is currently in the metropolitan region. India is expected to add 404 million urban residents by 2050 (UN, 2019). The rate of urbanization in India during the last decade has risen to double its value during the preceding decade. A noticeable uptick in Kerala's urban population in Kerala (i.e., 25.96–47.70%) during 2001–2011 is a notable illustration of fast urbanization (Census of India, 2011). Urban areas have experienced significant changes in their land use, land cover, population, and population density as a result of the high rate of urbanization (Vidyarthi, 2021). These modifications dramatically change the microclimate of the urban and nearby suburban regions.

One of the well-known urban climate modifications is the urban heat island (UHI), which is characterized by a warmer temperature in urban areas compared to the countryside (Landsberg, 1981; Ren et al., 2020). Urban geometry within the urban canopy layer is one of the most important factors that cause the microscale heat island intensity and intra-urban air temperature differences (Voogt, 2002; Yang et al., 2021). The microclimate of metropolitan areas is significantly altered when pervious surfaces are replaced with impervious counterparts, such as construction materials, artificial pavements, and roadways. The majority of building materials have a low albedo surface, which increases solar radiation absorption throughout the day. The heat energy that has accumulated throughout the day will gradually begin to be released from the pavements and buildings at night. However, the low sky view factor and denser building clusters in urban regions reduce the ability of building mass to cool and eventually lead to more heat retention at night. The artificial heat produced by anthropogenic activity, commercial, and vehicular combustion also amplifies UHI intensity.

Solar radiation is the major source of energy and it contributes to most of the radiation reaching the Earth's surface. The energy input's into the Earth's surface must either be released from the surface (output) or stored as sensible or latent heat and be released at a later time. Solar radiation can reach the Earth's atmosphere as a direct or short wave, or it can heat the atmosphere or be scattered before being directed as long-wave radiation toward the Earth's surface. The incoming solar radiation may be instantaneously reflected back in the form of short-wave radiation or stored and then reradiated (long wave) to the atmosphere.

The energy balance between solar incident radiation, long-wave and short-wave emission, and sensible heat transfer controls the diurnal cycle of heating and cooling of the Earth's surface and atmospheric boundary layer. An energy budget accounts for the equilibrium of incoming and outgoing energy fluxes. The variation in the land cover, building, and surface morphology of urban areas and rural surroundings leads to different surface energy budgets. This discrepancy in heat generation and transfer results in the elevation of temperature between urban and rural environments. Consider a shallow layer at the surface containing air and surface elements in order to examine the UHI. The energy fluxes for this layer are solar radiation. The magnitude of shortwave and longwave radiation receiving and escaping the layer determines the net radiative energy. The net sum of the upwelling and downwelling solar shortwave radiation flux and longwave radiation determine the radiative energy budget. The net radiative energy (Q_{net}) is given in eq 10.1.

$$Q_{net} = S_d + S_u + L_d + L_u \tag{10.1}$$

where S_u and S_d refer to upwelling and downwelling solar shortwave radiation flux, and L_d and L_u refer to downwelling and upwelling infrared radiation—L_d is long-wave radiation emitted by the Sun and the atmosphere toward the surface of the Earth and L_u is the long-wave radiation emitted by the Earth's surface. The surfaces with low albedo absorb more energy and emit less solar energy into the atmosphere. Hence, upwelling longwave radiation from the surface depends on the albedo, water content, thermal conductivity, and the temperature of the surface. The materials with low albedo used in the urban regions enhance the upwelling infrared (longwave) radiation. The temperature of the air near the surface rises with the increase of Q_{net} and reduces when Q_{net} decreases. The mass and heat capacity of the layer, as well as the rate at which energy is lost and absorbed, determine how much energy is stored. The quantity of energy stored in the shallow layer will determine the ambient temperature there. Natural heating and cooling processes are altered by the introduction of anthropogenic heat from sources like industries and factories, ventilation systems, and internal combustion. These modifiers lead to comparatively slower nocturnal cooling rates in urbanized environments. As a result, average temperatures in urban areas are higher than in the adjacent countryside. These lead to the phenomenon of UHI.

10.1.1 PARADIGM SHIFT IN THE DEFINITION OF URBAN HEAT ISLAND

Urban heat island is a local-scale phenomenon that is characterized by the elevation of the atmospheric and surface temperature of urban regions relative to their surrounding non-urbanized areas. Urban heat islands can be categorized based on methodology, the factors that cause them to develop, and the equipment used to detect them. There are three different types of UHIs: surface, subsurface, and atmospheric. Urban heat islands are surface-level phenomena that can be detected using thermal infrared (remote sense) data that allows extracting land surface temperatures. It is characterized by variations in temperature between the materials in the urban and rural environment. A subsurface heat island exists beneath the city surface and conducts heat down into the ground. Consequently, the temperature distribution of the surface above determines the subsurface temperature (Benz et al., 2022). The third type of UHI is atmospheric, in which the air in urban areas is warmer than the air in adjoining rural areas. It is further classified into two, namely boundary layer urban heat islands and canopy layer UHIs (Oke, 1976; Wang, 2022). Boundary layer UHIs begin from the tops of the trees and buildings and extend up to the region where the urban landscape is unaffected. Canopy layer UHIs exist in the atmosphere's layer above the ground where human influence is greatest and extends up to the tops of trees and roofs. Consequently, the urban canopy layer heat island is essentially a microclimate phenomenon.

The comprehensive research of UHI was started in the early 19th century. There are three types of scientific studies on changes to urban microclimates: observational studies, mitigation studies, and implementation studies. In 1806, Luke Howard (Howard, 1833) conducted the first scientific investigation of urban microclimate. The UHI magnitude was determined by measures of daily maximum and minimum temperature from a small network of common thermometers from urban–rural regions. From the middle of the 19th century, research focused on using micrometeorological theory to understand the mechanisms that result in urban effects. The UHI was interpreted as a consequence of modifications in urban geometry and atmospheric composition. A statistical connection between UHI intensity and meteorological parameters was first investigated by Sundborg in 1950 (Oke, 1995). He correlated UHI intensity with air temperature (T), absolute humidity (e), wind speed (U), and cloud cover (N) as shown in eq 10.2.

$$\Delta T = 2.8 - 0.10N - 0.38U - 0.02T + 0.03e \qquad (10.2)$$

Several studies on various aspects of UHI intensity, including remote sensing and modeling have been conducted all over the world, including India. However, the variation in the definition of urban region from country to country and within country over time causes discrepancies in the comparison of UHI intensity of cities in different regions. This lack of uniformity in the delineation of urban areas was overcome by the introduction of Local Climate Zone (LCZ) classification for the city put forward by Oke, which was modified by Stewart (Stewart and Oke, 2012). Local climate zones are defined as regions of uniform surface-air temperature distribution at horizontal scales of 10^2–10^4 m (Stewart and Oke, 2012).

10.1.2 A REVIEW OF LOCAL CLIMATE ZONE CLASSIFICATION

The LCZ classification is based on canopy aspect ratio, pervious and impervious surface fraction, sky view factor, and anthropogenic heat flux. Stewart and Oke classify the urban–rural built into a hierarchy of 10 climate zones, including compact highrise (CHR), compact idrise (CMR), compact lowrise (CLR), open highrise (OHR), open midrise (OMR), open lowrise (OLR), Large Lowrise (LLR), lightweight lowrise (LWLR), heavy industry (HI), and sparsely built (SB) (Stewart and Oke, 2012).

Three compact zones (CHR, CMR, and CLR) are characterized by sets of buildings and narrow streets with a low sky view factor. These zones use heavy, thick, and well-insulated building materials and have less permeable streets that are paved in concrete or asphalt. Openset zones (OHR, OMR, and OLR) are featured with scattered buildings on a high natural and pervious surface. There is abundant vegetation with less traffic in these zones. Skyline buildings fall under highrise zones of more than 10 stories tall. The height of the buildings in midrise and lowrise zones range of 3–8 stories and 1–3 stories, respectively.

Flat and horizontal lowrise buildings, well separated by paved and open surfaces and extending outward rather than upward, come under the LLR zone. Sparse pervious surface cover with low demand for space heating and cooling and moderate-to-high traffic also feature this zone. Detached and semi-detached single-story buildings with lightweight construction materials come under the LWLR category. This zone is also characterized by unpaved surfaces with abundant vegetation with low traffic flow. The HI zone consists of a large number of small- and large-scale industries and factories with a substantial discharge of excess heat and pollutants. This zone is characterized by a mix of heavy and lightweight construction materials with a high demand for space heating/cooling. Sparsely built zones consist of small or medium buildings scattered across a natural or agricultural landscape with plentiful pervious surfaces. Roads and pavements are narrow with light-moderate traffic density. The previous fraction is greater than 60%, and the average sky view factor is higher than 0.8 in this zone.

10.1.3 RESEARCH OBJECTIVES

The constraints of field measurements can be resolved owing to the use of microclimatic simulation in urban microclimate studies. It is hard to simultaneously measure the meteorological parameters of urban regions as it requires multiple instruments (Sharmin et al., 2017). The introduction of LCZ classification in urban studies imparts the potential to incorporate various modeling tools and simulations in urban microclimate studies. The integration of field measurement data into modeling is made simple by well-defined LCZs with distinctive characteristics. Thus, the use of suitable microclimate models brings an upper edge in urban microclimate studies which leads to policy-making and mitigation strategies (Wong et al., 2011; Tsoka et al., 2018).

This study aims to investigate the responsiveness of ENVI-met, a three-dimensional (3D) microclimatic model with a high temporal and spatial resolution to assess the impact of urban geometry (LCZ zones) on an urban thermal environment in a tropical humid climate (Huttner and Bruse, 2009). This study also examines the outcomes of the ENVI-met model simulation of two distinct zones with diverse building and surface morphology in the urban region of Kochi, a tropical coastal city on the southwest coast of India. The primary data from two locations come under the compact midrise zone (CMZ) (Kochi City Centre) and openset midrise zone (OMZ) (Kakkanadu) selected for simulation in the present study (Thomas et al., 2014). These classes were so chosen to represent a typical urban morphology (e.g., CMR) with dense buildings and excess impervious surface fraction and a second zone with detached buildings and abundant vegetation (OMR).

10.2 METHODOLOGY

The methodology involved in the present study was a combination of field data collection from the LCZs in the study area and simulation using ENVI-met. Field measurements were carried out at CMR and OMR zones at the city of Kochi in the Ernakulum district to measure the diurnal variability of the meteorological parameters, namely, temperature, humidity, and wind speed on 12 and 13 March 2022. The ENVI-met V 5.0.3 was used to run the simulations. The input settings were provided by the area input file, configuration file, and database. Area input files created for the CMR and OMR zones were used in the simulations. ENVI-met Leonardo 5.0 was used to analyze the simulated data. The general methodological framework of the study is provided in Figure 10.1.

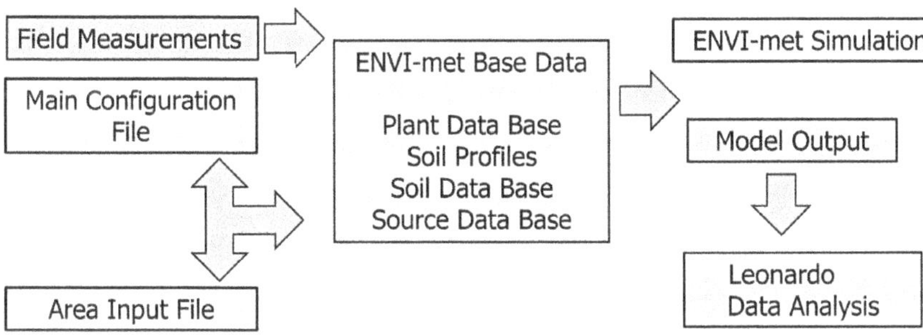

FIGURE 10.1 Methodological framework of the study.

10.3 ENVI-MET MODEL OVERVIEW

The ENVI-met V 5.0.3 fluid dynamics non-hydrostatic model was used for the urban microclimate simulations in the present study. This model is used to simulate the surface-vegetation-air interactions in urban environments and to investigate the spatiotemporal variation of the ambient air temperature. The input parameters for the ENVI-met model consist of meteorological conditions, surface and building morphology, and vegetation. The model can calculate the mean radiant temperature, ambient air temperature at different heights, wind velocity and direction, specific and relative humidity (RH), leaf temperature plant CO_2 flux, etc. This model is designed to simulate the urban characteristics and microclimate of most of the cities, irrespective of geographical features (Rahul et al., 2020; Liu et al., 2021; Cortes et al., 2022).

10.3.1 ENVI-MET SIMULATION

Two sets of simulations with the area input file attributes of the CMZ and the OMZ were used in the current study. The input parameters for the ENVI-met model were given through the configuration file, area input file, and database

(Fig. 10.1). The geographic information for the study area was provided in the area input file using a graphical user interface. 50 ? 50 ? 30 grid cells with a 1-m resolution along the *x*- and *y*-axes were used in this study. For the vertical *z*-axis, 25 cells with a 1 m resolution and a telescopic grid with a 10% telescoping factor after 10 m were used. To enhance the bottom grid's resolution, the lowest grid box was divided into five smaller cells. Building constructions were created using the model's default roof and wall materials like burned bricks and stones and heavy concrete. The vegetation part included grass with an average density of 25 cm, 20 m of very dense grass, 4 m of dense hedging, and 2 m of dense hedging plants that are appropriate for the study region. The simulation also incorporated the loamy soil surface, the asphalt road, and the grey concrete pavement of the current building morphology. A 3D view of the area input file with CMR zone and OMR zone characteristics is shown in Figures 10.2 and 10.3.

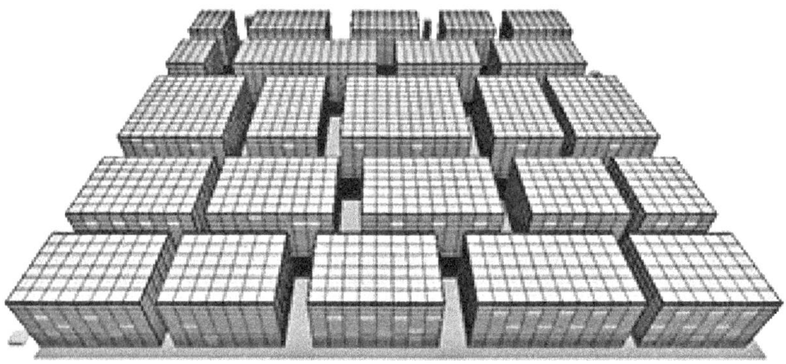

FIGURE 10.2 3D view of area input file with CMR zone properties.

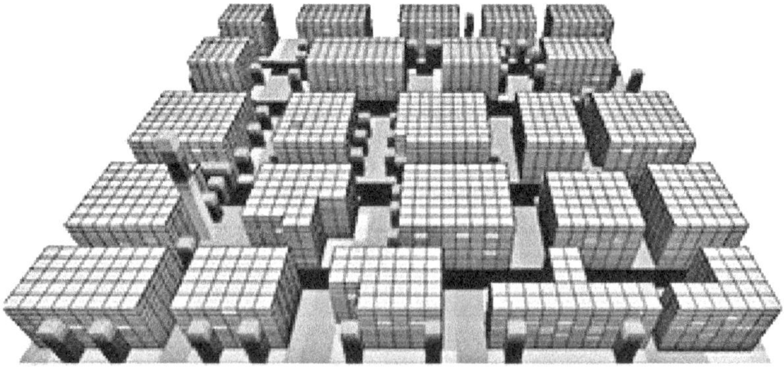

FIGURE 10.3 3D view of area input file with OMR zone properties.

The configuration file provided the ENVI-met simulation settings. The ENVI-met typically has a temporal resolution of 10 s and a spatial resolution of 0.5–10 m (2.0 m in the present investigation). The simulations were run for 48 h and began just before sunrise to follow the daily variation of solar energy. The field measurements and the simulations were conducted on the same days. The measurements were carried out on sunny days with clear sky conditions. Simple forced boundary conditions without a nested grid were used in this investigation. The screenshot of the configuration file is shown in Figure 10.4.

The details of the meteorological input parameters for simulation are given in Table 10.1. Data from the RH-temperature data logger (MadgTech USA, Model: RTDTemp 101) deployed in the study area during field measurements was used to simulate air temperature and RH. The air temperature was measured using automatic temperature recorders with 0.01-K resolution and 0.1-K accuracy. RH was measured with an accuracy of ±3.0% RH and a resolution of 0.1%. A digital anemometer was used to gauge the average wind speed.

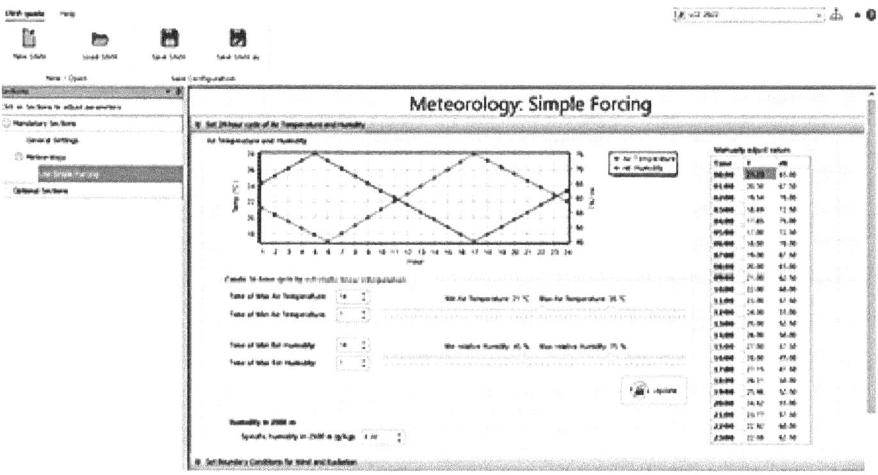

FIGURE 10.4 ENVI-met configuration file.

The simulated data was analyzed by ENVI-met Leonardo 5. The simulation settings used in this study are given in Table 10.1. The results of the simulations with CMR and OMR zones were compared to assess the accuracy and representation of the diurnal variability of the ambient air temperature at the LCZs in the tropical region. ENVI-met Leonardo 5 interface to analyze the output of stimulation is shown in Figure 10.5.

TABLE 10.1 General Simulation Settings for CMR and OMR.

Simulation settings	CMR	OMR
Start date	12.03.2022	12.03.2022
Start time	06:00 am	06:00 am
Total simulation time (h)	48	48
Minimum temperature (°C)	21	20
Maximum temperature (°C)	36	34
Minimum relative humidity (%)	65	50
Maximum relative humidity (%)	85	80
Average wind speed (m/s)	1.6	1.7
Wind direction	N	N
Roughness element in m	15	15

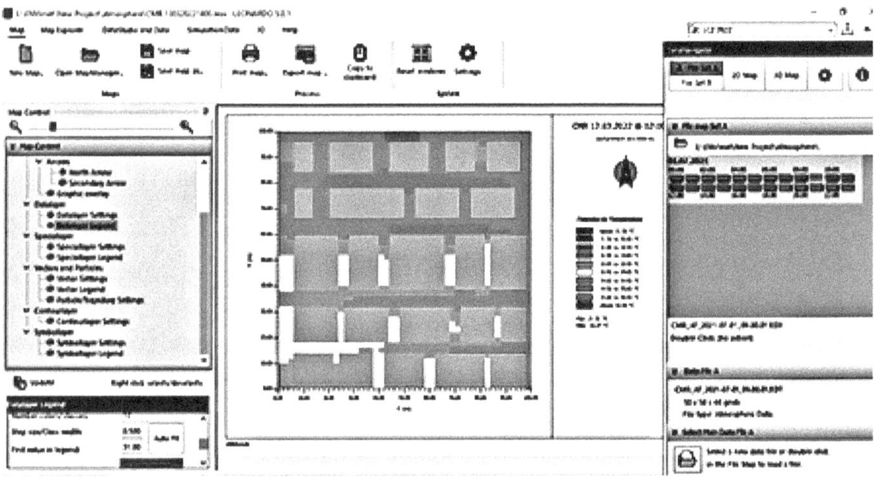

FIGURE 10.5 ENVI-met Leonardo interface.

10.4 RESULTS AND DISCUSSION

The spatiotemporal variability of the ambient air temperature was simulated for 48 h on the days of observations. The outcomes of the simulation imply that the models reasonably reflected the diurnal variations of temperature in both zones. The diurnal variation of ambient air temperature at CMR and OMR zones during simulation and observation is shown in Figure 10.6. CMR (sim) and OMR (sim) indicate the simulated values and CMR (obs) and OMR (obs) denote the observed values of air temperature, respectively.

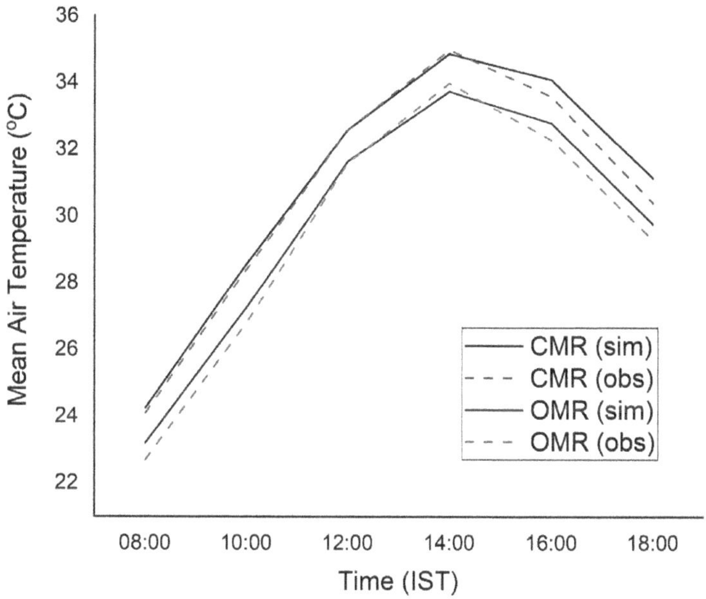

FIGURE 10.6 Observed and simulated diurnal variation of ambient air temperature at CMR and OMR zones.

The accuracy of the simulation was evaluated with error metrics shown in Table 10.2. The pairwise comparison of the observed and simulated air temperature data using a *t*-test at 95% confidence level showed insignificant differences between the observed and simulated temperatures. Therefore, it is clear from the mean and the data spread between observed and simulated values that the model simulations well captured the actual diurnal patterns in the ambient air temperature. The error matrices, including the mean absolute error (MAE), root mean squared error (RMSE), percent error in peak (PEP), coefficient of determination (R2), and mean relative error (MRE) were used to estimate the error in the simulation model predictions.

TABLE 10.2 Error in the Simulations With CMR and OMR Zones.

Zones	Error metrics				
	MAE (?C)	RMSE (?C)	PEP	R2	MRE
CMR	0.81	0.64	0.69	0.94	0.01
OMR	0.98	0.82	0.44	0.88	0.02
Ideal	*0*	*0*	*0*	*1*	*0*
Worst	∞	∞	±∞	*0*	±∞

The estimated error metrics for the zones are typically nearer to their conceptual ideal values, emphasizing that the ENVI-met accurately predicted the hourly variability of the air temperature (Dawson et al., 2007). The simulation results for 07:00, 10:00, 14:00, and 18:00 hours were investigated in detail for brevity. The ENVI-met model was capable of distinguishing two zones in a tropical humid climate with a noticeable variability in ambient air temperature. The summary statistics of ambient air temperature in the two zones is shown in Table 10.3.

TABLE 10.3 Summary Statistics of Ambient Air Temperature in Two Zones During Simulations.

Zones	Time (IST)	Ambient air temperature (?C)			
		Low	High	Mean	Standard deviation
CMR	07:00	21.5	23.0	22.3	0.7
	10:00	27.0	30.1	28.6	1.5
	14:00	33.5	36.3	34.9	1.4
	18:00	30.7	31.6	31.2	0.4
OMR	07:00	20.0	21.5	20.8	0.7
	10:00	26.0	28.5	27.3	1.2
	14:00	32.0	35.5	33.8	1.7
	18:00	29.3	30.2	29.8	0.5

The CMR zone with compact midrise tall buildings with high impervious surface fraction displayed higher temperatures throughout the simulation compared to OMR with tall buildings in open and natural surroundings. The spatial variation of the air temperature ranges between 21.5 and 23.0?C in the CMR zones and it ranges between 20.0 and 21.5?C in the OMR zone at 07:00 h. The mean value for the CMR and OMR zones was 22.3 and 20.8?C, respectively. As the day advances, the ambient air temperature of both zones has risen to 28.6?C (CMR) and 27.3?C (OMR) at 10:00 h. The heating rate was 2.1?C\h and 2.2?C\h in the CMR and OMR zones respectively, from 7:00 h to 10:00 h. The open regions in the OMR get heated up quickly compared to CMR, which consists of compact buildings with narrow streets, resulting in high heating rates in the OMR (Thomas and Zachariah, 2020). Additionally, the OMR zone receives more solar radiation than the CMR zone due to its higher sky view factor. Simulated spatial variability of the ambient air temperature in two zones at 07:00 h and 10:00 h is shown in Figure 10.7.

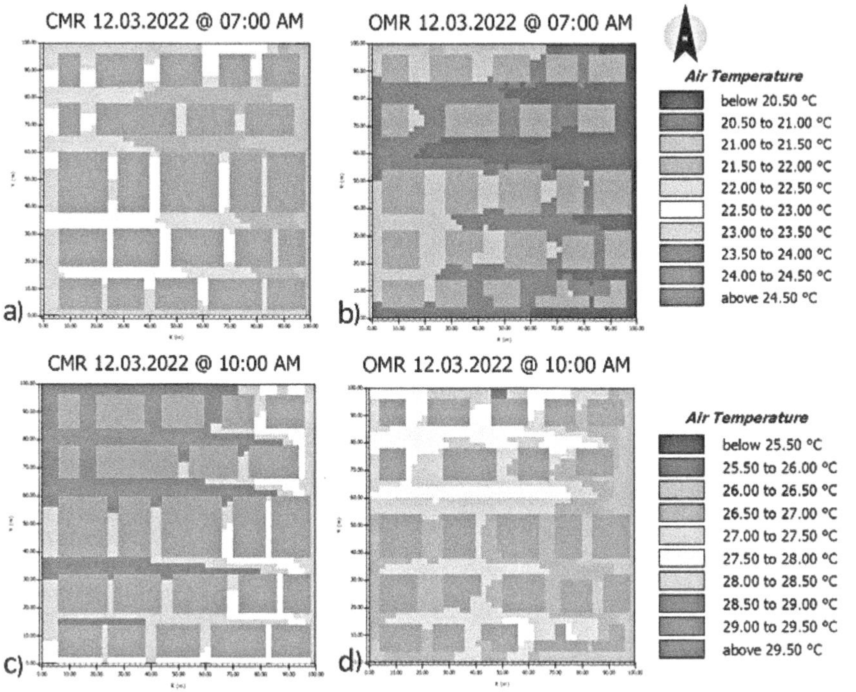

FIGURE 10.7 Simulated spatial variability of the ambient air temperature in the CMR (a, c) and OMR (b, d) zones at 07:00 h and 10:00 h.

At 14:00 h, there was a substantial difference in the mean air temperature between the two zones. The mean temperature of the ambient air was 34.9 and 33.8?C, respectively. The CMR zone attained a maximum temperature of 36.3?C, while OMR reached a maximum temperature of 35.5?C. Between 10:00 and 14:00, the heating rates for CMR and OMR were 1.58?C/h and 1.62?C/h, respectively. However, the cooling phase was initiated in two zones after 14:00 hours. In the CMR and OMR zones, the mean cooling rates during the initial cooling phase were 0.9?C/h and 1.0?C/h, respectively. The cooling rate at OMR is slightly faster compared to the CMR zone. The markedly different urban geometry makes the cooling rates of LCZs differ widely and the growth of the heat island intensity varies as the night advances (Ansar et al, 2012). At 18:00 hours, the mean temperatures in the CMR and OMR zones were 31.2 and 29.8?C, respectively. Simulated spatial variability of the ambient air temperature in two zones at 14:00 h and 18:00 h is shown in Figure 10.8.

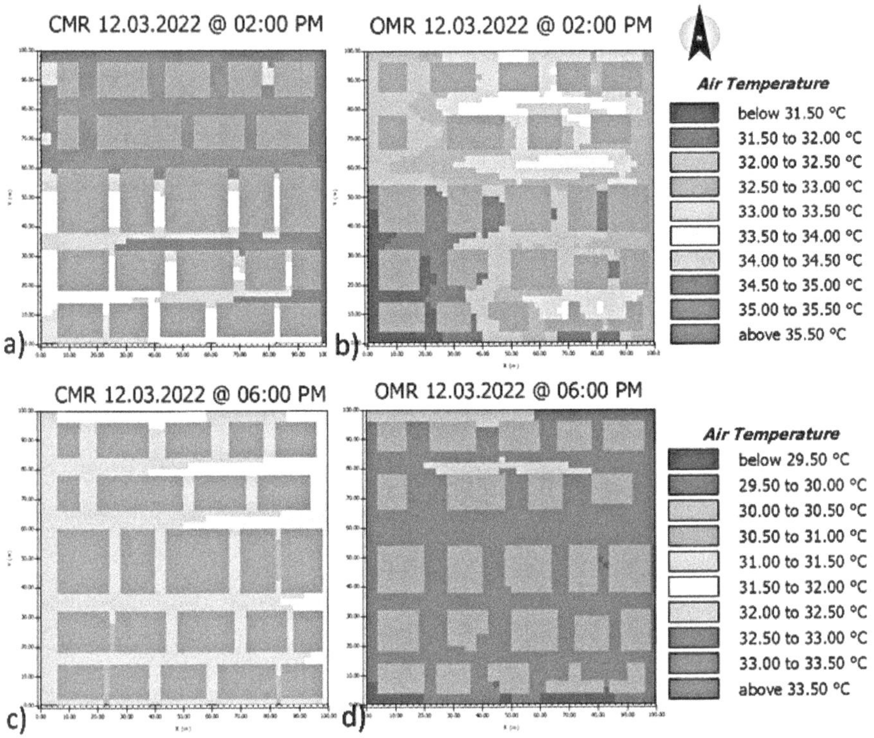

FIGURE 10.8 Simulated spatial variability of the ambient air temperature in the CMR (a, c) and OMR (b, d) zones at 14:00 h and 18:00 h.

The CMR zone with dense built-up and impervious surfaces restores the energy received and released slowly as time advances (Thomas et al., 2014). However, the presence of vegetation in the OMR fastens the cooling level to some extent during the evening. In the late evening, the variation in the cooling level increases, and the temperature differences become prominent leading to the phenomenon called UHI. Thus, urban geometry plays a major role in the variation of temperature in urban regions. Zones with a dense built-up and impervious fraction (e.g., CHR, CMR) enhance the intensity of UHI in the urban environment.

10.5 CONCLUSIONS

The role of urban geometry in the development of thermal gradient between the LCZs was successfully simulated by ENVI-met microclimate model in the tropical humid climate. The simulation results show a good correlation with observed data in the CMZ and CLZs. The model simulations captured well the actual diurnal patterns in the ambient air temperature. The thermal gradient between different zones and cooling rates in the zones were computed, which validates the LCZ classification. The estimated error metrics for the zones are often closer to their ideal values, indicating that the ENVI-met accurately predicted the diurnal variability of the ambient air temperature. CMR zone consists of compact building structures with narrow streets and heavy construction material that showed higher temperatures during simulation, mirroring the trend seen during field measurement. The integration of LCZ classification and ENVI-met modeling the urban microclimate studies resolved the constraints in the field measurements in the urban regions, especially in the Indian subcontinent where most of the cities have evolved from small urban sprawls.

ACKNOWLEDGMENT

The authors are grateful to the Principal, Research Council, and Management of Catholicate College, Pathanamthitta for the encouragement and support extended for this study.

KEYWORDS

- **urban microclimate**
- **ENVI-met**
- **local climate zone**
- **urban geometry**

REFERENCES

Ansar, S.; Dhanya, C. R.; Thomas, G.; Chandran, A.; John, L.; Prasanthi, S.; ... Zachariah, E. J. A Study of Urban/Rural Cooling Rates in Thiruvananthapuram, Kerala. *J. Ind. Geophys. Union* **2012,** *16* (1), 29–36.

Benz, S. A.; Menberg, K.; Bayer, P.; Kurylyk, B. L. Shallow Subsurface Heat Recycling is a Sustainable Global Space Heating Alternative. *Nat. Commun.* **2022,** *13* (1), 1–11.

Census of India. *Urban Agglomerations/Cities having Population 1 Million and Above*; Office of Registrar General of India, Government of India: New Delhi, 2011.

Cortes, A.; Rejuso, A. J.; Santos, J. A.; Blanco, A. Evaluating Mitigation Strategies for Urban Heat Island in Mandaue City Using ENVI-met. *J. Urban Manag.* **2022,** *11* (1), 97–106.

Dawson, C. W.; Abrahart, R. J.; See, L. M. HydroTest: A Web-based Toolbox of Evaluation Metrics for the Standardised Assessment of Hydrological Forecasts. *Environ. Model. Softw.* **2007,** *22* (7), 1034–1052.

Howard, L. *The Climate of London*; London: Dalton, 1833.

Huttner, S.; Bruse, M. In *Numerical Modeling of the Urban Climate—A Preview on ENVI-met 4.0*, 7th International Conference on Urban Climate ICUC-7, Yokohama, Japan, June, 2009; Vol. 29.

Landsberg, H. E. *The Urban Climate. Int. Geophy. Ser.*, Vol. *28*; Academic Press: New York and London, 1981.

Liu, Z.; Cheng, W.; Jim, C. Y.; Morakinyo, T. E.; Shi, Y.; Ng, E. Heat Mitigation Benefits of Urban Green and Blue Infrastructures: A Systematic Review of Modeling Techniques, Validation and Scenario Simulation in ENVI-met V4. *Build. Environ.* **2021,** *200,* 107939.

Oke, T. R. The Distinction Between Canopy and Boundary-layer Urban Heat Islands. *Atmosphere* **1976,** *14* (4), 268–277.

Oke, T. R. Classics in Physical Geography Revisited: Sundborg, Å. 1951: Climatological studies in Uppsala with special regard to the temperature conditions in the urban area. Geographica 22. *Prog. Phys. Geogr.* **1995,** 19 (1), 107–113.

Rahul, A.; Mukherjee, M.; Sood, A. Impact of Ganga Canal on Thermal Comfort in the City of Roorkee, India. *Int. J. Biometeorol.* **2020,** *64* (11), 1933–1945.

Ren, T.; Zhou, W.; Wang, J. Beyond Intensity of Urban Heat Island Effect: A Continental Scale Analysis on Land Surface Temperature in Major Chinese cities. *Sci. Total Environ.* **2021,** *791,* 148334.

Sharmin, T.; Steemers, K.; Matzarakis, A. Microclimatic Modelling in Assessing the Impact of Urban Geometry on Urban Thermal Environment. *Sustain. Cities Soc.* **2017,** *34,* 293–308.

Stewart, I. D.; Oke, T. R. Local Climate Zones for Urban Temperature Studies. *Bull. Am. Meteorol. Soc.* **2012,** *93* (12), 1879–1900.

Thomas, G.; Sherin, A. P.; Ansar, S.; Zachariah, E. J. Analysis of Urban Heat Island in Kochi, India, Using a Modified Local Climate Zone Classification. *Procedia Environ. Sci.* **2014,** *21,* 3–13.

Thomas, G.; Zachariah, E. J. In *Urban Climate and Local Climate Zone Classification in the City of Kochi in India*, AIP Conference Proceedings, Vol. 2287, No. 1, p. 020008; AIP Publishing LLC; 2020. DOI: 10.1063/5.0029887

Tsoka, S.; Tsikaloudaki, A.; Theodosiou, T. Analyzing the ENVI-met Microclimate Model's Performance and Assessing Cool Materials and Urban Vegetation Applications—A Review. *Sustain. Cities Soc.* **2018,** *43,* 55–76.

United Nations. Department of Economic and Social Affairs, Population Division. World Urbanization Prospects: The 2018 Revision (ST/ESA/SER.A/420). United Nations: New York, 2019.

Vidyarthi, S. Spatial Plans in Post-liberalization India: Who's Making the Plans for Fast-growing Indian Urban Regions? *J. Urban Affa.* **2021,** *43* (8), 1063–1080.

Voogt, J. Urban Heat Island. In *Encyclopedia of Global Environmental Change*, Vol. 3; Munn, T., Ed., John Wiley and Sons: Chichester, 2002.

Wang, Z. H. Reconceptualizing Urban Heat Island: Beyond the Urban-rural Dichotomy. *Sustain. Cities Soc.* **2022,** *77,* 103581.

Wong, N. H.; Jusuf, S. K.; Tan, C. L. Integrated Urban Microclimate Assessment Method as a Sustainable Urban Development and Urban Design Tool. *Landsc. Urban Plan.* **2011,** *100* (4), 386–389.

Yang, J.; Menenti, M.; Wu, Z.; Wong, M. S.; Abbas, S.; Xu, Y.; Shi, Q. Assessing the Impact of Urban Geometry on Surface Urban Heat Island Using Complete and Nadir Temperatures. *Int. J. Climatol.* **2021,** *41,* E3219–E3238.

CHAPTER 11

Pharmacokinetic Aspects of Biotechnology Products: Interaction with Artificial Drugs

LALI KIRVALIDZE[1], NINO LOMINADZE[1], MANUCHAR GVARAMIA[1], MANONI KURTANIDZE[1], NINO KOKIASHVILI[1], MAKA ALEXISHVILI[2], NATELA OKUJAVA[3], and MARINA RUKHADZE[1]

[1]*Faculty of Exact and Natural Sciences, Javakhishvili Tbilisi State University, Tbilisi, Georgia*

[2]*Department of Medical Chemistry, Tbilisi State Medical University, Tbilisi, Georgia*

[3]*Department of Neuromedicine, Tbilisi State Medical University, Tbilisi, Georgia*

ABSTRACT

Influence of caffeine (Caff) on the pharmacokinetics of other drugs is especially important due to the presence of Caff in coffee, tea, and other beverages and juices. Hence the present research aimed to study the pharmacokinetic interaction of Caff and risperidone (Risp) in rabbits.

Drugs, Caff, and Risp were administered as single oral doses as well as simultaneously with an interval of 1 h. The sequence of administration of the drugs was varied. Concentrations of Caff and Risp in blood plasma were measured with a high-performance liquid chromatography (HPLC) method. Multiple peaks of Risp appeared in mixtures under the influence of Caff. Considerable changes in absorption and elimination rates, k_{el}, MRT, and $T_{1/2el}$ of Risp are found. Multiple peaks of Caff were observed in mixtures under the influence of Risp. Increasing the rates of both elimination on the first

Application of Engineering Principles and Practices in Biotechnology.
Ann Rose Abraham, Leonardo Sepúlveda Torre, Tamara Tatrishvili, and A. K. Haghi (Eds.)

peaks and terminal elimination takes place. Suppression of the formation of theophylline (Th), one of the metabolites of Caff, occurred in the initial stages of the process.

Thus, suppression of absorption and elimination of Risp takes place under the influence of Caff, also enhancement of elimination of Caff is observed under the influence of Risp. This may be explained by both the competition of these drugs for the enzyme CYP3A4 and the activation of CYP1A2, the principal enzyme for Caff metabolism. In conclusion, our results indicate that different changes in the absorption, distribution, and elimination of the mentioned drugs are considerably influenced by the sequence of drug administration.

11.1 INTRODUCTION

Risperidone (Risp) is an antipsychotic drug, which is widely used in the treatment of schizoaffective and bipolar disorders. It represents a benzisoxazole derivative and acts as a selective antagonist of serotonin $5HT_2$ and dopamine D_2 receptors (Janssen et al., 1998; Leysen et al., 1988; Farde et al., 1995; Nyberg et al., 1996; Sajatovic et al., 2006). Risp is rapidly absorbed, its oral bioavailability is about 70%, and binding with plasma proteins equals 90%. The maximum concentration in plasma is reached in approximately 1 h, but the steady-state concentration is established in 1–5 days. The elimination period ($T_{1/2\ el}$) of Risp is changed within 3–20 h depending on the different factors. Risp undergoes intensive first-pass effect (Mannens et al., 1993; Borison et al., 1994; Heykants et al., 1994). Clearance of Risp is mainly performed by metabolism. Its major metabolite is 9-hydroxyrisperidone (9-OH-Risp), which has an antipsychotic activity similar to that of the parent drug (De Vane, 1995; Daniel, 1995; Aravagiri and Marder, 2002). Risp is metabolized by CYP2D6 and CYP3A4 enzymes (Bozina, 2006; Scordo et al., 1999; Mahatthanatrakul et al., 2007). CYP2D6 plays a predominant role in (+)-9-hydroxylation of Risp and CYP3A catalyzes the formation of the (-)-9-OH-Risp (Yasui-Furukori et al., 2001; Trevor et al., 2003). There are the data about inhibition of CYP2D6 enzymes by Risp (Trevor et al., 2003).

Caffeine (Caff) is a strong stimulator of the central nervous system. Stimulation of metabolic processes in different organs and tissues, as well as secretory action of the stomach, proceed under the influence of Caff.

Caff is absorbed well in the gastrointestinal tract, is permeated easily through tissues, and undergoes demethylation and hydroxylation in the liver (Kot and Daniel, 2009). Metabolism of Caff is realized basically by CYP1A2 enzyme; however, other enzymes also participate in its conversion process (Kot and Daniel, 2009). Caff is considered a validated marker of CYP1A2 enzymes (Kot and Daniel, 2009; Doude van Troostwijk et al., 2003). Some drugs inhibit the biotransformation of Caff, for example, fluvoxamine (Jeppesen et al., 1996; Rasmussen et al., 1998), omeprazole (Rost et al., 1999; Rost and Roots, 1994), ephedra alkaloids (Haller et al., 2002), verapamil (Smits et al., 1986; Stockey, 1996), but some drugs cause induction of Caff, for example, rifampin (Wietholtz et al., 1995). Caff influences renal clearance of lithium (Jefferson, 1988; Mester et al., 1995), the pharmacokinetics of carbamazepine and sodium valproate (Vaz et al., 1998), reduces significantly seizure protective ability of antiepileptic drugs: phenylhydantoin, diazepam, phenobarbitone, and carbamazepine (Kulkarni et al., 1989; Kulkarni et al., 1991).

Study of the drug interaction is topical at the polytherapy because drug interaction may be caused by considerable changes in the processes of absorption, biotransformation, excretion, drug-protein binding, influence on the receptors, etc.

Caff enters the human organism during the consumption of beverages like tea, coffee, colas, carbonated beverages, etc. because Caff is a naturally occurring constituent of many plants used for beverages. Therefore, the study of the influence of Caff on the pharmacokinetics of other drugs is important. The pharmacokinetic interaction of Caff and promethazine was studied by our group previously (Kokiashvili et al., 2012). The goal of our work was the study the pharmacokinetic interaction of Caff and Risp in the organism of rabbits.

11.2 MATERIALS AND METHODS

11.2.1 *EXPERIMENTS IN RABBITS*

The experiments were conducted in full accordance with the legal and statutory acts applicable in Georgia and international agreements ratified by the country, such as the Law of Georgia on Health Care and the European Convention for the Protection of Vertebrate Animals Used for Testing and Other Scientific Purposes. The blood samples were collected from the external ear of the rabbit (with a body weight of 1.7 kg) at several subsequent time points. The ear conches were treated with 70° alcohol. The butterfly was attached to a blood capillary to collect blood samples. The interval between experiments was at least 10 days. Doses of Risp and Caff were administered separately to the rabbit as a single oral dose. Drugs also were administered sequentially with an interval of 1.0 h. The sequence of the administration of drugs was varied.

11.2.2 SAMPLE PRETREATMENT

Extraction of drugs from blood plasma was carried out by liquid-liquid extraction procedure. A 0.15 mL of azaleptin solution (20 μg/mL; internal standard), 1 mL of 2 M sodium hydroxide, and 3 mL hexane-isoamyl alcohol (with ratio 98:2) were added to 0.5 mL of plasma for the determination of Risp. A 0.2 mL of 0.5 M hydrochloric acid, 0.5 mL p-nitroaniline (50 μg/mL), and 3 mL chloroform were added to 0.2 mL of plasma for the determination of Caff. The extraction mixtures were agitated by hand for 1 min and centrifuged for 10 min at 3000*g*. The organic layer was filtered, the filter was washed with 1 mL chloroform and then evaporated to dryness at ambient temperature with a gentle flow of air. The residue was dissolved in 50 μL of the mobile phase and 30–40 μL were injected for HPLC analysis.

11.2.3 CHROMATOGRAPHIC CONDITIONS

The analyses of Risp and Caff were carried out using a microcolumn high-performance liquid chromatograph Milichrom (Nauchpribor, Oryol, Russia) with an ultraviolet (UV) detector. The column (62 × 2 mm, i.d.) used was a Silasorb C_{18} (Lachema, Brno, Czechia) with particle size 5 m. The mobile phase was delivered with a flow rate of 50 μL/min.

The mobile phase used for the determination of Risp was a mixture of methanol-0.05M K_2HPO_4 (pH native 3.6) at a ratio of 35:65 (v/v). As an ion-pairing agent, 0.3% triethylamine (v/v) is added to the mobile phase. Detection was performed at a wavelength of 280 nm.

The mobile phase used for the determination of Caff and Th (theophylline) was a mixture of methanol–water at a ratio of 10:90 (v/v). Water pH is adjusted to 3 with acetic acid. A UV detector was operated at 280 nm.

11.2.4 CALCULATION OF PHARMACOKINETIC PARAMETERS

Pharmacokinetic parameters were calculated by the noncompartment analysis method.

Calculations are based on the area under the plasma concentration vs time curve [area under the curve (AUC)] and on the area under the $C \times t$ vs time curve [area under the first moment curve (AUMC)]. They were calculated by the trapezoidal rule.

The mean residence time (MRT) was calculated by the equation

$$\text{MRT} = \text{AUMC}/\text{AUC} \quad (11.1)$$

The MRT can be related to the average elimination rate constant by the equation

$$k_{el} = 1/\text{MRT} \quad (11.2)$$

$$k_{el} = \text{AUC/AUMC} \quad (11.3)$$

Clearance (CL), specific clearance ($\dot{C}L$) steady-state volume of distribution V_{ss}, and specific steady-state volume of distribution $\dot{V}_{ss}$ are calculated by following equations:

$$\text{CL} = \text{Dose/AUC} \quad (11.4)$$

$$\dot{C}L = \text{CL/m} \quad (11.5)$$

$$V_{ss} = \text{CL} \times \text{MRT} \quad (11.6)$$

$$\dot{V}_{ss} = V_{ss}/\text{m} \quad (11.7)$$

11.3 RESULTS

11.3.1 PHAMACOKINETICS OF CAFF AND RISP IN ORGANISM OF RABBIT

The pharmacokinetic (C_{plasma} – time) curve after administration of 80-mg Caff to the rabbit with a body weight of 1.7 kg is shown in Figure 11.1. The multiple peaks are observed on this curve, herewith the first C_{max} is reached after 3 h, but the second one after 6 h. Theophilline one of the metabolites of Caff reaches its maximum concentration on the second peak of Caff, then C_{Th} diminishes (Fig. 11.1). The conversion degree of Caff into Th (C_{Th}/C_{Caff}, %) is increased per time and reaches approximately 17% (Fig. 11.1).

The pharmacokinetic curve after administration of 10-mg Risp to the rabbit with a body weight of 1.7 kg is shown in Figure 11.2. Similarly, Caff, the concentration of Risp in plasma reaches a maximum twice at 0.6 and 7 h. The calculated values of AUC, AUMC, MRT, k_{el}, $T_{1/2\,el}$, CL, and V_{SS} of Caff and Risp are illustrated in Tables 11.1 and 11.2.

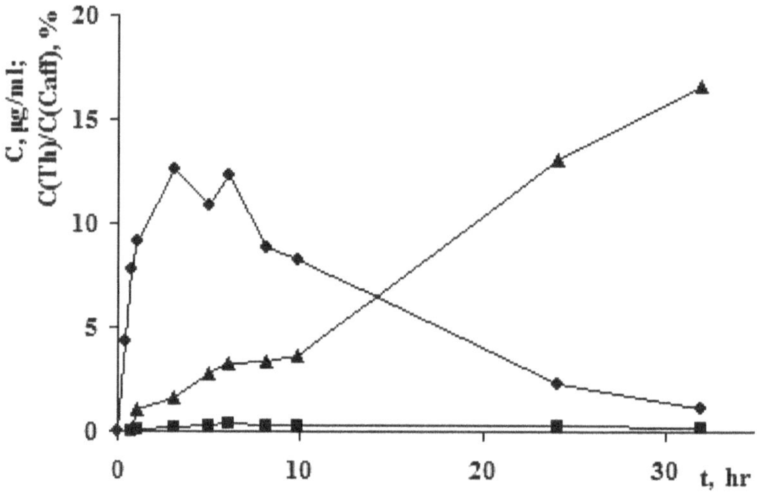

FIGURE 11.1 Plasma concentration–time curves of Caff and Th in the rabbit after oral administration of 80-mg Caff. (-●-) Concentration of Caff; (-■-) Concentration of Th; (-▲-) Dependence of C_{Th}/C_{Caff} ratio in percentage from time.

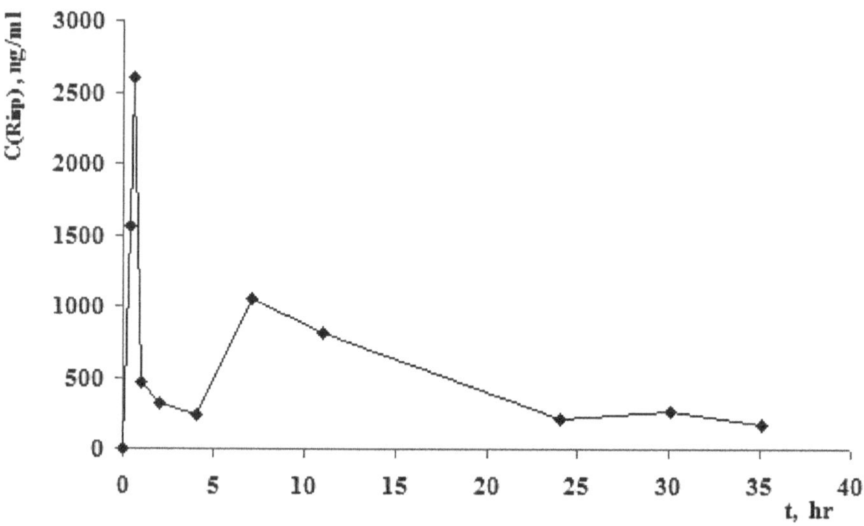

FIGURE 11.2 Plasma concentration–time curve of Risp in the rabbit after oral administration of 10-mg Risp.

TABLE 11.1 Pharmacokinetic Parameters of Caff by Oral Administration of Drugs to Rabbits.

Doses of drugs	AUC (μg/mL) × h	AUMC (μg/mL) × h^2	MRT, h	k_{el}, h^{-1}	$T_{1/2\ el}$, h	CL, l/h	$\dot{C}L$, l/h × kg	V_{ss}, L	V_{SS} l/kg
80-mg Caff	188.43	1847	9.8	0.102	6.79	0.424	0.249	4.156	2.445
80-mg Caff + 10-mg Risp	245	3216.45	13.13	0.076	9.12	0.326	0.192	4.287	2.522
10-mg Risp + 80-mg Caff	195	2141.22	10.98	0.091	7.62	0.41	0.241	4.505	2.65

TABLE 11.2 Pharmacokinetic Parameters of Risp by Oral Administration of Drugs to Rabbits.

Doses of drugs	AUC, (μg/mL)× h	AUMC (μg/mL) × h^2	MRT, h	k_{el}, h^{-1}	$T_{1/2\ el}$, h	CL, l/h	ĊL, l/h × kg	V_{ss}, l	V_{SS} l/kg
10-mg Risp	17,288.8	105,975	6.13	0.163	4.25	0.578	0.34	3.543	2.085
80-mg Caff + 10-mg Risp	18,701	365,973	19.57	0.051	13.59	0.535	0.314	10.47	6.159
10 mg Risp + 80-mg Caff	34,762.6	609,696	17.54	0.057	12.15	0.288	0.169	5.227	3.075

11.3.2 INTERACTION OF RISP AND CAFF IN RABBITS

The sequence of administration of drugs was varied in experiments for investigation of the pharmacokinetic interaction of Risp and Caff: (1) 80-mg Caff was orally administered to rabbit with body weight of 1.7 kg and 10-mg Risp 1 h later (Fig. 11.3). This case is called (Caff + Risp) mixture; (2) 10-mg Risp and 80-mg Caff after 1 h were administered to the rabbit (Fig. 11.4). This case will be designated further as "Risp + Caff" mixture.

The mutual arrangement of pharmacokinetic curves is strongly influenced by the sequence of administration of drugs (Figs. 11.3 and 11.4), namely, the curves are symbate only within time periods 5/11 and 30/48 h in (Caff + Risp) mixture, whereas curves of Risp and Caff are mainly symbate in Risp

+ Caff mixture except intervals of time 3.2/4.6 and 11/24 h, where they are antibate. Besides both drugs reveal four maxima in (Caff + Risp), but three maxima are observed in Risp + Caff mixture.

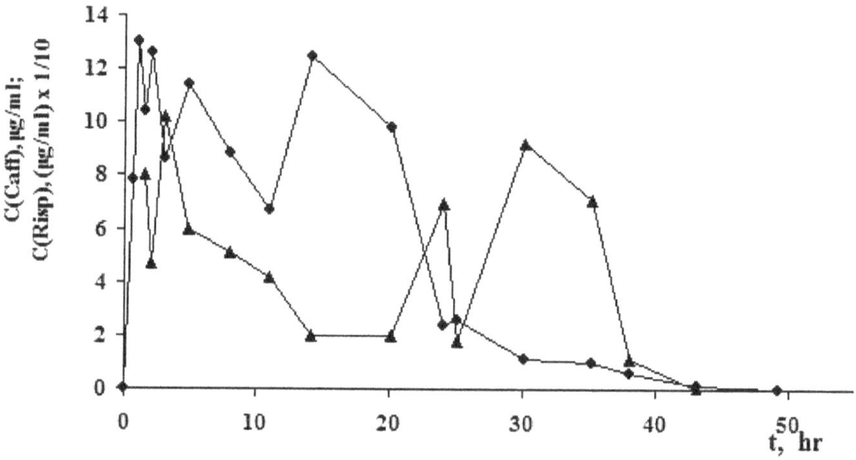

FIGURE 11.3 Plasma concentration–time curves of Caff and Risp in the rabbit after oral administration of 80-mg Caff + 10-mg Risp. (-•-) Concentration of Caff; (-▲-) Concentration of Risp.

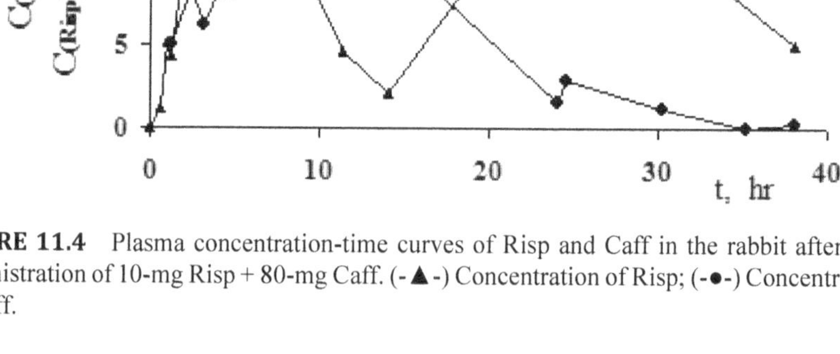

FIGURE 11.4 Plasma concentration-time curves of Risp and Caff in the rabbit after oral administration of 10-mg Risp + 80-mg Caff. (-▲-) Concentration of Risp; (-•-) Concentration of Caff.

11.3.3 INFLUENCE OF RISP ON PHARMACOKINETICS OF CAFF

Dependence of plasma concentration vs time curves for Caff in cases of Caff only, mixtures Caff + Risp and Risp + Caff are given in Figure 11.5.

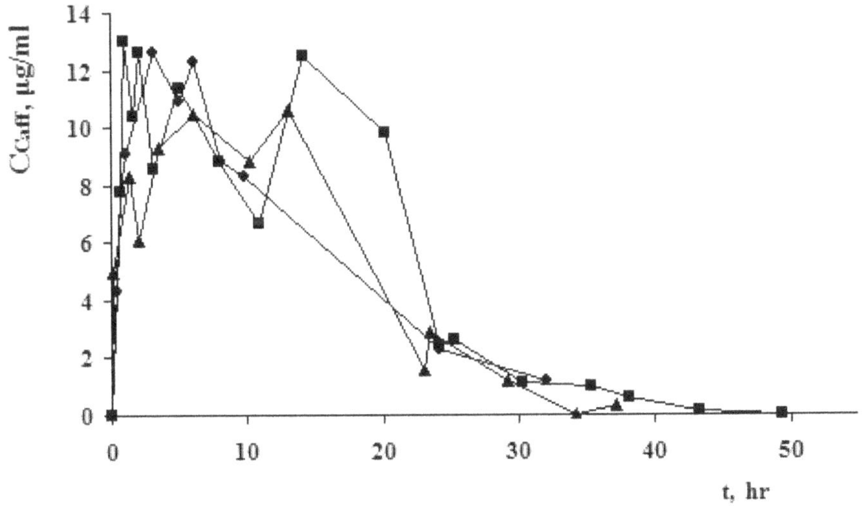

FIGURE 11.5 Plasma concentration–time curves of Caff in the rabbit after oral administration of (-●-) 80-mg Caff; (-■-) 80-mg Caff + 10-mg Risp; (-▲-) 10-mg Risp + 80-mg Caff.

Multiple peaks of Caff are formed under the influence of Risp in both mixtures. Their number reaches four when Caff enters in organism first, but the number of peaks of Caff is equal to three in the case when Risp enters first. The additional peaks of Caff are formed under the influence of Risp in both mixtures. Their number reaches four, where Caff enters into the organism first, but the number of peaks of Caff, where Risp enters first is equal to three. The time for reaching the first peaks is diminished in comparison with Caff only. It should be stressed that pharmacokinetic curves of Caff are symbate in mixtures after approximately 3 h. This means, that the pharmacokinetics of Caff are affected by the sequence of drug administration basically during the first 3 h.

The absorption rates (W_{abs}) of Caff are practically the same in Caff and mixtures and are equal to approximately 12.4/14 (μg/mL)/h. The rates of terminal elimination ($W_{el.term}$) and elimination rates on the first peak ($W_{el.init}$) are increased significantly in the presence of Risp (Fig. 11.6).

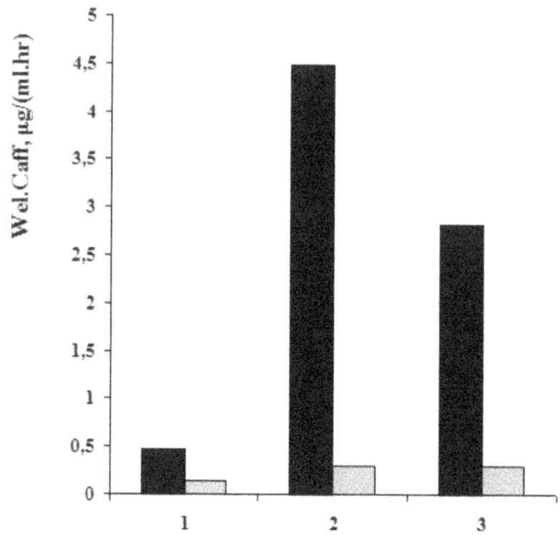

FIGURE 11.6 Initial (■ $W_{el.in}$) and terminal (□ $W_{el.term}$) elimination rates of Caff after oral administration of (1) 80-mg Caff; (2) 80-mg Caff + 10-mg Risp; (3) 10-mg Risp + 80-mg Caff.

The values of all pharmacokinetic parameters in both mixtures and Caff only are close to each other, as illustrated in Table 11.1.

Plasma concentration of Th, one metabolite of Caff, and conversion degree of Caff into Th in mixtures and Caff only are given in Figures 11.7 and 11.8. The suppression of metabolism of Caff in the direction of Th takes place in mixtures, especially in Risp + Caff mixture at the beginning of the process: the time of appearance of Th in plasma is increased, concentration and conversion degree of Th decrease. The concentration of Th later is increased and becomes not only equal but exceeds even the concentration of Th in Caff only (Figs. 11.7 and 11.8).

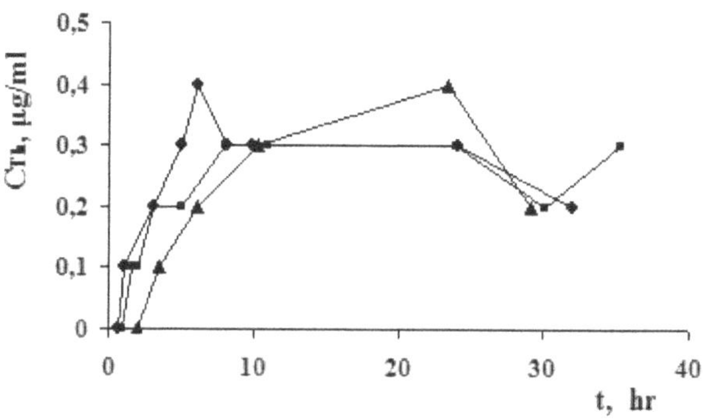

FIGURE 11.7 Plasma concentration–time curves of Th in the rabbit after oral administration of (-●-) 80-mg Caff; (-■-) 80 mg Caff + 10-mg Risp; (-▲-) 10-mg Risp + 80-mg Caff.

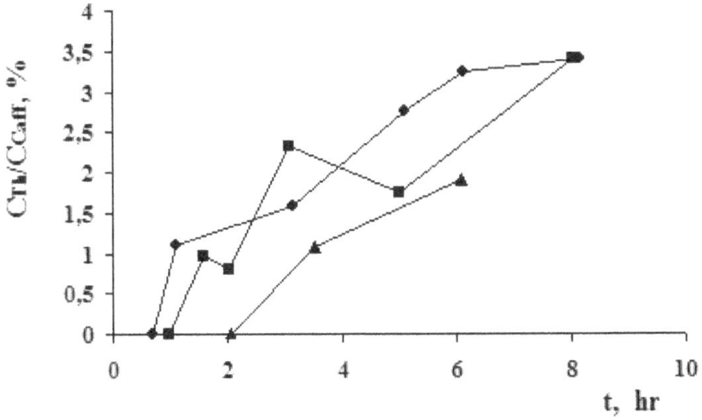

FIGURE 11.8 Curves of conversion degree of Caff into Th (C_{Th}/C_{Caff}, %) vs time in the rabbit after oral administration of (-●-) 80-mg Caff; (-■-) 80-mg Caff + 10-mg Risp; (-▲-) 10-mg Risp + 80-mg Caff.

11.3.4 INFLUENCE OF CAFF ON PHARMACOKINETICS OF RISP

The pharmacokinetic curves of Risp in both mixtures Caff + Risp and Risp + Caff, as well as in the case of administration of Risp only are shown in Figure 11.9. Multiple peaks of Risp are appeared in mixtures as shown in Figure 11.9. Four peaks of Risp are presented in Caff + Risp mixture, but three peaks are observed in Risp + Caff mixture. Besides the first C_{max} in the case of Risp only exceeds considerably all other C_{max} of Risp in mixtures.

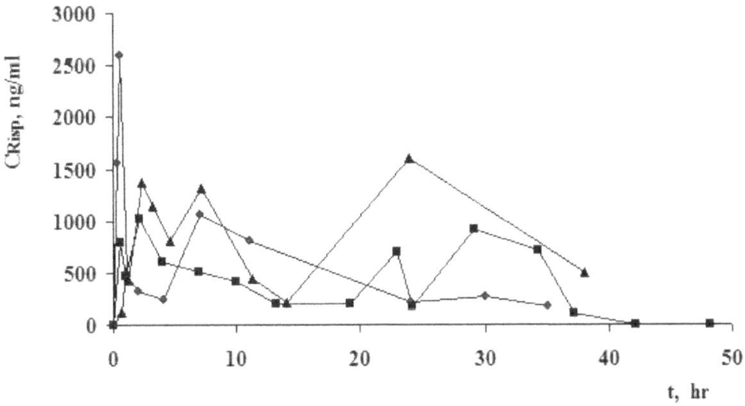

FIGURE 11.9 Plasma concentration-time curves of Risp in the rabbit after oral administration of (-●-) 10-mg Risp; (-■-) 80-mg Caff + 10-mg Risp; (-▲-) 10-mg Risp + 80-mg Caff.

The calculated pharmacokinetic parameters of Risp are illustrated in Table 11.2. As shown in Table 11.2, in mixtures the values of k_{el} are reduced approximately 3-fold, but the values of MRT and $T_{1/2\,el}$ are increased 3 times. The value of AUC 2 times exceeds and CL is 2 times less in Risp + Caff mixture in comparison with Risp only. However, the values of AUC and CL are the same in Caff + Risp mixture as well as in the case of Caff only.

The elimination and absorption rates on the first peaks are sharply decreased in mixtures (Fig. 11.10). The rate of terminal elimination of Risp has the same value in both Caff only and Caff + Risp mixture. As to Risp + Caff mixture, the calculation of the elimination rate was impossible because of a deficiency of terminal points.

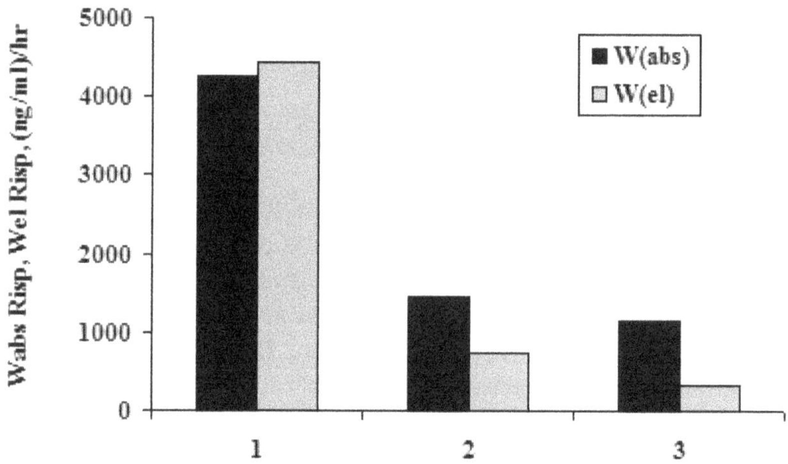

FIGURE 11.10 Absorption and elimination rates of Risp on the first peaks after oral administration of (1) 10-mg Risp; (2) 80-mg Caff + 10-mg Risp; (3) 10-mg Risp + 80-mg Caff.

11.4 DISCUSSION

The formation of additional peaks at the initial stages in both Caff + Risp and Risp + Caff mixtures (Figs. 11.5 and 11.9), also the antibate character of pharmacokinetic curves of Caff and Risp (Figs. 11.3 and 11.4) and a sharp decreasing of absorption rate of Risp (Fig. 11.10) indicates that the competition of Caff and Risp for absorption sites takes place. The competition is stronger in Caff + Risp mixture than in Risp + Caff mixture. In these mixtures, the dosage of Caff was 80 mg and the dosage of Risp was 10 mg. Therefore, in case when Caff enters first an organism, it occupies a significant part of absorption sites and impedes absorption of Risp. As a result, the complex mutual relation of pharmacokinetic curves of Caff and Risp is obtained (Fig. 11.3). However, in the case, where Risp enters first, it occupies some part of the absorption sites and competition gains the softer character (Fig. 11.4). It is possible, that the distinguished affinity of these drugs to the occupation of absorption sites plays some role in this process. The values of absorption rates are affected by the aforementioned competition, namely, absorption rate of Risp is sharply decreased under the influence of Caff (Fig. 11.10), but Risp does not affect the value of the absorption rate of Caff. Thus, the suppression of absorption of Risp under the influence of Caff takes place.

It should be mentioned, that a decrease of plasma concentration of Risp as well as Caff within 5/11 h is observed in Caff + Risp mixture (Fig. 11.3). The concentration of drugs decreases within 7/11 h in Risp + Caff mixture (Fig. 11.4). Such prolonged elimination is followed by the significant increase of concentration of drugs and hence formation of new peaks occurs. It is possible, that drugs within 5/11 hours pass through those segments of intestine, where absorption is strongly limited. Then they reach so-called "absorption window" where absorption intensity increases (Rukhadze et al., 2002).

The curves of Caff and Risp are antibate at intermediate stages of the process, viz. within 14/30 and 11/24 h for Caff + Risp and (Risp+Caff) mixtures respectively (Figs. 11.3 and 11.4). This antibate character is mainly determined by the competition of drugs for elimination. The elimination of Caff from the last peak in both mixtures begins at the same time after 14 h from the beginning of the process when its concentration is within 10.6–12.5 μg/mL. Enhanced elimination of Risp begins when the sharp phase of elimination (24–30 h) from the last peak of Caff is completed and where the concentration of Caff is low (Figs. 11.3 and 11.4). Thus, a competition of Risp and Caff proceeds not only in absorption but also in terminal elimination. Besides Caff suppresses Risp in both cases.

As to the elimination of Risp and Caff at the initial stages, a sharp decrease in the elimination rate of Risp under the influence of Caff (Fig. 11.10) and also a sharp increase of the elimination rate of Caff in the presence of Risp (Fig. 11.6) take place. At the same time, Risp suppresses the elimination of Caff in the direction of Th, namely, Th appears in plasma later and its concentration is smaller in mixtures (especially in the case when Risp enters first in an organism) in comparison with Caff only (Fig. 11.7). Also, the conversion degree of Caff into Th decreases (Fig. 11.8).

It should be mentioned, that Caff has four metabolites: paraxanthine, theobromine, Th, and 1,3,7-trimethyluric acid. Several enzymes participate in the metabolism of Caff. Its metabolism proceeds differently in various species of animals, for example, Caff is converted on five enzymes CYP1A2, CYP3A4, CYP2C8/C9, and CYP2E1 in humans, but four enzymes CYP1A2, CYP2C, CYP2C11, and CYP3A2 are responsible for its conversion in rats (Kot and Daniel, 2009). Herewith the basic metabolite in humans is paraxanthine (70%), but 1,3,7-trimethyluric acid (70%) represents the main metabolite in rats. It should be stressed, that metabolites of Caff are obtained from two or three enzymes in both humans and rats. Vice versa, one enzyme may participate in the formation of different metabolites, for example, CYP 1A2 takes part in the formation of all metabolites in both humans and rats (Kot and Daniel, 2009). Metabolism of Risp proceeds comparatively simply because only two CYP2D6 and CYP3A4 enzymes participate in its conversion (CYP3A4 enzyme determines the system elimination of Risp).

Thus, the CYP3A4 enzyme is common for Caff and Risp, on which they are converted and on which Th is formed. It may be supposed, that a competition for CYP3A4 enzyme takes place in mixtures. This resulted in the inhibition of the metabolism of Caff in the direction of Th on the one hand, and in the suppression of the metabolism of Risp on the other hand. There are data about inhibition of CYP3A4 enzyme by Risp in case of interaction with carbamazepine (Mula and Monaco, 2002).

As to increasing of elimination rate of Caff under the influence of Risp, it is possible that Risp modifies the system of enzymes so, that the conversion of Caff into the other metabolites proceeds more easily with the modified system of enzymes. It is known, that induction and inhibition of enzymes may be caused not only by the compound, which is metabolized by these enzymes but also by the compound, which does not undergo conversion on these enzymes, for example, significant increase of content and activity of CYP1A2 enzyme (main enzyme of metabolism of Caff) is observed in rats after administration of Risp (also promazine, perazine, and clozapine) during two weeks (Daniel, 2005; Rane et al., 1995). Finally, it may be concluded, that inhibition of one direction of metabolism of Caff (conversion into Th) and induction of the other directions proceeded under the influence of Risp.

The mutual arrangement of pharmacokinetic curves is influenced significantly by sequence of drug administration, namely, curves are symbate only within time periods 5–11 and 30–48 h in Caff + Risp mixture

(Fig. 11.3), whereas curves of Risp and Caff are mainly symbate in Risp + Caff mixture, but they are antibate within time periods 3–5 and 11–24 h (Fig. 11.4). Moreover, both drugs have four maxima in Caff + Risp mixture, but three maxima are observed in Risp + Caff mixture. Thus, the different changes in absorption, distribution, and elimination take place according to the sequence of drug administration. It should be mentioned that pharmacokinetic curves of Caff are symbate in the mixture after approximately 3 h from the beginning of the process. This means, that the pharmacokinetics of Caff are basically affected by the sequence of drug administration during the first 3 h.

11.5 CONCLUSIONS

The competition of Risp and Caff for occupation of absorption sites takes place by simultaneous administration of Caff and Risp to the rabbit. Caff diminishes sharply the absorption rate of Risp, but Risp has a slight influence on the absorption rate of Caff.

The competition of Caff and Risp for elimination is observed in mixtures within a time period of 11–30 h. Elimination of Risp is suppressed by Caff: The intensive elimination of Risp begins when the elimination of the basic mass of Caff is already completed and its concentration in blood plasma is low. In mixtures, the value of the terminal elimination constant of Risp is reduced 3-fold, but the same value for Caff decreases only by 34%.

The elimination rate of Risp is sharply decreased and the elimination rate of Caff is increased in mixtures at the initial stages of the process.

The inhibition of the formation of Th and induction of the other directions of metabolism of Caff take place in mixtures under the influence of Risp.

The mutual arrangement of the pharmacokinetic curves is considerably affected by the sequence of drug administration. The different changes in absorption, distribution, and elimination are observed depending on the sequence of drug administration.

ACKNOWLEDGMENT

The research was supported by Shota Rustaveli National Science Foundation Georgia (No.GNSF/ST09_964_4_510).

STATEMENT OF ETHICS

The experiments were conducted in full accordance with the legal and statutory acts applicable in Georgia and international agreements ratified by the country, such as the Law of Georgia on Health Care and European Convention for the Protection of Vertebrate Animals Used for Testing and Other Scientific Purposes.

KEYWORDS

- **caffeine**
- **risperidone**
- **drug interaction**
- **CYP enzymes**

REFERENCES

Aravagiri, M.; Marder, S. R. Brain, Plasma and Tissue Pharmacokinetics of Risperidone and 9-hydroxyrisperidone After Separate Oral Administration to Rats. *Psychopharmacology (Berl)* **2002,** *159* (4), 424–431.

Borison, R. L.; Dimond, B.; Pathiraja, A.; Meibach, R. C. Pharmacokinetics of Risperidone in Chronic Schizophrenic Patients. *Psychopharmacol. Bull.* **1994,** *30* (2), 193–197.

Bozina, N. Interactions of Antiepileptic and Psychotropic Drugs-Pharmacogenetics of CYP Enzymes and P-glycoprotein Transporter. *Paediatr. Croat.* **2006,** *50* (2), 41–48.

Daniel, W. Metabolism of Psychotropic Drugs: Pharmacological and Clinical Relevance. *Pol. J. Pharmacol.* **1995,** *47* (5), 367–379.

Daniel, W. A. The Influence of Long-Term Treatment with Psychotropic Drugs on Cytochrome P450: The Involvement of Different Mechanisms. *Expert Opin. Drug Met.* **2005,** *1* (2), 203–217.

De Vane, C. L. Brief Comparison of the Pharmacokinetics and Pharmacodynamics of the Traditional and Newer Antipsychotic Drugs. *Am. J. Health Syst. Pharm.* **1995,** *52* (3 Suppl. 1), S15–S18.

Doude van Troostwijk, L. J.; Koopmans, R. P.; Guchelaar, H. J. Two Novel Methods for the Determination of CYP1A2 Activity Using the Paraxanthine/Caffeine Ratio. *Fundam. Clin. Pharmacol.* **2003,** *17* (3), 355–362.

Farde, L.; Nyberg, S.; Oxenstierna, G.; Nakashima, Y.; Halldin, C.; Ericcson, B. Positron Emission Tomography Studies on D_2 and 5-HT_2 Receptor Binding in Risperidone-treated Schizophrenic Patients. *J. Clin. Psychopharmacol.* **1995,** *15* (1), 19S–23S.

Haller, C. A.; Jacob, P. V.; Benowitz, N. L. Pharmacology of Ephedra Alkaloids and Caffeine After Single-dose Dietary Supplement Use. *Int. J. Clin. Pharmacol. Ther.* **2002,** *71* (6), 421–432.

Heykants, J.; Huang, M. L.; Mannens, G.; Meuldermans, W.; Snoek, E.; Van Beijsterveldt, L.; et al. The Pharmacokinetics of Risperidone in Humans: A Summary. *J. Clin. Psychiatry.* **1994,** *55,* 13–17.

Janssen, P. A. J.; Niemegeers, C. J. E.; Awouters, F.; Schellekens, K. H. L.; Megens, A. A. H. P.; Meert, T. F. Pharmacology of Risperidone (R64 766) a New Antipsychotic with Serotonin-S_2 and Dopamine-D_2 Antagonistic Properties. *J. Pharmacol. Exp. Ther.* **1988,** *244* (2), 685–693.

Jefferson, J. W. Lithium Tremor and Caffeine Intake. *J. Clin. Psychiatry* **1988,** *49* (2), 72–73.

Jeppesen, U.; Loft, S.; Poulsen, H. E.; Brosen, K. A Fluvoxamine-Caffeine Interaction Study. *Pharmacogenetics* **1996,** *6* (3), 213–222.

Kokiashvili, N.; Alexishvili, M.; Gonashvili, M.; Okujava, N.; Titvinidze, G.; Rukhadze, M. Revealing of Pharmacokinetic Peculiarities of Surface Active Drug Promethazine in Its Interaction with Caffeine in Rabbits. *Colloid Surf. A* **2012,** *413,* 169–173.

Kot, M.; Daniel, W. A. Caffeine as a Marker Substrate for Testing Cytochrome P450 Activity in Human and Rat. *Pharmacol. Rep.* **2009,** *60* (6), 789–797.

Kulkarni, C.; Joseph, T.; David, J. Inhibition of Anticonvulsant Action of Carbamazepine by Aminophylline and Caffeine in Rats. *Indian J. Exp. Biol.* **1989,** *27* (12), 1048–1051.

Kulkarni, C.; Joseph, T.; David, J. Influence of Adenosine Receptor Antagonists, Aminophylline and Caffeine on Seizure Protective Ability of Antiepileptic Drugs in Rats. *Indian J. Exp. Biol.* **1991,** *29* (8), 751–754.

Leysen, J. E.; Gommeren, W.; Eens, A.; De Chaffoy de Courcelles, D.; Stoof, J. C.; Janssen, P. A. J. Biochemical Profile of Risperidone, a New Antipsychotic. *J. Pharmacol. Exp. Ther.* **1988,** *247* (2), 661–670.

Mahatthanatrakul, W.; Nontaput, T.; Ridtitid, W.; Wongnawa, M.; Sunbhanich, M. Rifampin a Cytochrome P450 3A Inducer, Decreases Plasma Concentrations of Antipsychotic Risperidone in Healthy Volunteers. *J. Clin. Pharm. Ther.* **2007,** *32* (2), 161–167.

Mannens, G.; Huang, M. L.; Meuldermans, W.; Hendricks, J.; Woestenborghs, R.; Heykands, J. Absorption, Metabolism and Excretion of Risperidone in Humans. *Drug Metab. Dispos.* **1993,** *21* (6), 1134–1141.

Mester, R.; Toren, P.; Mizrachi, I.; Wolmer, L.; Karni, N.; Weizman, A. Caffeine Withdrawal Increases Lithium Blood Levels. *Biol. Psychiat.* **1995,** *37* (5), 348–350.

Mula, M.; Monaco, F. Carbamazepine-Risperidone Interactions in Patients with Epilepsy. *Clin. Neuropharmacol.* **2002,** *25* (2), 97–100.

Nyberg, S.; Nakashima, Y.; Nordström, A. L.; Halldin, C.; Farde, L. Positron Emission Tomography of In-Vivo Binding Characteristics of Atypical Antipsychotic Drugsm Review of D_2 and 5-HT_2 Receptor Occupancy Studies and Clinical Response. *Br. J. Psychiatry Suppl.* **1996,** *168* (29), 40–44.

Rane, A.; Liu, Z.; Henderson, C. J.; Wolf, C. R. Divergent Regulation of Cytochrome P450 Enzymes by Morphine and Pethidine: A Neuroendocrine Mechanism? *Mol. Pharmacol.* **1995,** *47* (1), 57–64.

Rasmussen, B. B.; Nielsen, T. L.; Brosen, K. Fluvoxamine is a Potent Inhibitor of Caffeine In Vitro. *Pharmacol. Toxico.* **1998,** *83* (6), 240–245.

Rost, K. L.; Fuhr, U.; Thomsen, T.; Zaigler, M.; Brockmoller, J.; Bohemeier, H.; Roots, I. Omeprazole Weakly Inhibits CYP1A2 Activity in Man. *Int. J. Clin. Pharmacol. Ther.* **1999,** *37* (11), 567–574.

Rost, K. L.; Roots, J. Accelerated Caffeine Metabolism After Omeprazole Treatment. *Int. J. Clin. Pharmacol. Ther.* **1994,** *55* (4), 402–411.

Rukhadze, M.; Alexishvili, M.; Gonashvili, M.; Sidamonidze, N. Influence of Dose on the Pharmacokinetics of Promethazine in Rabbits. Comparison of Pharmacokinetics of Promethazine and Chlorpromazine. *J. Biol. Phys. Chem.* **2002,** *2* (3/4), 85–88.

Sajatovic, M.; Madhusoodanan, S.; Fuller, M. A. Risperidone in the Treatment of Bipolar Mania. *Neuropsych. Dis. Treat.* **2006,** *2* (2), 127–138.

Scordo, M. G.; Spina, E.; Facciola, G.; Avenoso, A.; Johansson, I.; Dahl, M. L. Cytochrome P450 2D6 Genotype and Steady State Plasma Levels of Risperidone and 9-hydroxyrisperidone. *Psychopharmacology (Berl).* **1999,** *147* (3), 300–305.

Smits, P.; Thien, T.; van't Laart, A. Influence of Slow Calcium-Channel Blockade on the Vascular Effects of Coffee. *Eur. J. Clin. Pharmacol.* **1986,** *30* (2), 171–175.

Stockey, I. H. *Drug Interactions*, 4th Ed.; Pharmaceutical Press: London, 1996.

Trevor, I.; Prior, M. D.; Baker, G. B. Interactions Between the Cytochrome P450 System and the Second-Generation Antipsychotics. *J. Psychiatry Neurosci.* **2003,** *28* (2), 99–112.

Vaz, J.; Kulkarni, C.; David, J.; Joseph, T. Influence of Caffeine on Pharmacokinetic Profile of Sodium Valproate and Carbamazepine in Normal Human Volunteers. *Indian J. Exp. Biol.* **1998,** *36* (1), 112–114.

Wietholtz, H.; Zysset, T.; Marschall, H. U.; Generet, K.; Matern, S. The Influence of Rifampin Treatment on Caffeine Clearance in Healthy Man. *J. Hepatol.* **1995,** *22* (1), 78–81.

Yasui-Furukori, N.; Hidestrand, M.; Spina, E.; Facciola, G. F.; Scordo, M. G.; Tybring, G. Different Enantioselective 9-hydroxylation of Risperidone by the Two Human CYP2D6 and CYP3A4 Enzymes. *Drug Metab. Dispos.* **2001,** *29* (10), 1263–1268.

CHAPTER 12

Biosensors Technology: The Future of Bio-Informational Engineering

BANKOLE OLUWATOSIN EMMANUEL[1], JOSE SANDOVAL[2], and CRISTOBAL N. AGUILAR[3]

[1]*Department of Chemical Sciences, Faculty of Science and Science Education, Anchor University, Ipaja, Lagos State, Nigeria*

[2]*Departamento de Química Analítica, Facultad de Ciencias Químicas, Universidad Autónoma de Coahuila, Saltillo, México*

[3]*Bioprocesses and Bioproducts Research Group. Food Research Department. Universidad Autónoma de Coahuila, Saltillo, México*

ABSTRACT

Food production is an approach with significant challenges, which considers growing human population and providing clean resources and food qualities caused by various effects of chemicals and biological contaminants, such as bacteria.

For the safety of the food industries and also to ensure human health, this chapter devoted on using biosensors, which are smart, quick, and reliable for the screening of both food biological or microbial (e.g. pathogens) and chemical contaminants that adversely affect the food quality and safety.

12.1 INTRODUCTION

Food and its wholesomeness are pertinently indispensable to human lives and survival (Arora et al., 2011). However, food production is currently

---

Application of Engineering Principles and Practices in Biotechnology.
Ann Rose Abraham, Leonardo Sepúlveda Torre, Tamara Tatrishvili, and A. K. Haghi (Eds.)

accosted with great challenges, which include growing human population and maintaining clean resources and food qualities caused by adverse effects of chemicals and biological contaminants, especially, bacteria (Garnett, 2013).

Bacteria are present in all living things including plants due to the vital role they play in ecology of the planet and in daily activities. Good bacteria are used for food products such as yogurt, cheese, and fermented sausages, while those that are harmful to health and must be avoided are referred to as "pathogen" (FMPRE). It is important to note and understand that natural toxins from microorganisms and substances produced when food is heated are of major interest (Schrenk, 2004), and therefore should be of great focus. According to Schrenk, satisfactorily formulated food quality control, food toxicology, and nutritional knowledge are main requirements for results-oriented scientific risk assessment and implementation of regulations (Schrenk, 2004). To safeguard the food industries' reputation and also ensure human health sustenance after food consumption, food allergens, microbial sampling, and analysis are very important. The ever-*increasing demand* to stop the sudden occurrence of microorganism causing diseases and ensuring food safety are global public health issues of great concerns as well as incontrovertible in the food industry (Shaibani et al., 2018; Zhang, 2019). For instance, it was reported that food recalls cost an average of $15 million per incident and caused remarkable harm to brands' reputation and credibility. Also, foodborne illnesses caused 48 million sick and was responsible for 3000 fatalities annually (Ghorashi). Foods devoid of microorganism-causing disease and other contaminants enhance and increase hygienic and nutritive values. Microbial analysis of foods or food products is a worldwide issue due to daily growing spread of infectious diseases through foods which is deadly for numerous people in the world (Arora et al., 2011). Also, early discovery of food products that contain microorganisms that have potential to cause diseases is pivotal for keeping them away from being consumed by the people (Shaibani et al., 2018).

The routine traditional detection methods of microbial identification (e.g. *Salmonella, E. Coli., Listeria monocytogenes etc.*) in contaminated foods basically include morphological evaluation of the pathogen and experiment to predict its growing potential in different media under varying conditions (Washington, 1996; Pividori and Alegret, 2010). This conventional diagnostic methods are restricted by delayed analysis times, expensive, and laborious sample preparation, the need for skilled or technical-know-how workers (Davis et al., 2013; Mishra et al., 2018), and can only be performed on previously produced foods (Vidic et al., 2019). Moreover, the regular methods of extracting and identifying bacteria in food substances depend on the four major steps, listed as follows (Tietjen and Fung, 1995):

1. Pre-enrichment,
2. Selective enrichment in selective and varying media,
3. Biochemical screening, and
4. Serological confirmation

Consequent to the reality of the life-threatening effect of unwholesome food or food products and their potential as an infectious agent of many familiar diseases (Arora et al., 2011), the new emerging researches are now devoting efforts on using biosensors, which are smart, quick, and reliable for the screening of both food biological or microbial (e.g. pathogens) and chemical contaminants that adversely affect the food quality and safety (Scognamiglio et al., 2014). Also, analysis of food pathogens using modern tools is very pertinent in research because of the rapid expansion of food trade, especially to meet hygienic and pathogen-free foods by the growing world population that may exceed nine billion by 2050 (Viswanathan et al., 2009; Busemeyer et al., 2013).

12.2 BIOSENSORS AND COMPONENTS

Historically, the beginning of the applications of biosensors can be traced to the remarkable work done on the continuous monitoring of blood oxygen levels during cardiovascular surgery in 1962 (Clark and Lyons, 1962). Biosensors are analytical devices used for the detection of chemical substances. They change a biotic response into an understandable and simple electrical indicator (Di Lorenzo, 2016; Mehrotra et al., 2016). The main parts of a common biosensors comprise: (1) bioreceptors or biomolecules; and (2) physical transducer or physicochemical like electrode.

12.2.1 TYPES OF BIOSENSORS FOR ANALYSIS

Biosensors can be grouped on the basis of the device known as transducer or biorecognition elements (bioreceptors) involved in their configurations as shown in Figure 12.1. Based on the device, biosensors are further grouped as calorimetric, electrochemical, optical, piezoelectric, and thermal biosensors (Di Lorenzo, 2016; Sawant, 2017; Girigoswami and Akhtar, 2019).

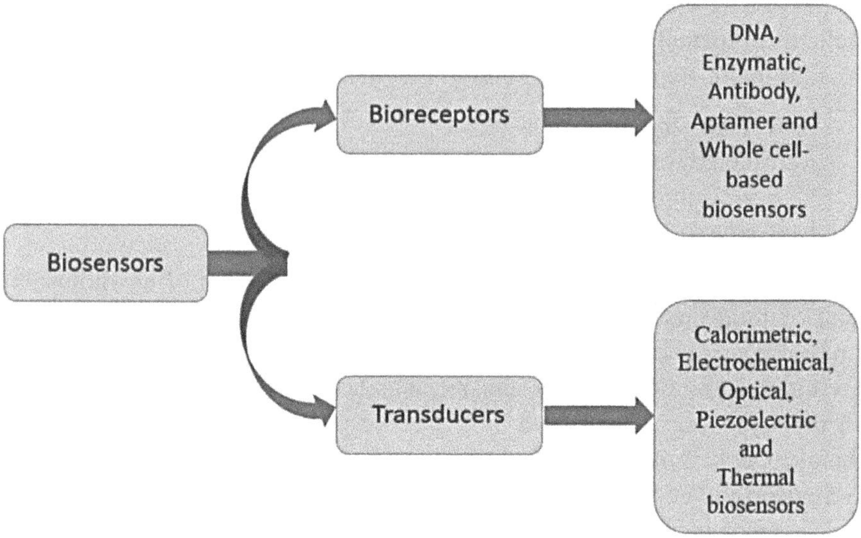

FIGURE 12.1 Types of biosensors based on the devices and bioreceptors.

12.2.1.1 BIORECEPTOR-BASED BIOSENSORS

The bioreceptor is the sensitive component which identifies and interacts directly with desired chemical substance. On the basis of the bioreceptor or biorecognition elements unit used for the fabrication, biosensors can be classified further as antibody-based, aptamer-based, and others, as listed in Figure 12.1 (Sawant, 2017). Further information about the first-four mentioned will be given with their uses in the detection and identification of pathogen in food substances.

12.2.1.1.1 Antibody-Based Biosensor (Immunosensor)

Antibody-based biosensors (immunosensors) ensure rapid and sensitive analysis for the detection of many microorganisms causing diseases and related harmful chemicals (Byrne et al., 2009; Kang et al., 2009). Antibodies are also referred as immunoglobulin produced in the body in defense of foreign antigen or invading pathogen (Banada and Bhunia, 2007). They are standard bioreceptors that give elevated specificity and sensitivity to sensors for pathogen detection (Byrne et al., 2009; Sharma et al., 2016). The applications of these biosensors include a hand-held device designed for the immunomagnetic identification and analysis of *Escherichia coli* present in food and biological samples (Mujika et al., 2009). An enzyme-linked immunosorbent assay (ELISA) and SPR biosensor platform were also fabricated for studying antigen–antibody interactions (Wei et al., 2007). Moreover, an antibody-based biosensor referred as magneto-elastic immunosensors has also been fabricated to identify bacteria causing diseases and other harmful chemicals (Menti et al., 2016).

12.2.1.1.2 Aptamer-Based Biosensor

Aptamer-based biosensors are the most powerful techniques in biosensing. Modification of chemical substance plays vital roles in excellent aptamer biosensor platform, which enhances efficient aptamer immobilization on the surface (Pol et al., 2019). Deoxyribonucleic acid (DNA) or ribonucleic acid (RNA) is the aptamer that selectively link to substances of interest, similar to antigen–antibody interaction (Zhou et al., 2014; Zhang et al., 2018). They can be chosen by a method known as systematic evolution of ligands through exponential enrichment (SELEX) (Teng et al., 2016). Moreover, aptamers possess many advantages compared to traditional antibodies. The merits are small in size, chemical stability, cost effectiveness, remarkable flexibility in design, high sensitivity, and selectivity (Song et al., 2008). Aptamer-based biosensors have been applied in the food industry, especially for water and food pathogens detection due to their extremely high affinity and specificity. The applications include the testing of the effectiveness of an aptamer-based biosensor by a potentiometer for the detection of *Escherichia coli* cells present in apple juice (Zelada-Guillén et al., 2010); impedimetric aptasensor to identify human pathogen *Staphylococcus aureus* (*S. aureus*) (Reich et al., 2017) and *E. coli* O78:K80:H11 in water, juices, and milk samples (Kaur et al., 2017). Meanwhile, a comprehensive preparation and application of aptamer-based biosensors in rapid detection of *E. coli* has been reviewed (Zhao et al., 2018).

12.2.1.1.3 DNA-Based Biosensor

The development and application of biosensors in food industry is solely for rapid and exact identification of foodborne pathogens to avert the spread of foodborne diseases. This goal is achievable by the use of low cost and highly sensitive electrochemical DNA biosensors (Wu et al., 2019). A lot of researches have been performed on applications of DNA and/or gp120 aptamer biosensors (John et al., 2014; Song et al., 2018; Singh et al., 2013; Singh et al., 2010). The DNA-biosensors such as DNA nanopyramids platform has been used for the identification of *E. coli* lipopolysaccharides and lysate (Giovanni et al., 2015) and *Salmonella* (Suryapratiwi et al., 2017; Savas et al., 2018). Besides, a DNA-based piezoelectric biosensor has been considered specific for the identification of the mecA gene of *Staphylococcus aureus* (Tombelli et al., 2006).

12.2.1.1.4 Enzymed-Based Biosensor

Enzymes are biological catalysts produced within the living organisms, specifically to increase the rate (about 10^{17}-fold or more) of biochemical reactions by lowering the activation energy (Miller and Wolfenden, 2002; Mäntsälä and Niemi, 2009; Ashrafi et al., 2019). Enzymatic biosensors have been used in food analysis with high sensitivity, good detection limit, and high reproductive report (Monosik et al., 2012). Example of enzyme-based biosensors is a 2D lactate electrochemical biosensor designed for lactace determination (Parra-Alfambra et al., 2018). According to Sharma et al., labeled antibody with enzymes can be employed for identification of *Campylobacteria jejuni, E Coli.*, and *Listeria monocytpogenes* (Sharma et al., 2013). Generally, ELISA is the most commonly used immunodiagnostic technique (Kokoskova and Janse, 2009; Vashist and Luong, 2018).

12.2.1.2 TRANSDUDERS-BASED BIOSENSORS

The transducer is the physicochemical like electrode, which transforms the biological interaction received into the electronic or bio-electrochemical signals. The information from the transducer is further amplified, processed, and then displayed by the detector in the course of analysis. Examples of transducers include optical fiber, vibrating quartz, and others (Di Lorenzo, 2016; Bănică, 2012; Dincer et al., 2019). Specifically, the most commonly used biosensor systems based on their transducer properties for the detection of pathogens in foods and drinks are surface plasmon resonance, potentiometric, etc. (Leonard et al., 2003). Electrochemical biosensor and its group (amperometric and potentiometric-based) and optical-based biosensors will be discussed, providing information about their applications in food pathogen detection.

12.2.1.2.1 Electrochemical Biosensors

The electrochemical biosensors are better than other analytical transducing systems because they are very sensitive and have prospect of miniaturization (Palchetti and Mascini, 2008). Besides, electrochemical biosensors have a wide range of linear response, excellent stability, and reproducibility (Tutulea et al., 2012). Further grouping of electrochemical biosensors are conductometric, amperometric, and potentiometric (Girigoswami and Akhtar, 2019; Palchetti and Mascini, 2008; Terry et al., 2005). The signal measurement and elucidation for biological samples are usually electrochemical in nature, where the transducer used is bio-electrochemical element (Mishra et al., 2018). Examples of these biosensors already exploited for the identification and analysis of food pathogens are indicated in Table 12.1. The typical set-up of an electrochemical biosensor for food pathogens detection is shown in Figure 12.2.

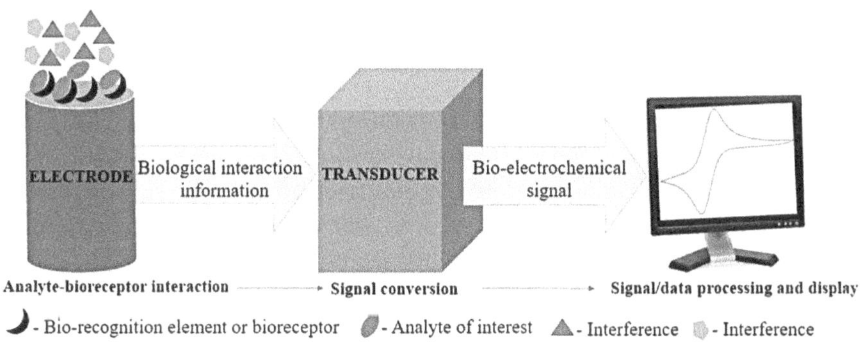

FIGURE 12.2 Typical electrochemical biosensor for food pathogens detection, showing the features.

12.2.1.2.1.1 Amperometric Biosensors

Amperometric biosensor is one of the electrochemical detection method that has been extensively researched for identification of food and water pathogen. (Sharma et al., 2013; Leonard et al., 2003; Palchetti and Mascini, 2008). Amperometric biosensors usually measure the current resulting from redox reaction that biologically active substance undergoes for identified signal quantification (Sadeghi, 2013). The use of amperometric biosensor in food pathogen analysis includes the detection of *E. coli* O157:H7 (Rochelet et al., 2015; Dhull et al., 2019).

12.2.1.2.1.2 Optical-Based Biosensors

Optical-based biosensors are another transducer-based biosensors with can be used for the detection of pathogens in food substances. The types of optical-based biosensors are surface plasmon resonance (SPR), fluorescence, and bioluminescent optical fibre etc (Damborský et al., 2016). The optical-based biosensors have the excellence of portability, label-free detection of biological and chemical substances, direct and real-time measurement, highly sensitive, specificity, and cost effectiveness (Singh, 2017; Peltomaa et al., 2018). However, optical biosensors have been considered suitable for repetitive analysis or continuous monitoring. (Ligler, 2008). Optical-based biosensors can detect *Listeria monocytogene* (Vizzini et al., 2019; Ohk and Bhunia, 2013) as well as *Salmonella typhimurium* (Seo et al., 1999). Also, oligomers of acylated lysines (OAKs) optical biosensors, capable of providing various possible sequence combinations for fabricating new detection platforms have been used for preferential capture of *E. coli* cell (Tenenbaum and Segal, 2015).

12.2.1.2.1.3 Potentiometic Biosensors

Potentiometric biosensors as subdivision of electrochemical biosensors are devices incorporating a biological sensing element connected to an electrochemical potential transducer (Yunus et al., 2013). The biosensors measure the potential difference between two electrodes under the condition no current flows and use the potential measured for analytical quantification of the component of interest in solution (Cosio et al., 2012). Potentiometric biosensors can detect the level of bacteria present in food substances by measuring changes in the pH of the medium (Jiang et al., 2018). Potentiometric biosensors can be used for the detection of *E. coli* (Shaibani et al., 2018; Massad-Ivanir et al., 2016). Additionally, *Salmonella typhimurium* was detected using a potentiometric magnetic immunoassay according to Silva et al. (2015).

12.3 PATHOGENS OF FOCUS IN FOODS USING BIOSENSORS

The pathogens of serious concerns in the food substances include-*Salmonella* (*Salmonella Typhimurium Salmonella enterica, Salmonella enteritidis*), *E. coli* O157:H7, etc. *Salmonella* and *E. coli* O157:H7 will be discussed, while Table 16.1 gives summary of some other pathogens detected using biosensors.

12.3.1 SALMONELLA

Salmonella species are the main pathogens common to both animals and humans. There are two different species of *Salmonella* such as *Salmonella enterica and Salmonella bongor*. *Salmonella enterica* is further split into six subspecies (Creative-Biolabs). *Salmonella* is a Gram-negative bacilli, responsible for most of the foodborne pathogens around the world, especially for more than millions of illness annually in the United States alone (Bell et al., 2016; Ricke et al., 2018). Low numbers of *Salmonella* cells in foods can be infectious. This necessitates the need for serious food safety and safeguarding measures through earlier, brisk, proven detection, and recognition of the microorganisms causing disease at all stages in the food systems (Tietjen and Fung, 1995; Bell et al., 2016; Ricke et al., 2018), especially by improved method of analysis.

12.3.2 ESCHERICHIA COLI O157:H7

Escherichia coli (E. coli) is among the most recurrent pathogens found in human bacterial infections (Pividori and Alegret, 2010), causing several major outbreaks in the past (Dhull et al., 2019). Primarily, the bacteria normally lives in lower intestines and also in the gut of some animals (vertebrates), predominantly as aerobic organism, living in symbiosis with its host (Tenaillon et al., 2010). E. coli strain are harmless, but some strains of *E. coli* can cause diarrhea if contaminated foods and fouled water are eaten and drank, respectively (WebMD LLC). There are many reports on *E. coli* outbreaks due to consumption food processing inadequacy or contaminated foods. For instance, there was an *E coli* O157:H7 spread due to mistake made during meat processing and cooking. The report revealed that the epidemic was due to the fast food eaten earlier (Bell et al., 1994). The spread of *E. coli* O157:H7 among the residents due to consumption of contaminated ground beef products was reported by the Department of Health of Colorado in 2002 (Centers for Disease Control and Prevention, 2002). Also, the spread of *E. coli* O157:H7 was linked to eating infectious ground beef according to Vogt in 2005 (Vogt and Dippold, 2005). According to Hussein, eating beef products containing Shiga toxin as well as ground beef not properly cooked has been causing wide spread human infections in the world since many years now (Hussein, 2007). Moreover, *E. coli* O157:H7 has been reported as an emerging cause of foodborne illness, and also identified as the leading cause of post-diarrheal hemolytic-uremic syndrome (HUS) and acute renal failure in infancy and childhood (Peacock et al., 2001).

TABLE 12.1 Examples of Food Products Pathogens Detected by Biosensors.

Pathogens	Food sample	Biosensor	Detection limit	References
Campylobacter jejuni	Broiler	SPR	1×10^3 CFU/mL	Wei et al., 2007
E. coli	Orange	Potentiometric	1×10^2 CFU/mL	Shaibani et al., 2018
E. coli	Apple Juice	Potentiometic aptamer-based	1×10^4 CFU/mL	Zelada-Guillén et al., 2010
E. coli	Water, juice and milk samples	Impedimetric aptasensor	1×10^1–10^6 CFU/mL	Kaur et al., 2017
E. coli	RTE meat	Multiplex fiber optic	1×10^3 CFU/mL	Ohk and Bhunia, 2013
E. coli	Water	Optical	$>10^7$ CFU/mL	Massad-Ivanir et al., 2016
E. coli	Vegetable food	Antibody-based	1–2 × 101 CFU/mL	Ercole et al., 2003
E. coli	Water	MSMC	1×10^5 CFU/mL	Fu et al., 2010
E. coli	Chicken	MSPR	14 CFU/25 g (mL)	Zhang et al., 2017
Listeria monocytogenes	RTE meat	Multiplex fiber optic	1×10^3 CFU/mL	Ohk and Bhunia, 2013
Listeria monocytogenes	Chicken	MSPR	28 CFU/25 g (mL)	Zhang et al., 2017
Salmonella	Chicken	Microfluidic-based fluorescence	1×10^3 CFU/mL	Kim et al., 2015
Salmonella	RTE turkey	Impedance-based	8 cells/mL	Liu et al., 2018
Salmonella	RTE turkey	Microfluidic-based impedance	300 cells/mL	Liu et al., 2019
Salmonella	Poultry	Impedance-based	7 cells/mL	Jasim et al., 2019
Salmonella typhimurium	Chicken	Microfluidic-based impedance	10 cells/mL	Abdullah et al., 2019
Salmonella enterica	RTE meat	Multiplex fiber optic	1×10^3 CFU/mL	Ohk and Bhunia, 2013
Salmonella enteritidis	Chicken	MSPR	6 CFU/25 g (mL)	Zhang et al., 2017
Staphylococcus aureus	NS	SWCNT-based	1×10^4 CFU/mL	Choi et al., 2017

CFU, colony forming units; MSMC, magnetostrictive microcantilever; RTE, ready-to-eat; SEB, simultaneous enrichment broth; MSPR, multichannel surface plasmon resonance; SPR,surface plasmon resonance; SWCNT, single-walled carbon nanotube; NS, not specific.

12.4 CONCLUSION

Food and its wholesomeness are indispensable to human lives and survival. The presence of pathogens or microorganisms in any food substance (liquid, solid, or semi-liquid) will make it unhealthy for human consumption, leady to foodborne outbreaks. Considering the life-threat involved in eating contaminated food, the limited conventional diagnostic methods cannot provide the urgency demands in food microbial analysis. Instead, more efforts must be devoted to improving on the use of biosensors, which are smart, rapid, and reliable for screening both food biological or microbial and chemical contaminants that adversely affect the food quality and safety.

KEYWORDS

- **biosensors technology**
- **microorganisms**
- **food substance**
- **microbial analysis**
- **chemical contaminants**

REFERENCES

Abdullah, A.; Dastider, S. G.; Jasim, I.; Shen, Z.; Yuksek, N.; Zhang, S.; Dweik, M.; Almasri, M. Microfluidic Based Impedance Biosensor for Pathogens Detection in Food Products. *Electrophoresis* **2019,** *40* (4), 508–520.

Arora, P.; Sindhu, A.; Dilbaghi, N.; Chaudhury A. Biosensors as Innovative Tools for the Detection of Food Borne Pathogens. *Biosens. Bioelectron.* **2011,** *28,* 1–12.

Ashrafi, A. M.; Sýs, M.; Sedláčková, E.; Farag, A. S.; Adam, V.; Přibyl, J.; Richtera, L. Application of the Enzymatic Electrochemical Biosensors for Monitoring Non-Competitive Inhibition of Enzyme Activity by Heavy Metals. *Sensors* **2019,** *19* (13), 2939.

Banada, P. P.; Bhunia, A. Antibodies and Immunoassays for Detection of Bacterial Pathogens. In *Principles of Bacterial Detection: Biosensors, Recognition Receptors, and Microsystems*, 2007. DOI: 10.1007/978-0-387-75113-9_21

Bănică, F.-G. *Chemical Sensors and Biosensors: Fundamentals and Applications*; John Wiley & Sons: Chichester, UK, 2012; p 576.

Bell, B. P.; Goldoft, M.; Griffin, P. M.; Davis, M. A.; Gordon, D. C.; Tarr, P. I.; Bartleson, C. A.; Lewis, J. H.; Barrett, T. J.; Wells, J. G.; et al. A Multistate Outbreak of *Escherichia coli* O157:H7- Associated Bloody Diarrhea and Hemolytic Uremic Syndrome from Hamburgers. The Washington Experience. *JAMA* **1994,** *272* (17), 1349–1353.

Bell, R. L.; Jarvis, K. G.; Ottesen, A. R.; McFarland, M. A.; Brown, E. W. Recent and Emerging Innovations in *Salmonella* Detection: A Food and Environmental Perspective. *Microb. Biotechnol.* **2016,** *9* (3), 279–292.

Busemeyer, L.; Mentrup, D.; Möller, K.; Wunder, E.; Alheit, K.; Hahn, V.; Maurer, H. P.; Reif, J. C.; Würschum, T.; Müller, J.; Rahe, F.; Ruckelshausen A. Breed Vision-A Multi-sensor Platform for Non-destructive Field-based Phenotyping in Plant Breeding. *Sensors* **2013,** *13* (3), 2830–2847.

Byrne, B.; Stack, E.; Niamh Gilmartin, N.; O'Kennedy, R. Antibody-Based Sensors: Principles, Problems and Potential for Detection of Pathogens and Associated Toxins. *Sensors (Basel)* **2009,** *9* (6), 4407–4445.

Centers for Disease Control and Prevention (CDC). Multistate Outbreak of Escherichia coli O157:H7 Infections Associated with Eating Ground Beef—United States, June-July 2002. *MMWR Morb. Mortal. Wkly Rep.* **2002,** *51* (29), 637–639.

Choi, H. K.; Lee, J.; Park, M. K.; Oh, J. H. Development of Single-walled Carbon Nanotube-based Biosensor for the Detection of *Staphylococcus aureus*. *J. Food Qual.* **2017,** *2017,* 8.

Clark, L. C.; Lyons, C. Electrode Systems for Continuous Monitoring in Cardiovascular Surgery. *Ann. N Y Acad. Sci.* **1962,** *102,* 29–45.

Cosio, M. S.; Scampicchio, M.; Benedetti, S. Chapter 8 - Electronic Noses and Tongues. In *Chemical Analysis of Food: Techniques and Applications,* 2012; pp 219–247.

Creative-Biolabs (CB). Antibody Development for *Salmonella [Online*]. https://www.creative-biolabs.com/adc/antibody-development-for salmonella.htm? (*accessed Jan 16, 2020).*

Damborský, P.; Švitel, J.; Katrlík, J. Optical Biosensors. *Essays Biochem.* **2016,** *60* (1), 91–100.

Davis, D.; Guo, X.; Musavi, L.; Lin, C. S.; Chen, S.; Wu, V. C. H. Gold Nanoparticle-modified Carbon Electrode Biosensor for the Detection of *Listeria monocytogene*. *Indian Biotechnol.* **2013,** *9* (1), 31–36.

Dhull, N.; Kaur, G.; Jain, P.; Mishra, P.; Singh, D.; Ganju, L.; Gupta, V.; Tomar M. Label-free Amperometric Biosensor for *Escherichia coli* O157:H7 Detection. *Appl. Surf. Sci.* **2019,** *495,* 143548.

Di Lorenzo, M. 11 - Use of Microbial Fuel Cells in Sensors. In *Microbial Electrochemical and Fuel Cells*, 2016; pp 341–356.

Dincer, C.; Bruch, R.; Costa-Rama, E.; Fernández-Abedul, M. T.; Merkoçi, A.; Manz, A.; Urban, G. A.; Güder F. Disposable Sensors in Diagnostics, Food, and Environmental Monitoring. *Adv. Materials* **2019,** *31* (30), 1806739.

Ercole, C.; Del Gallo, M.; Mosiello, L.; Baccella, S.; Lepidi A. Escherichia Coli Detection in Vegetable Food by a Potentiometric Biosensor. *Sens. Actuators B* **2003,** *91,* 163–168.

Foundation for Meat and Poultry Research and Education (FMPRE). Microbiological Testing [Online]. https://www.meatpoultryfoundation.org/fact-sheets/microbiological-testing (accessed Jan 10, 2020).

Fu, L.; Zhang, K.; Li, S.; Wang, Y.; Huang T.-S.; Zhang, A.; Cheng Z.-Y. In Situ Real-time Detection of *E. coli* in Water Using Antibody-coated Magnetostrictive Microcantilever. *Sens. Actuat. B: Chem.* **2010,** *150,* 220–225

Garnett T. Food Sustainability: Problems, Perspectives and Solutions. *Proc. Nutr. Soc.* **2013,** *72,* 29–39.

Ghorashi, M. Technology's Role in Eradicating Foodborne Illness [Online]. https://www.foodsafetymagazine.com/signature-series/technologye28099s-role-in-eradicating-foodborne-illness (accessed Jan 1, 2020).

Giovanni, M.; Setyawati, M. I.; Tay, C. Y.; Qian, H.; Kuan, W. S.; Leong, D. T. Electrochemical Quantification of *Escherichia coli* with DNA Nanostructure. *Adv. Func. Mater.* **2015,** *25,* 3840–3846.

Girigoswami, K.; Akhtar, N. Nanobiosensors and Fluorescence based Biosensors: An Overview. *Int. J. Nano Dimens.* **2019,** *10* (1), 1–17.

Hussein, H. S. Prevalence and Pathogenicity of Shiga Toxin-producing *Escherichia coli* in Beef Cattle and their Products. *J. Anim. Sci.* **2007,** *85* (13 Suppl), E63–E72.

Jasim, I.; Shen, Z.; Mlaji, Z.; Yuksek, N. S.; Abdullah, A.; Liu, J.; Dastider, S. G.; El-Dweik, M.; Zhang, S.; Almasri, M. An Impedance Biosensor for Simultaneous Detection of Low Concentration of Salmonella Serogroups in Poultry and Fresh Produce Samples. *Biosens. Bioelectron.* **2019,** *126,* 292–300.

Jiang, Y.; Liu, X.; Dang, T. C.; Huang, X.; Feng, H.; Zhang, Q.; Yu, H. A High-sensitivity Potentiometric 65-nm CMOS ISFET Sensor for Rapid *E. coli* Screening. *IEEE Trans. Biomed. Circuits Syst.* **2018,** *12* (2), 402–415.

John, S. V.; Rotherham, L. S.; Khati, M.; Mamba, B. B.; Arotiba, O. A. Towards HIV Detection: Novel poly(propylene imine) Dendrimer-streptavidin Platform for Electrochemical DNA and gp120 Aptamer Biosensors. *Int. J. Electrochem. Sci.* **2014,** *9,* 5425–5437.

Kang, J.; Kim, S.; Kwon Y. Antibody-based Biosensors for Environmental Monitoring. *Toxicol. Environ. Health. Sci.* **2009,** *1,* 145–150.

Kaur, H.; Shorie, M.; Sharma, M.; Ganguli, A. K.; Sabherwal, P. Bridged Rebar Graphene Functionalized Aptasensor for Pathogenic E. coli O78:K80:H11 Detection. *Biosens. Bioelectron.* **2017,** *98,* 486–493.

Kim, G.; Moon, J. H.; Moh, C. Y.; Lim, J. A Microfluidic Nano-biosensor for the Detection of Pathogenic Salmonella. *Biosens. Bioelectron.* **2015,** *67,* 243–247.

Kokoskova, B.; Janse, J. D. Enzyme-linked Immunosorbent Assay for the Detection and Identification of Plant Pathogenic Bacteria (in Particular for Erwinia Amylovora and Clavibacter michiganensis subsp. Sepedonicus). *Meth. Mol. Biol.* **2009,** *508,* 75–87.

Leonard, P.; Hearty, S.; Brennan, J.; Dunne, L.; Quinn, J.; Chakraborty, T.; O'Kennedy, R. Advances in Biosensors for Detection of Pathogens in Food And Water. *Enzyme Microb. Technol.* 2003, *32* (1), 3–13.

Ligler, F. S. Fluorescence-Based Optical Biosensors. In *Biophotonics. Biological and Medical Physics, Biomedical Engineering*, Pavesi, L., Fauchet P. M., Eds.; Springer: Berlin, Heidelberg, 2008.

Liu, J.; Jasim, I.; Abdullah, A.; Shen, Z.; Zhao, L.; El-Dweik, M.; Zhang, S.; Almasri, M. An Integrated Impedance Biosensor Platform for Detection of Pathogens in Poultry Products. *Sci. Rep.* **2018,** *8* (1), 16109.

Liu, J.; Jasim, I.; Shen, Z.; Zhao, L.; Dweik, M.; Zhang, S.; Almasri, M. A Microfluidic Based Biosensor for Rapid Detection of *Salmonella* in Food Products. *PLoS One* **2019,** *14* (5), e0216873.

Mäntsälä, P.; Niemi, J. Enzymes: The Biological Catalysts of Life. *Physiol. Maintanance.* **2009,** *2,* 1–9.

Massad-Ivanir, N.; Shtenberg, G.; Raz, N.; Gazenbeek, C.; Budding, D.; Bos, M. P.; Segal, E. Porous Silicon-based Biosensors: Towards Real-time Optical Detection of Target Bacteria in the Food Industry. *Sci. Rep.* **2016,** *6,* 38099.

Mehrotra, P. Biosensors and Their Applications-A Review. *J. Oral Biol. Craniofac. Res.* **2016,** *6* (2), 153–159.

Menti, C.; Henriques, J. A.; Missell, F. P.; Roesch-Ely, M. Antibody-based Magneto-elastic Biosensors: Potential Devices for Detection of Pathogens and Associated Toxins. *Appl. Microbiol. Biotechnol.* **2016,** *100* (14), 6149–6163.

Miller, B. G.; Wolfenden, R. Catalytic Proficiency: the Unusual Case of OMP Decarboxylase. *Annu. Rev. Biochem.* **2002,** *71,* 847–885.

Mishra, G. K.; Barfidokht, A.; Tehrani, F.; Mishra, R. K. Food Safety Analysis Using Electrochemical Biosensors. *Foods* **2018,** *7,* 141.

Monosik, R.; Stredansky, M.; Tkac, J.; Sturdik E. Application of Enzyme Biosensors in Analysis of Food and Beverages. *Food Anal. Methods* **2012,** *5* (1), 40–53.

Mujika, M.; Arana, S.; Castaño, E.; Tijero, M.; Vilares, R.; Ruano-López, J. M.; Cruz, A.; Sainz, L.; Berganza, J. Magnetoresistive Immunosensor for the Detection of *Escherichia coli* O157:H7 Including a Microfluidic Network. *Biosens. Bioelectron.* **2009,** *24* (5), 1253–1258.

Ohk, S. H.; Bhunia, A. K. Multiplex Fiber Optic Biosensor for Detection of Listeria Monocytogenes, *Escherichia coli* O157:H7 and Salmonella Enterica from Ready-to-eat Meat Samples. *Food Microbiol.* **2013,** *33* (2), 166–171.

Palchetti, I.; Mascini, M. Amperometric Biosensor for Pathogenic Bacteria Detection. In *Principles of Bacterial Detection: Biosensors, Recognition Receptors and Microsystems*; Zourob, M., Elwary, S., Turner A., Eds.; Springer: New York, NY, 2008; pp 299–312.

Parra-Alfambra, A. M.; Casero, E.;Vázquez, L.; Quintana, C.; de Pozo, M.; Petit-Domínguez M. D. MoS2 Nanosheets for Improving Analytical Performance of Lactate Biosensors. *Sens. Actuators B: Chem.* **2018,** *274,* 310–317.

Peacock, E.; Jacob, V. W.; Fallone, S. M. *Escherichia coli* O157:H7: Etiology, Clinical Features, Complications, and Treatment. *Nephrol. Nurs. J.* **2001,** *28* (5), 547–550, 553–555; quiz 556–557.

Peltomaa, R.; Glahn-Martínez, B.; Benito-Peña, E.; Moreno-Bondi, M. C. Optical Biosensors for Label-free Detection of Small Molecules. *Sensors* **2018,** *18* (12), 4126.

Pividori, M. I.; Alegret, S. Electrochemical Biosensors for Food Safety. *Contribut. Sci.* **2010,** *6* (2), 173–191.

Pol, L.; Acosta, L. K.; Ferré-Borrull, J.; Marsal, L. F. Aptamer-based Nanoporous Anodic Alumina Interferometric Biosensor for Real-time Thrombin Detection. *Sensors* **2019,** *19* (20), 4543.

Reich, P.; Stoltenburg, R.; Strehlitz, B.; Frense, D.; Beckmann, D. Development of an Impedimetric Aptasensor for the Detection of *staphylococcus aureus*. *Int. J. Mol. Sci.* **2017,** *18* (11), pii: E248.

Ricke, S. C.; Kim, S. A.; Shi, Z.; Park, S. H. Molecular-based Identification and Detection of Salmonella in Food Production Systems: Current Perspectives. *J. Appl. Microbiol.* **2018,** *125* (2), 313–327.

Rochelet, M.; Solanas, S.; Betelli, L.; Chantemesse, B.; Vienney, F.; Hartmann, A. Rapid Amperometric Detection of *Escherichia coli* in Wastewater by Measuring β-D Glucuronidase Activity with Disposable Carbon Sensors. *Anal. Chim. Acta* **2015,** *892,* 160–166.

Sadeghi, S. J. Amperometric Biosensors. In *Encyclopedia of Biophysics*, Roberts, G. C. K., Eds.; Springer: Berlin, Heidelberg, 2013.

Savas, S.; Aylin Ersoy, A.; Gulmez, Y.; Kilic, S.; Levent, B.; Altintas, Z. Nanoparticle Enhanced Antibody and DNA Biosensors for Sensitive Detection of *Salmonella. Mater. (Basel)* **2018,** *11* (9), 1541.

Sawant, S. N. 13-Development of Biosensors from Biopolymer Composites. In *Biopolymer Composites in Electronics,* 2017; pp 353–383.

Schrenk, D. Chemische Lebensmittelkontaminanten. *Bundesgesundheitsbl-Gesundheitsforsch – Gesundheitsschutz* **2004,** *47,* 841–847.

Scognamiglio, V.; Arduini, F.; Palleschi, G.; Rea, G. Biosensing Technology for Sustainable Food Safety. *TrAC Trends Anal. Chem.* **2014,** *62,* 1–10.

Seo, K. H.; Brackett, R. E.; Hartman, N. F.; Campbell, D. P. Development of a Rapid Response Biosensor for Detection of *Salmonella Typhimurium. J. Food Prot.* **1999,** *62* (5), 431–437.

Shaibani, P. M.; Etayash, H.; Jiang, K.; Sohrabi, A.; Hassanpourfard, M.; Naicker, S.; Sadrzadeh, M.; Thundat, T. Portable Nanofiber-Light Addressable Potentiometric Sensor for Rapid *Escherichia coli* Detection in Orange Iuice. *ACS Sens.* **2018,** *3* (4), 815–822.

Sharma, H.; Agarwal, M.; Goswami, M.; Sharma, A.; Roy, S. K.; Rai, R.; Murugan, M. S. Biosensors: Tool for Food Borne Pathogen Detection. *Vet. World* **2013,** *6* (12): 968–973.

Sharma, S.; Byrne, H.; Richard, J.; O'Kennedy, R. J. Antibodies and Antibody-derived Analytical Biosensors. *Essays Biochem.* **2016,** *60* (1), 9–18.

Silva, N. F. D.; Magalhaes, J. M. C. S.; Oliva-Teles, M. T.; Delerue-Matos, C. A Potentiometric Magnetic Immunoassay for Rapid Detection of *Salmonella typhimurium. Anal. Methods* **2015,** *7* (9), 4008–4011.

Singh, A.; Sinsinbar, G.; Choudhary, M.; Kumar, V.; Pasricha, R.; Verma H. N.; Singh S. P.; Arora K. Graphene Oxide-chitosan Nanocomposite based Electrochemical DNA Biosensor for Detection of Typhoid. *Sens. Actuators B* **2013,** *185,* 675–684.

Singh, P. Surface Plasmon Resonance: A Boon for Viral Diagnostics. *Reference Module Life Sci.* **2017**. DOI: 10.1016/B978-0-12-809633-8.12245-9

Singh, R.; Sumana, G.; Verma, R.; Sood, S.; Pandey, M. K.; Gupta, R. K.; Malhotra, B. D. DNA Biosensor for Detection of Neisseria Gonorrhoeae Causing Sexually Transmitted Disease. *J. Biotechnol.* **2010,** *150* (3), 357–365.

Song, S.; Wang, L.; Li, J.; Fan, C.; Zhao, J. Aptamer-based Biosensors. *TrAC Trends Anal. Chem.* **2008,** *27* (2), 108–117.

Song, W.; Zhang, N.; Luan, Z.; Zhang, X.; He, P. Application of a Cation-exchange Reaction of CuS Nanoparticles and Fluorescent Copper Nanoparticles in a DNA Biosensor. *RSC Adv.* **2018,** *8,* 15248–15252.

Suryapratiwi, W. N.; Paat, V. I.; Gaffar, S.; Hartati, Y. W. DNA Biosensor for Detection of *Salmonella typhi* from Blood Sample of Typhoid Fever Patient Using Gold Electrode Modified by Self-assembled Monolayers of Thiols. *AIP Conf. Proc.* **2017,** *1848,* 030005.

Tenaillon, O.; Skurnik, D.; Picard, B.; Denamur, E. The Population Genetics of Commensal *Escherichia coli. Nat. Rev. Microbiol.* **2010,** *8* (3), 207–217.

Tenenbaum, E.; Segal, E. Optical Biosensors for Bacteria Detection by a Peptidomimetic Antimicrobial Compound. **Analyst 2015, 140**, 7726–7733.

Teng, J.; Yuan, F.; Ye, Y.; Zheng, L.; Yao, L.; Xue, F.; Chen, W.; Li, B. Aptamer-based Technologies in Foodborne Pathogen Detection. *Front. Microbiol.* **2016,** *7,* 1426.

Terry, L. A.; White, S. F.; Tigwell, L. J. The Application of Biosensors to Fresh Produce and the Wider Food Industry. *J. Agric. Food Chem.* **2005,** *53,* 1309–1316.

Tietjen, M.; Fung, D. Y. C. *Salmonella* and Food Safety. *Crit. Rev. Microb.* **1995,** *21,* 53–83.
Tombelli, S.; Minunni, M.; Santucci, A.; Spiriti, M. M.; Mascini, M. A DNA-based Piezoelectric Biosensor: Strategies for Coupling Nucleic Acids to Piezoelectric Devices. *Talanta*. **2006,** *68* (3), 806–812.
Tutulea, M. D.; Cretescu, I.; Sibiescu, D.; Stan C. Electrochemical Sensors for Heavy Metal Ions Detection from Aqueous Solutions. *Environ. Eng. Manag. J.* **2012,** *11* (2), 463–470.
Vashist, S. K.; Luong, J. H. T. Chapter 5 - Enzyme-Linked Immunoassays. In *Handbook of Immunoassay Technologies. Approaches, Performances, and Applications*; 2018, pp 97–127.
Vidic, J.; Vizzini, P.; Manzano, M.; Kavanaugh, D.; Ramarao, N.; Zivkovic, M.; Radonic, V.; Knezevic, N.; Giouroudi, I.; Gadjanski, I. Point-of-Need DNA Testing for Detection of Foodborne Pathogenic Bacteria. *Sensors (Basel)* **2019,** *19* (5), 1100.
Viswanathan, S.; Radecka, H.; Radecki, J. Electrochemical Biosensors for Food Analysis. *Monatsh. Chem.* **2009,** *140* (8), 891–899.
Vizzini, P.; Braidot, M.; Vidic, J.; Manzano, M. Electrochemical and Optical Biosensors for the Detection of *Campylobacter* and *Listeria monocytogene*: An Update Look. *Micromachines* **2019,** *10,* 500.
Vogt, R. L.; Dippold, L. *Escherichia coli* O157:H7 Outbreak Associated with Consumption of Ground Beef, June-July 2002. *Public Health Rep.* **2005,** *120* (2), 174–178.
Washington, J. A. Principles of Diagnosis. In *Medical Microbiology,* 4th ed.; University of Texas Medical Branch at Galveston: Galveston, TX, chapter 10; 1996.
WebMD LLC. What is E. Coli? [Onlin]. https://www.webmd.com/food-recipes/food-poisoning/what- -is-e-coli#1 Information (accessed Jan 16, 2020).
Wei, D.; Oyarzabal, O. A.; Huang, T. S.; Balasubramanian, S.; Sista, S.; Simonian A. L. Development of a Surface Plasmon Resonance Biosensor for the Identification of *Campylobacter jejuni*. *J. Microbiol. Methods* **2007,** *69* (1), 78–85.
Wu, Q.; Zhang, Y.; Yang, Q.; Yuan, N.; Zhang, W. Review of Electrochemical DNA Biosensors for Detecting Food Borne Pathogens. *Sensors* **2019,** *19* (22), 4916.
Yunus, S.; Jonas, A. M.; Lakard, B. Potentiometric Biosensors. In *Encyclopedia of Biophysics*, Roberts, G. C. K., Eds.; Springer: Berlin, Heidelberg, 2013.
Zelada-Guillén, G. A.; Bhosale, S. V.; Riu, J.; Rius, F. X. Real-time Potentiometric Detection of Bacteria in Complex Samples. *Anal. Chem.* **2010,** *82* (22), 9254–9260.
Zhang, W.; Liu, Q. X.; Guo, Z. H.; Lin, J. S. Practical Application of Aptamer-based Biosensors in Detection of Low Molecular Weight Pollutants in Water Sources. *Molecules* **2018,** *23* (2), 344.
Zhang, X.; Tsuji, S.; Kitaoka, H.; Kobayashi, H.; Tamai, M.; Honjoh, K. I.; Miyamoto, T. Simultaneous Detection of *Escherichia coli* O157:H7, *Salmonella enteritidis,* and *Listeria monocytogenes* at a Very Low Level Using Simultaneous Enrichment Broth and Multichannel SPR Biosensor. *J. Food Sci.* **2017,** *82* (10), 2357–2363.
Zhang, Z.; Zhou, J.; Du, X. Electrochemical Biosensors for Detection of Foodborne Pathogens. *Micromachines (Basel)* **2019,** *10* (4), pii: E222.
Zhao, Y. W.; Wang, H. X.; Jia, G. C.; Li, Z. Application of Aptamer-Based Biosensor for Rapid Detection of Pathogenic *Escherichia coli*. *Sensors (Basel)* **2018,** *18* (8), 2518.
Zhou, W.; Huang, P. J. J.; Ding, J.; Liu, J. Aptamer-based Biosensors for Biomedical Diagnostics. *Analyst* **2014,** *139,* 2627–2640.

CHAPTER 13

Advanced Energy Materials Derived from Microorganisms, Plants, and Animals

DARIEO THANKACHAN[1] and NEHA KANWAR RAWAT[2]

[1]*Department of Materials Science and Engineering, National Taiwan University of Science and Technology, Taipei, Taiwan, ROC*

[2]*Materials Research Laboratory, Department of Chemistry, Jamia Millia Islamia, New Delhi, India*

ABSTRACT

As a result of the growing need for sustainable green energy, renewable energy globally has moved to the forefront by creating sustainable energy storage and transfer materials.

On the other hand, for the production of nanomaterials, which are applied extensively in energy sectors, biomass is considered as a better substitute.

This chapter reports the latest progress and achievements in application of novel energy materials.

13.1 INTRODUCTION

Because of their applicability, broad range of applications, and international commitment to progress toward cleaner energy sources, power storage and conversion components have reached the pinnacle of contemporary civilization. The ever-increasing demand for energy has necessitated the quest for environmental sustainable and cost-effective energy storage options. (Ma et al., 2020) Renewable energy has moved to the forefront as a result of the growing need for sustainable green energy. Furthermore, creating high-performance energy storage and transfer materials is a trend in the field of sustainability. Biomass are considered as a better substitute

Application of Engineering Principles and Practices in Biotechnology.
Ann Rose Abraham, Leonardo Sepúlveda Torre, Tamara Tatrishvili, and A. K. Haghi (Eds.)

for the production of nanomaterials which are used to energy applications. Carbon black, for example, a petroleum-based substance utilized in lithium-ion batteries (LIBs), has little use in sodium-ion batteries (SIBs). Effective options for materials and products which are developed from petroleum-based compounds must be identified in order to change the standard toward materials which are scalable and biological in origin. Waste biomass may be used to turn waste material like coffee grinds into societally useful goods. (Liu et al., 2020) Because biomass is readily available and biological samples have a variety of microstructural features, a wide spectrum of biomass may be examined, allowing for great material design flexibility.

Taking cues from nature, scientists and researchers have addressed energy-related challenges during the last several decades. For example, the inherent composition of some biomass are perhaps very beneficial for biological material layout. Particularly exciting for waste products is the transformation of biomass into nanoparticles generated from living organisms for energy storage transfer applications. In terms of waste minimization, objectives connected to energy and carbon capture, developing technology to turn the current enormous amount of trash into valuable goods is very advantageous to society. Waste materials have a lot of potential and can be reused. Nanocarbons may be created in one step rather than two by basically carbonizing biomass, and they don't require template removal following synthesis. (Bhat et al., 2020) Scalability depends on minimizing the number of processes and using reasonably priced precursors since converting biomass to carbon consumes a lot of energy. Research into these materials is particularly broad since there are so many distinct biological starting points; as a result, an evaluation is required to further ongoing research in the field. Animals, plants, certain viruses and fungi, protists, and bacteria have all directly or indirectly produced nanomaterials (Sidhu, 2001; Zhang et al., 2019; Qu et al., 2020; Krikstolaityte et al., 2018; Wang et al., 2018; Mujib et al., 2020; Ghouri et al., 2017). The diverse structures, which are formed from a range of templates, each have their own set of features that may aid in the enhancement of the material created (Fang et al., 2019).

13.2 ENERGY MATERIALS DERIVED FROM MICROORGANISMS

Numerous microorganisms exhibit surface properties that are advantageous for bio-templating and are easy to cultivate in large amounts, and have structures that are especially beneficial for the creation of nanoparticles; therefore they have a lot of potential for bio-templating nanomaterials. There are more ways to change these features to better suit a particular application. The most often employed study subjects are the bacterium *Escherichia coli*, the bacteriophage M13, and occasionally Tobacco Mosaic Virus (TMV), since they have the right surface features and are frequently used in a variety of research domains. Prominent viral templates utilized to manufacture respective nanostructures for energy applications comprise M13 and Fd-virus as nanowires, CIV virus as nanospheres, and TMV virus as nanorods. Bacterial templates are employed as microorganisms in nanostructures like nanorods for bacteria such as Subtilis, *E. coli*, and Bulgaricus. Bacteria like *E. coli* flagella and Salinarum were also employed in the nanowire structure. In the nanorod structure, Theromophilus bacteria are employed, whereas in the nanosheet structure, Subtilis bacteria are used (Zhang et al., 2019; Shim et al., 2011; Kumara et al., 2007; Beznosov et al., 2015; Zhou et al., 2007). Yeast as a hollowsphere and microsphere are two microorganism fungus that have been employed as a bio-template for generating diverse nanostructures for energy purposes (Beznosov et al., 2015; Ren et al., 2005); conidia (Fan et al., 2011) as nanowire and bran (Liang et al., 2015) as nanocube are also used. Figure 13.1 depicts the microbial cells producing wide variety of by-products from renewable feed stocks. The utilization of microbes and their enzymes to transform carbohydrates, lignins, and glycerol into other renewable resources, such as the generation of bioenergy, is known as microbial biotechnology (Ramamurthy et al., 2021).

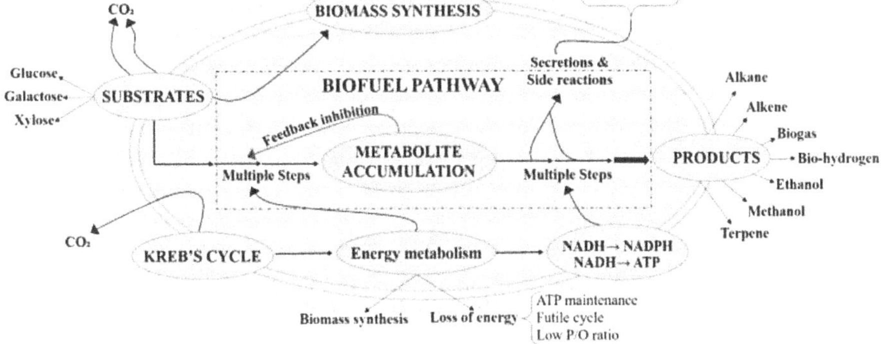

FIGURE 13.1 Microbial cells producing wide variety of by-products from renewable feed stocks.

Source: Reprinted with permission from Ramamurthy et al., 2021. https://creativecommons.org/licenses/by/4.0/

13.2.1 VIRUSES

Viruses are commonly used as a biological-template in the production of nanomaterials which are used in energy applications. Virus populations produce well-ordered, homogenous structures that may be altered with regularly accessible solutions. Genetic techniques can be used to modify or functionalize a viral structure. Virus structures are also helpful as bio-templates because they don't have a membrane and have well-defined forms. These topologies are typically appropriate for nanomaterial manufacturing. It is simple to remove viral remnants from bio-templated materials, and since viral structures can withstand changes in pH as well as temperature (Wen and Steinmetz, 2016; Royston et al., 2008; Radloff et al., 2005). Numerous techniques may be used to grow viruses, and they can organize and multiply in homogenous populations while still in solution (Brown et al., 2013; Culver et al., 2015). The process of producing bacteriophages in *E. coli* bacterial strains (described as virus-like particles at times, or VLPs) is the most common way to produce viral structures. This method was chosen because it enables for speedy production and scalability. TMV-like viruses may be replicated by heterologous expression, which entails genetically modifying *E. coli* to create viral structures (Hwang et al., 1994). TMV, an elongated rod shaped virus, as a bio-template being looked at due to its ability to mineralize both its inner as well as outer channels, enabling control over the variety of materials produced. Each of the virus's 2100 coat proteins is 300 nm long, 18 nm wide on the outside, and 4 nm wide on the inside (Bromley et al., 2008; Chen et al., 2010). Due of TMV's ability to mineralize both its internal and external channels, it has been examined as a bio-template since it allows control over the range of materials that may be created from it (Bromley et al., 2008; Knez et al., 2003). Each of the virus's 2100 coat proteins is 300 nm long, 18 nm wide on the outside, and 4 nm thick on the inside (Chen et al., 2010). TMV VLPs may be mineralized to generate semiconducting and insulating nanowires, which can be used to make energy-related materials (Brown et al., 2013). It is simple to purify TMV nanorods, have a long shelf life, and have a number of modifications made to them to improve functionality. Because of hydrophobic contacts at the rod ends, TMV nanorods will align self, head-to-tail in an acidic environment, enabling nanowire templating (Shenton et al., 1999). An intriguing potential for bio-templating nanomaterials is viruses. It is possible to create VLPs in both research and business using well-known techniques for creating and isolating viral structures. The resultant particle populations are monodispersed, and the structures are frequently chemically and mechanically robust. There are a range of surfaces and structures that are all adaptable without materially affecting the regular production procedure. Viral architecture-derived bio-templated nanomaterials, particularly current collectors and battery electrodes, exhibit fascinating electrical and chemical characteristics for energy applications.

13.2.2 BACTERIA

Bacteria is a different potential being looked into as a microorganism bio-template for the creation of energy nanomaterials. Bacteria are easily grown, have regular sizes, and morphologies, and can be genetically modified (Zhang et al., 2019). Bacterial mass production is also not environmentally hazardous. Additionally, bacteria are capable of self-assembly, enabling the production of monodispersed nanomaterials (Kumara et al., 2007; Zhou et al., 2007). The rod-shaped, gram-positive bacterium phosphate, teichoic acids, and carbonyl are functional groups found in the cell wall of the peptidoglycan of the bacterium Subtilis. The electrostatic interactions between metal oxides and the cell surface are made possible by the negative charge of the phosphate groups (Shim et al., 2011). Metal oxides may adhere to cells thanks to surface reduction, and when they spontaneously oxidize, they create bacterial metal hybrids. The hybrid material is then calcined to eliminate the organic component, leaving behind a metal oxide nanorod with porous hollow structure. The bio-form template is secured by the metal oxide product (Shim et al., 2011). To regulate pore size, redesigned polystyrene (PS) spheres with amine substituent can also be employed. To alter the pore size, the PS spheres' diameter can be changed (Gao et al., 2016). The rod-shaped, gram-negative bacterium *E. coli* measures 1.4 μm in length and 0.6 μm in width. Hydrolysis was used by nanomaterials will be produced using an *E. coli* bio-template by Zhang et al. as well as by Nomura et al. In order to create nanorod hybrids, the bacterial colony was treated with alcohol and zirconium butoxide, according to Nomura et al. The hybrids are then calcined to destroy the bacterial template (Zhang et al., 2019; Nomura et al., 2013). Flagella can also be utilized as a bio-template in place of complete *E. coli* cells. The flagella of *E. coli* measure 10–15 μm and 12–25 nm in width, S. flagella's length is about 10 μm from 10–15 nm (Kumara et al., 2007). Instead of employing the complete cell as a biological template, the E. flagella should constantly be improved by the addition of peptide loops to help metal-ion nanoparticles stick to the surface and produce nanotubes. The flagellin can be genetically altered to modify the amino acid chains' order in order to create a more functional biological template (Rebentrost et al., 2009). As a possible bio-template with a variety of features, the archaebacterium Salinarum is being researched. Salinarum is known to flourish in challenging environments, which is helpful for bio-templating as it allows the system to function in very acidic or basic conditions without modifying the composition of the template. The bacterium S. flagella has a diameter of 10–15 nm and it has an average length of 10 μm. There is no DNA in the flagella, which are entirely composed of proteins. Aspartate or glutamate should undergo genetic modification to produce carboxyl groups in the flagella. When metal ions connect to flagella, nanowires are created, and these groupings act as their binding sites (Beznosov et al., 2015). The gram-positive bacteria Lactobacillus (LB) has peptidoglycan, teichoic acid, and teichuronic acid in its cell walls. Streptococcus theromophilus (theromophilus) and Bulgaricus were the two LB types employed by Zhou and his associates as bio-templates. Theromophilus has a diameter of 0.5–0.9 μm and it also is a spherical form. Bulgaricus, on either side, has a rod form with dimensions that range from 0.3–0.8 μm in width and 1–5 μm in length (Zhou et al., 2007).

13.2.3 FUNGI

While metal oxide nanospheres have been made using baker's yeast as a bio-template, additional fungal applications rely on other fungal structural properties. The majority of battery electrodes have been made using nanomaterials with fungus-templated surfaces. Baker's yeast cells have a positive surface charge and are eukaryotic, elliptical, and 3–4.5 μm in diameter (Zhao et al., 2018). Electrostatic interactions involving carboxyl group, phosphate group, and amide group on the surface allow for surface functionalization (Zhang et al., 2012). Through the biomineralization of yeast cells, mesoporous silicate and mesoporous zirconium phosphate air electrode electrocatalysts were also created. During the synthesis process, the size and shape of the pores were controlled by changing the reaction mixtures. Disilicate was unable to attach to the cell wall of the yeast because of its negative surface charge, which allowed silica to cover the surface in its place. After the yeast template was removed from the nanoparticle, a mesoporous silica/carbon air electrode material was remained (Cui and Liu, 2017). From the conidia of several fungi, Sugunan et al. developed gold microwires. In fungus, cellular mitosis creates a spore called a conidium (Shaheen et al., 2021). A solution containing glutamate and gold nanoparticles was administered to live cultures of Aspergillus niger, Aspergillus nidulans, and Neurospora crassa. When the fungus utilizes glutamate to produce conidia, there are changes to the local charge setup, allowing gold nanoparticles to adhere to the growth surface. Fungal samples that were either dead or lacked a growing substrate did not exhibit this phenomena (Sugunan et al., 2007; Osherov and May, 2001). The chitin-rich bran of the common forest litter fungus is a significant source of nitrogen. N-doped carbon molecules are created through the carbonization of forest bran. Researchers used a carbon matrix with a fungal bran template to make zinc-manganese oxide (ZMO) nano-cubes. This technique involves washing the fungal bran, carbonizing it, and then activating it with potassium hydroxide. To produce nano-cubes, the activated carbon matrix is annealed in a ZMO-containing solution. This material outperformed other regularly used materials in supercapacitors in terms of cycle stability. ZMO has no impact on the volumetric expansion of this substance (Qu et al., 2020). Biomineralization and deposition are two fungi-templating strategies. In deposition techniques, the template's surface charge is utilized, but it must be active. Although biomineralization avoids agglomeration, it is limited by the cell wall's functional groups.

13.3 ENERGY MATERIALS DERIVED FROM PLANTS

Particularly in the realm of rechargeable battery systems, biochar derived from various biomass sources that are pyrolyzed have recently been employed frequently for energy storage applications, either directly or as a model (Jensen et al., 2009; Xia et al., 2013; Li et al., 2021). Due to its high energy and power density as well as outstanding energy efficiency when compared to other secondary batteries like lead-acid, Ni-Cd, and Ni-MH batteries, the rechargeable lithium-ion battery (LIB) is one of the most popular electrochemical power sources (Li et al., 2007; Zheng et al., 2008; Zhang et al., 2010). Earth's abundant plant life makes it possible to build a wide range of structures that can serve as materials for energy storage and conversion. Over the past several years, numerous research teams have focused on creating nanoparticles from plant matter utilizing a variety of methods. Plant material may be used to create a variety of morphologies since plant microstructures come in a wide variety and material synthesis processes. As an effective bio-template for the production of nanoscale particles, E. cognata phytochemicals, for instance, have been employed (Shaheen et al., 2021; Shaheen et al., 2020). Thermal conversion of biomass to carbon is often utilized to use plant-based biomass for energy storage/conversion material applications. Although biomass may be easily calcined to get carbon, this process can be changed in a number of ways, producing a wide range of carbon matter with noticeably with various electrochemical characteristics. No matter how it is changed, calcining biomass by thermal decomposition to carbon has the advantages of being affordable, straightforward, and time-consuming. However, because of the high energy needs for big batches, pyrolysis' scalability is typically a problem. The capacity to scale up these processes may benefit from strategies like using the by-products of pyrolysis as fuel to assist maintain the high temperatures needed or producing biochar using solar energy. Small molecules generated from biomass might be utilized to create binders or electrolytes, two components of sustainable batteries. When these materials are used together to create energy storage devices, the entire carbon cycle is maintained. (Fig. 13.2) (Liedel, 2020).

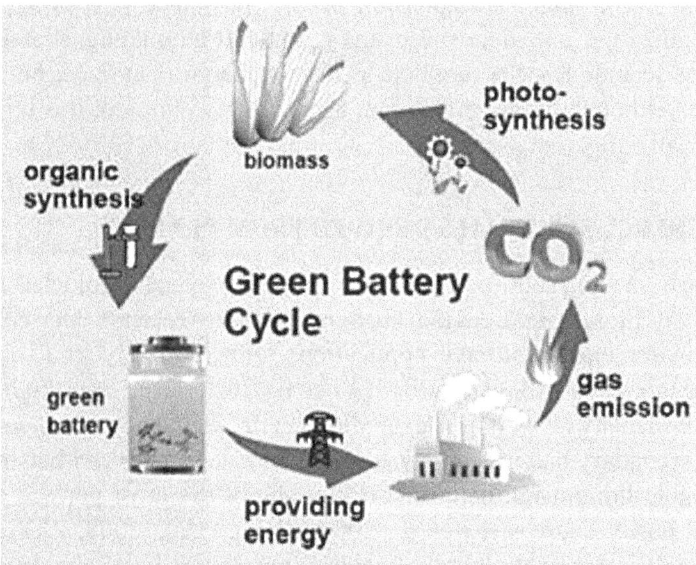

FIGURE 13.2 Ideal cycle for green batteries.

Source: Reprinted with permission from Liedel 2020. https://creativecommons.org/licenses/by/4.0/

13.3.1 WOOD

Wood has a porous hierarchical structure and is a renewable resource, excellent mechanical characteristics, and a diverse set of physicochemical features. The use of wood-based materials and derivatives in innovative materials for energy storage, flexible electronics, and renewable energy sources has a lot of potential. As a result of billions of years of development, wood has a delicate and sophisticated structure that serves a variety of purposes. For multilayer pore architectures, it could serve as a predecessor. There are multiple little vertically oriented grooves found in wood. There are also many fibers and tracheids with sizes ranging from 20 to 140 μm, which are used to transport nutrients, water, and ions. Lignin, hemicellulose, and cellulose are the primary components of wood cell walls. Crystalline basic filaments with diameters of 3–5 nm and lengths of 30–60 nm are tightly packed with cellulose molecules. The filaments and layers of the wood cell wall give it outstanding mechanical properties. Active materials, particularly high-mass-loading electrodes, may delaminate from current collectors in energy storage devices, and high electrode tortuosity may limit the use of active materials by preventing ion transport and extending the ion diffusion channel. Additionally, the binder could impair electron flow and create "dead" regions that can't support electrochemical processes (Bresser et al., 2013). The many open channels in the hierarchically porous and low-tortuosity structure of wood make it feasible for solution penetration, ion transport, and gas bubble desorption (Song et al., 2018; Che et al., 2019). Several different structural forms of wood-derived materials, including high density wood, transparent wood, and sponge-like wood, are created through a series of physical/chemical treatments on wood.

13.3.2 SUPERCAPACITOR APPLICATIONS USING WOOD

The electrode, electrolyte, current collector, diaphragm, and shelf are the main SC parts. A wide-operating temperature range, quick charge-discharge, high energy and power densities, a very long life cycle, they are both safe and environmentally friendly (Muzaffar et al., 2019). The electrode materials have a considerable impact on the electrochemical performance of the SCs. Wood may considerably boost ion and electron transmission due to its 3D straight channel structure, making it a potential natural electrode material (Zhu et al., 2017).

13.3.3 HETEROATOM-DOPED ELECTRODE MADE OF WOOD

Due to their competitive electrochemical activity, high conductivity, cost effectiveness, and outstanding durability, heteroatom-doped carbon materials have become viable metal-free catalysts for accelerating the oxygen reduction process (Hu et al., 2017; Pei et al., 2017). Meanwhile, carbon materials having a hierarchically porous structure may facilitate fast mass transfer and provide a high number of active sites due to their dimensional design (Shang et al., 2016; Shinde et al., 2017; Xu et al., 2016). Tang et al. carbonized delignified basswood impregnated with trithiocyanuric acid to form an N, S co-doped carbon skeleton (TARC-N) for the SC electrode (TA) (Tang et al., 2018). It has a gravimetric specific capacitance (Cs) of 704 F $g?^{-1}$ at 0.2 A g1 and an excellent gravimetric specific capacitance (Cs) of 704 F g1 at 0.2 A $g?^{1}$. At a current density of 2 A $g?^{1}$, the capacitance preserved 94% of its original capacitance after 5000 charge-discharge cycles. This is due to the multispace straight-channel structure of wood, which facilitates electrolyte ion transport and quick electrochemical kinetics. Heteroatom doping increases the hydrophilicity and polarity of wood carbons, enabling the insertion of functional groups to produce pseudocapacitive behavior.

13.3.4 WOOD-BASED LITHIUM BATTERY

Owing to its substantial theoretical specific capability (3860 mAh $g?^{1}$) along with a weak electrochemical potential (?3.04 V vs the typical hydrogen electrode), for the upcoming generation of energy storage technologies, the lithium (Li) metal anode is regarded as the “Holy Grail.” However, several issues with the Li metal anode exist, such as the creation of amorphous lithium dendrites and the need of electrolytes, decreased coulomb performance as a result of the ongoing electrolyte reaction, and SEI film breakage as a result of volume expansion, all have negative effects on safety and low cycle life, which limit the practical use of Li metal batteries (Zhang et al., 2020; Hu et al., 2020).

13.3.5 RICE HUSK DERIVED NANOSTRUCTURED SILICON AS AN INCREASED PERFORMANCE LI-ION BATTERY ANODE

Compared to typical materials for graphite anodes (372 mA h/g), for Li-ion batteries, silicon as a possible anode material might offer a specific capacity of up to 4200 mA h/g. Likewise, when Li is inserted and removed, Si undergoes a high-volume shift (>400%), causing the electrode to fracture and pulverize. Reduced silicon size to the nanoscale may be able to withstand the volume shift during Li insertion/extraction, allowing strain to be accommodated and even preventing breakage (Armand and Tarascon, 2008). Pyrolysis of silane, polysilane, and halosilane precursors at high temperatures and energies, or laser ablation of bulk materials are the only viable methods for generating nano-Si anode materials (Cui et al., 2008; Yao et al., 2011; Sotiropoulou et al., 2008). New production techniques for making nano-Si materials with graphite anode are urgently needed to fulfil industrial demand. And there is also a requirement for nano-silicon materials with graphite anode cost and scalability. Cui's team designed and synthesized pure silicon nanoparticles (SiNPs) from rice husks with a conversion yield of up to 5% by mass (RHs). Due to their tiny size (10–40 nm) and porous nature, these SiNPs are appropriate for use as Li-ion battery anodes (Liu et al., 2013). In attempt to develop nano-Si materials that are equivalent in price and scalability to graphite anodes, advanced manufacturing techniques are being developed. Rice, the second-most consumed crop in the world, produces a large amount of waste, primarily rice husks. The primary ingredients of rice husks are cellulose, lignin, and hydrated silica. The silicon was absorbed as silicates by the rice plant's root, which was then transported to the plant's surface. The primary structure of rice husks is connected by inorganic silica, with a small amount of silica also forming covalent bonds with the organic components. Silica, which had a concentration of around 20% and filled the gaps between the epidermal cells, made up the rough interlayer (epidermis) of the RHs. Rice husks are a possible source for products manufactured of silicon or carbon since they include the two primary species of carbon and silica. Currently, rice husks may be used to create silicon carbide (SiC), silicon nitride (SiN), pure silicon (Si), silicon tetrachloride ($SiCl_4$), silica (SiO_2), and zeolite ($Na[AlSi2O_6]\cdot H_2O$). Due to its outstanding stability and practical efficiency, Si has lately become a crucial component of solar cells. Owing to the use of silicon-based solar cells being hampered by their high cost due to silicon's shortage, the second and third generations of solar cells were created. If bio-residues were employed as the silicon source, the cost of solar cells may be significantly reduced. Rice husks are a viable source of silicon since they provide a silica and carbon by-product in large quantities and at a low cost. In order to employ Si in solar cells, research into this material first started on rice husks in 1982, and subsequent studies enhanced the synthesis techniques. Si produced with the best practices may have a purity of 99.95%, making it appropriate for solar cells usage (Shackley et al., 2012). Magnesiothermic reactions enable silicon to be produced at lower temperatures, giving them a practical way to harvest silicon from plants. In addition to rice husks, the synthesis approach may be used to additional silica-rich plants, such as poaceae, equisetaceae, and cyperaceae

13.3.6 A HYBRID PEANUT SHELL-BASED SODIUM ION CAPACITOR

Rechargeable battery and super-capacitor hybridization have been extensively pushed and explored with the goal of exploiting the improved energy density of the batteries and the high power of the capacitors to satisfy the requirements for fully electric cars (Cericola and Kötz, 2012; Conway and Pell, 2003; Ding et al., 2015; Park et al., 2014). Rechargeable batteries, the two primary electrochemical energy sources, employ a faradaic process to transform electrical energy into chemical energy, which they subsequently store. Due to the relatively high faradaic resistance, it performs poorly in terms of power performance even if it stores energy with a high energy density. Because the input electric energy is stored in the electric field of the electrochemical double layer at the active carbon/electrolyte interphase without any means of energy conversion or charge transmission, a supercapacitor—also known as an EDLC (double-layer electrochemical capacitor)—produces high power and a long lifespan but low energy density. The use of a supercapacitor for high-power discharge and a battery for high-energy density storage is idealized by the combination of the two aforementioned energy sources. The energy density and power density of the battery and capacitor combination are calculated using the weighted average of the battery and capacitor in terms of their mass ratio. When utilizing the same battery and capacitor, comparing parallel and hybrid configurations does not appear to increase energy or power density; however, internal configurations of the battery and capacitor electrodes have a distinct impact. The cathode limits the energy density and power output of a conventional lithium-ion battery because it slows down charge transfer in the bulk and at the cathode/electrolyte contact and has less capacity than the commonly used graphite anode. As a consequence, the asymmetric hybrid cell, which combines a lithium-ion battery's anode and a super-active capacitor's carbon electrode in a single energy storage system, has the potential to produce energy and power densities that are equivalent to both of these energy storage systems. The problem of energy density and power density in energy storage systems is therefore shown to have a potential answer in the hybrid ion capacitor. Because of its low cost and democratically dispersed reserves, sodium is becoming a viable alternative to existing commercial Li-ion systems. Na-ion capacitors and other Li-ion devices have significant material design problems. Through the use of bio nanotechnology, a simple yet adaptable method, the difficulties associated with creating high-performance materials utilizing sustainable biomass energy may be solved (Ding et al., 2015).

The production of peanuts annually amounts to roughly 20 million tons, making them a common food crop. As a result, the approximately 6 million tons of peanut shells produced as waste are no longer useful for commerce. Ding et al. demonstrated via bio nanotechnology that the carbon in peanut shells makes suitable anode and cathode materials for a Na-ion capacitor (Ding et al., 2015). The unique feature of this method is that it yields both the cathode and anode active materials (carbon) from a single precursor, peanut shell, making it both economical and ecologically responsible. Notably, for each of the material classes, the electrodes which developed from these carbon materials exhibit some of the finest sodiation capacity-rate, capability-cycling retention combinations ever recorded in the literature. This method employed the inner part of the shell as the anode precursor. It involved carbonizing the inner shell in argon at 1200 °C and activating it in air at a low temperature. This produced enough porosity while preserving the macroscopically sheet-like structure of the precursor. The outer rough shell was employed as a precursor for the cathode after hydrothermal treatment, which was then followed by chemical activation with KOH at 800–850 °C in argon. This approach is based on an understanding of the differences between the inner and outer shell structures, as well as how these variations may affect the microstructures of the final electrodes. The tissue that makes up the peanut shell is exceedingly diverse, with varying percentages and distributions in the inner and outer shells, despite the fact that the core of the peanut shell is made of cellulose, hemicellulose, and lignin. Because each electrode of a sodium ion capacitor necessitates carbon with inherently various levels of graphene ordering, surface area/porosity, and surface functionality, the microstructure of the peanut's inner and outer shells may be an ideal place to start when looking to develop these electrode materials. The intercalation anode and the adsorption cathode are additional components of this type of device. Environmental risks from synthetic material pollution are getting worse. Despite the fact that plastic and petroleum derivatives cannot decompose through microbial action and cannot biodegrade, they accumulate in the environment year after year due to the growing cost of fossil fuels, forcing us to use more biomaterials in daily life. Biodegradable polymers were found to be an alternative substance that may substitute synthetic polymers without compromising their physicochemical properties in the early 1980s. As a result, a lot of academics and businesses started concentrating on biodegradable polymers. However, a great number of biodegradable polymers have recently been synthesized and may be used in a range of applications. Natural polymers are numerous and can be manufactured from renewable resources (Rinaudo, 2006).

13.4 BIOPOLYMER-BASED ENERGY MATERIALS

In order to improve the electrical properties as well as chemical capabilities of bio composites, polysaccharides can also be categorized according to their ionic nature (neutral, anionic, or cationic). Animal protein and fat are generated from microorganisms, while another type of polysaccharide and polyesters are derived from bacteria. Polysaccharide, which contains polyphenol, is acquired from plants. Due to their numerous special qualities that are pertinent to the development of biological and electrochemical devices, polysaccharides have been used as composite matrix. Numerous research teams have used biopolymer starch with success in a variety of energy applications, including high-energy batteries, fuel cells, electrochromic displays, actuators, and solar cells; other applications include the food industry and artificial muscles (Sudhakar et al., 2018). The hydroxyl groups in the sugar rings make it easier to swap out different functional groups. Differences in sugar content and functional group substitution have an impact on the 3D packing of polysaccharides and their interactions with other polymers or salts. In comparison to polysaccharides with few hydrogen bonds, those with many hydrogen bonds tend to be more conductive. Electroactive materials' mobility and ion mobility are governed by the polymer's degree of crystallinity. Electroactive materials' moisture content fluctuates depending on the environment and how hydrophilic they are (Plackett and Hansen, 2012; Finkenstadt and Willett, 2005). Due to the characteristics described above, polysaccharides make an excellent material for bio-inspired energy devices. Biopolymers are biodegradable materials made with living things (such as microorganisms and plants). The distinction between natural and synthetic polymers refers to the fact that these polymers may be chemically synthesized from lipids, amino acids, proteins, or vegetable oils in addition to occurring naturally in our bodies. (Fig. 13.3) (Dziuba et al., 2021).

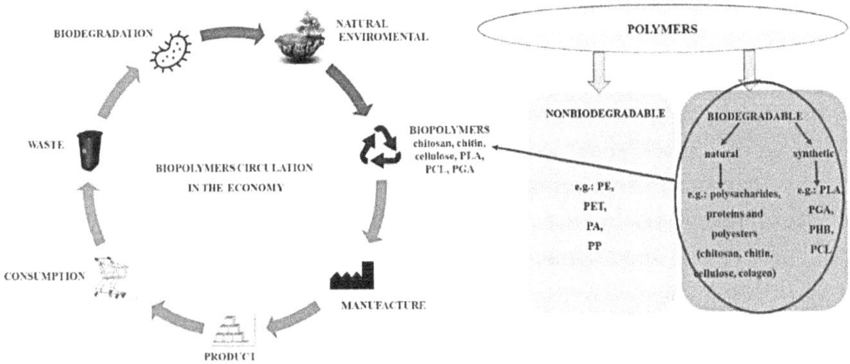

FIGURE 13.3 Biodegradable polymer life cycle in relation to the circular economy.

Source: Reprinted with permission from Dziuba et al., 2021. https://creativecommons.org/licenses/by/4.0/

13.4.1 ION-CONDUCTING MEMBRANES MADE OF AGAROSE/AGAR

Although agarose is a pure form of agar, agar is a type of marine algal biopolymer made from hydrophilic red seaweed polysaccharides. It is composed of linearly arranged -d-galactose and 1, 4-linked 3, 6-anhydro-l-galactose units that can form a long chain. However, depending on the kind of agarose (high or low EEO) used for synthesis, gel formation occurs at temperatures ranging from 32 °C to 45 °C. Agarose is typically insoluble in cold water but readily dissolves in hot water, generating a homogenous solution at temperatures ranging from 80 °C to 95 °C. Agarose dissolves quickly in a variety of dipolar aprotic solvents, including DMF, DMSO, DMAc, NMP, glycol, and orthophosphoric acid (Hsu et al., 2011). The capacity to create a macroporous matrix with thermoreversible hysteresis is the fundamental benefit of utilizing agarose in the manufacture of ion-conducting membranes. The agarose-based biopolymer's ionic conductivity varies from 10^{1}–$10?^{1}$ mS cm$?^{1}$. NaCl doped agarose has a very high level of ion conductivity with a conductivity of 10^{1} mS cm$?^{1}$ (Liew et al., 2019).

13.4.2 ION-CONDUCTING MEMBRANES MADE OF CARRAGEENAN

Red algae or seaweeds (Rhodophyceae) are the source of the water-soluble polysaccharide known as carrageenan powder; nevertheless, an anionic polymer has sulfated groups sparingly. It is composed of a linear galactan chain with linkages to (1 3)-D and (1 4)-d-galactopyranosyl (or 3, 6-anhydro-d-galactopyranosyl) through an ester sulfate linkage network.

A classification of carrageenan biopolymer is κ-carrageenan, ι-carrageenan, and λ-carrageenan based on the concentration of the sulfate group and the presence of 3, 6-anhydro-d-galactose (Stephen and Phillips, 2016).

Ion-conducting membranes based on acetic acid with 0.95 mS cm?[1] conductivity have been reported by a significant number of groups. Carrageenan-based ion-conducting membranes have previously been used by several researchers in the development of a variety of energy devices (fuel cell, battery, and supercapacitor). Ionic conductivity of LiI, NaI, and KOH based dopants exceeds 1 mS cm?[1] (Bella et al., 2015; Di Palma et al., 2017).

13.4.3 ION-CONDUCTING MEMBRANES MADE OF STARCH

Sago, potato, maize, arrowroot, peas, and rice are just a few examples of plants from which starch is frequently derived. According to the grade, starch is composed of two different kinds of polysaccharides, amylose and amylopectin, as well as a little amount of proteins and lipids (Lu et al., 2009). Several starch-based biopolymers, such as sago starch, rice starch, wheat starch, tamarind seed, pea starch, maize starch, potato starch, and arrowroot-based starch, were used to create ion-conducting membranes. One characteristic that all starch-based ion-conducting membranes have in common is that they have strong ionic conduction in the range of 10–10?[1] mS cm?[1]. Li^+, Na^+, K^+, and $NH4^+$ are common monovalent cations, with a variety of anion types such as Cl?, I?, Br?, SCN?, and ClO4? being used to create membranes that conduct ions and have low activation energies and high mobile ion concentrations.

13.4.4 MEMBRANES THAT CONDUCT ALGINATE IONS

Alginate is a kind of biopolymer derived from brown seaweeds and belongs to the Phaeophyceae family. A linear polysaccharide chain made up of β-d amannuronopyranosyl and α-L guluronopyranosyl units makes up the structure of alginate. Controlling the ratio of G-, M-, and MG-blocks, where M blocks contain mannuronopyranose residues and G blocks include remnants of guluronopyranose or combine MG blocks, can tailor the strength of the crosslink network (Stephen and Phillips, 2016). With G-blocks, alginate creates a reliable, top-notch gel; whereas, with calcium, M-blocks can quickly generate a complicated structure. It takes a long time to dissolve in water and forms a viscous solution, but it is found insoluble in ethanol solution and ether. At ambient temperature, LiClO4 has the greatest ion-conducting membrane conduction of 3.1 $10?^{1}$ mS $cm?^{1}$, whereas CH_3COOH has a conduction of 8.7 10^{2} mS $cm?^{1}$ (Iwaki et al., 2012).

13.5 ENERGY MATERIALS DERIVED FROM ANIMALS

Considered as probable precursors of electronic active materials for energy storage and conversion applications include animal bone, hair, and occasionally nails. Liu and colleagues used human hair as a source of fibrous carbon in their study in 2017 to develop fibre-based solid-state supercapacitors (Liu et al., 2017). This study emphasizes the benefits of using human hair, which has excellent tensile strength, elastic recovery qualities, and delayed degradation properties, as the material for flexible super capacitors. Additionally, following carbonization, the biological substance in the hair has higher quantities of intrinsic dopants, which results in fibres with beneficial properties. Because of the aforementioned properties of hair, solid-state super capacitors made using nanostructure MnO2 function very effectively (Liu et al., 2017). Being able to transform this waste product into something useful for future technologies is a great turning point to push the research in this subject of energy because the majority of people have hair and need frequent haircuts.

Another study produced porous cheese-like carbon for zinc air batteries using the hair protein keratin (Wang et al., 2018). The impacts and effects of nitrogen and sulfur co-doping on oxygen reduction processes are explored (ORR). An alternative viewpoint at the utilization of waste from the meat industry, primarily animal bones, in energy storage and conversion technologies. Bones have a unique composition that results in carbon that is generated from them having a large surface area and a particular hierarchically porous structure (Xie et al., 2017). Egg yolk has lately been the subject of research on materials for energy storage and conversion. An investigation on creating a powerful super capacitor material made from egg yolk was published in 2019 by Zhang et al. To synthesize iron-encapsulated nanoparticles in carbon nanotubes, an iron precursor is mixed with egg yolk, hydrothermally reacted, and then annealed (Zhao et al., 2019). The results of this study are significant because carbon nanotubes seem to form spontaneously during the procedure utilizing a simple, low-cost approach without any templating. A unique egg white gel polymer electrolyte and green solid-state supercapacitor were created by Na et al. using a novel cracked eggshell and rice husks (Fig. 13.4) (Mensah-Darkwa et al., 2019).

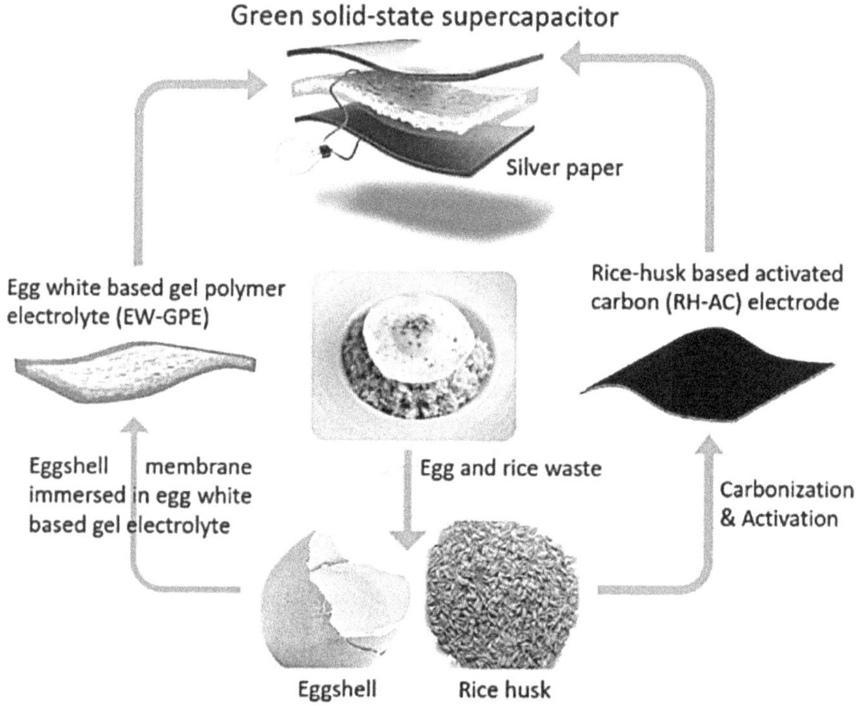

FIGURE 13.4 Schematic for making a green solid-state supercapacitor with leftover rice and broken eggshell.

Source: Reprinted with permission from Mensah-Darkwa et al., 2019. Copyright © 2019 by the authors. Licensee MDPI, Basel, Switzerland. https://creativecommons.org/licenses/by/4.0/

13.5.1 ENERGY MATERIALS MADE FROM CRAB SHELLS

The amine-containing polysaccharide chitin is widely present in shellfish shells, they're an excellent option for intrinsic nitrogen doping because of this property. Chemical methods and sometimes biological methods generally used in the isolation process of chitin polymer from oyster shells (Santos et al., 2020; Yadav et al., 2019). Chemical treatment methods such as acid washing remove minerals from the shells, such as calcium. After that, the proteins are eliminated using an alkali treatment, and the chitin is then isolated using washing. In biological techniques, treatment with enzymes including papain, trypsin, alcalase, protease, and pepsin are utilized. Deacetylation of chitin yield cationic polymer chitosan. In 2019, in their research on hierarchical porous carbon (HPC) compounds for application in supercapacitors,

Fu and colleagues employed crab shells as a chitosan-rich precursor (Li et al., 2019). To generate porous carbon, crab shells were primarily carbonized in a furnace, after that it is acid washed to completely remove different carbonates and create large pores. The carbon is then dried, cleaned with water, and heated to a high temperature before being activated with KOH. Which having a capacity retention rate of 94% even after 10,000 cycles, it illustrates how clam waste may be utilized to create high-performance supercapacitors (Li et al., 2019). Crab shells have been successfully used to create $Ca(OH)_2$-Carbon framework, which has been used in Li-S batteries and supercapacitor applications (Shao et al., 2016). Because crab shells contain calcium, it is possible to engineer special micro- and nanostructures. Crab shells are calcined at various temperatures to create the material mentioned, which the separator is made of by combining gelatin films (Shao et al., 2016).

13.5.2 ENERGY MATERIALS MADE FROM SHRIMP SHELLS

Due to the quantity of chitin and proteins they contain, porous carbon compounds may be found in large quantities in shrimp shells. Recently, mesoporous carbon networks made of shrimp shells were reported (Zheng et al., 2020). Zheng et al. saw the publication of a study on the catalytic activity of the carbon dioxide produced by using shrimp shell for microbial fuel cells. Interest in using non-platinum group metals in catalyst research and design has increased due to the potential cost savings. The intrinsically doped carbon in this study exhibits the essential electrocatalytic activity since nitrogen and phosphorous dopants were used (Liu et al., 2020).

KEYWORDS

- **advanced energy materials**
- **sustainable green energy**
- **nanomaterials**
- **microorganisms**
- **power storage**

REFERENCES

Armand, M.; Tarascon, J. M. Building Better Batteries. *Nature* **2008,** *451,* 652–657.

Bella, F.; Mobarak, N. N.; Jumaah, F. N.; Ahmad, A. From Seaweeds to Biopolymeric Electrolytes for Third Generation Solar Cells: An Intriguing Approach. *Electrochim. Acta* **2015,** *151,* 306–311.

Beznosov, S. N.; Veluri, P. S.; Pyatibratov, M. G.; Chatterjee, A.; MacFarlane, D. R.; Fedorov, O. V.; Mitra, S. Flagellar Filament Bio-templated Inorganic Oxide Materials–Towards an Efficient Lithium Battery Anode. *Sci. Rep.* **2015,** *5,* 1–7.

Bhat, V. S.; Jayeoye, T. J.; Rujiralai, T.; Sirimahachai, U.; Chong, K. F.; Hegde, G. Influence of Surface Properties on Electro-chemical Supercapacitors Utilizing Callerya Atropurpurea Pod Derived Porous Nanocarbons: Structure Property Relationship Between Porous Structures to Energy Storage Devices. *Nano Select* **2020,** *1,* 226–243.

Bresser, D.; Passerini, S.; Scrosati, B. Recent Progress and Remaining Challenges in Sulfur-based Lithium Secondary Batteries—A Review. *Chem. Commun.* **2013,** *49,* 10545–10562.

Bromley, K. M.; Patil, A. J.; Perriman, A. W.; Stubbs, G.; Mann, S. Preparation of High Quality Nanowires by Tobacco Mosaic Virus Templating of Gold Nanoparticles. *J. Mater. Chem.* **2008,** *18,* 4796–4801.

Brown, A. D.; Naves, L.; Wang, X.; Ghodssi, R.; Culver, J. N. Carboxylate-Directed in Vivo Assembly of Virus-like Nanorods and Tubes for the Display Of Functional Peptides and Residues. *Biomacromolecules* **2013,** *14,* 3123–3129.

Cericola, D.; Kötz, R. Hybridization of Rechargeable Batteries and Electrochemical Capacitors: Principles and Limits. *Electrochim. Acta* **2012,** *72,* 1–17.

Che, W.; Xiao, Z.; Wang, Z.; Li, J.; Wang, H.; Wang, Y.; Xie, Y. Wood-Based Mesoporous Filter Decorated with Silver Nanoparticles for Water Purification. *ACS Sustain. Chem. Eng.* **2019,** *7,* 5134–5141.

Chen, X.; Gerasopoulos, K.; Guo, J.; Brown, A.; Wang, C.; Ghodssi, R.; Culver, J. N. Virus-enabled Silicon Anode for Lithium-Ion Batteries. *ACS Nano* **2010,** *4,* 5366–5372.

Conway, B. E.; Pell, W. G. Double-layer and Pseudocapacitance Types of Electrochemical Capacitors and their Applications to the Development of Hybrid Devices. *J. Solid State Electrochem.* **2003,** *7,* 637–644.

Cui, J.; Liu, H. Mesoporous SiO2 Produced by Mineralization of Yeast Cells as an Efficient Electrocatalyst for Oxygen Reduction Reaction. *Russ. Chem. Bull.* **2017,** *66,* 969–974.

Cui, L. F.; Ruffo, R.; Chan, C. K. *Nano Lett.* **2008,** *8,* 491–495.

Culver, J. N.; Brown, A. D.; Zang, F.; Gnerlich, M.; Gerasopoulos, K.; Ghodssi, R. Plant Virus Directed Fabrication of Nanoscale Materials and Devices. *Virology* **2015,** *479,* 200–212.

Di Palma, T. M.; Migliardini, F.; Caputo, D.; Corbo, P. Xanthan and κ-Carrageenan Based Alkaline Hydrogels as Electrolytes for Al/air Batteries. *Carbohydr. Polym.* **2017,** *157,* 122–127.

Ding, J.; Wang, H.; Li, Z.; Cui, K.; Karpuzov, D.; Tan, X.; Kohandehghan, A.; Mitlin, D. Peanut Shell Hybrid Sodium Ion Capacitor with Extreme Energy-power Rivals Lithium Ion Capacitors. *Energy Environ. Sci.* **2015,** *8,* 941–955.

Dziuba, R.; Kucharska, M.; Madej-Kiełbik, L.; Sulak, K.; Wiśniewska-Wrona, M. Biopolymers and Biomaterials for Special Applications within the Context of the Circular Economy. *Materials* **2021,** *14,* 7704.

Fan, X.; Song, X.; Yang, X.; Hou, L. Facile Fabrication of ZrO2 Hollow Porous Microspheres with Yeast as Bio-templates. *Mater. Res. Bul.* **2011,** *46,* 1315–1319.

Fang, Y.; Yu, X.-Y.; Lou, X. W. D. Nanostructured Electrode Materials for Advanced Sodium-ion Batteries. *Matter* **2019,** *1,* 90–114.

Finkenstadt, V.; Willett, J. Preparation and Characterization of Electroactive Biopolymers. In *Macromolecular Symposia*; Wiley Online Library, 2005; pp 367–372.

Gao, L.; Liang, C. N.; Li, H. H.; Lu, Z. X. Hierarchically Templated Synthesis of Hollow Nanoporous Gold Rods and TiO2-Coated Gold Rods. *ChemNanoMat.* **2016,** *2,* 1098–1103.

Ghouri, Z. K.; Al-Meer, S.; Barakat, N. A.; Kim, H. Y. ZnO@ C (core@ shell) Microspheres Derived from Spent Coffee Grounds as Applicable Non-precious Electrode Material for DMFCs. *Sci. Rep.* **2017,** *7,* 1–8.

Hsu, H.-L.; Hsu, W.-T.; Leu, J. Effects of Environmentally Benign Solvents in the Agarose Gel Electrolytes on Dye-sensitized Solar Cells. *Electrochim. Acta* **2011,** *56,* 5904–5909.

Hu, C.; Dai, L. Multifunctional Carbon-Based Metal-Free Electrocatalysts for Simultaneous Oxygen Reduction, Oxygen Evolution, and Hydrogen Evolution. *Adv. Mater.* **2017,** *29,* 1604942.

Hu, Z.; Li, J.; Zhang, X.; Zhu, Y. Strategies to Improve the Performance of Li Metal Anode for Rechargeable Batteries. *Fronti. Chem.* **2020, 8.**

Hwang, D. J.; Roberts, I. M.; Wilson, T. Expression of Tobacco Mosaic Virus Coat Protein and Assembly of Pseudovirus Particles in *Escherichia coli*. *Proc. Natl Acad. Sci.* **1994,** *91,* 9067–9071.

Iwaki, Y. O.; Escalona, M. H.; Briones, J. R.; Pawlicka, A. Sodium Alginate-Based Ionic Conducting Membranes. *Mol. Cryst. Liq. Cryst.* **2012,** *554,* 221–231.

Jensen, M.; Keding, R.; Höche, T.; Yue, Y. Biologically Formed Mesoporous Amorphous Silica. *J. Am. Chem. Soc.* **2009,** *131,* 2717–2721.

Knez, M.; Bittner, A. M.; Boes, F.; Wege, C.; Jeske, H.; Maiβ, E.; Kern, K. Biotemplate Synthesis of 3-nm Nickel and Cobalt Nanowires. *Nano Lett.* **2003,** *3,* 1079–1082.

Krikstolaityte, V.; Joshua, O. E. Y.; Veksha, A.; Wai, N.; Lisak, G.; Lim, T. M. Conversion of Spent Coffee Beans to Electrode Material for Vanadium Redox Flow Batteries. *Batteries* **2018,** *4,* 56.

Kumara, M. T.; Tripp, B. C.; Muralidharan, S. Self-assembly of Metal Nanoparticles and Nanotubes on Bioengineered Flagella Scaffolds. *Chem. Mate.* **2007,** *19,* 2056–2064.

Li, J.; Zheng, J. M.; Yang, Y. Studies on Storage Characteristics of LiNi0.4Co0.2Mn0.4O2 as Cathode Materials in Lithium-Ion Batteries. *J. Electrochem. Soc.* **2007,** *154,* a427–a432.

Li, Y.; Fu, Z.-Y.; Su, B.-L. Hierarchically Structured Porous Materials for Energy Conversion and Storage. *Adv. Func. Mater.* **2012,** *22,* 4634–4667.

Li, Z.-X.; Yang, B.-L.; Zou, K.-Y.; Kong, L.; Yue, M.-L.; Duan, H.-H. Novel Porous Carbon Nanosheet Derived from a 2D Cu-MOF: Ultrahigh Porosity and Excellent Performances in the Supercapacitor Cell. *Carbon* **2019,** *144,* 540–548.

Liang, H.; Soref, R.; Mu, J.; Majumdar, A.; Li, X.; Huang, W.-P. Simulations of Silicon-on-Insulator Channel-Waveguide Electrooptical 2 × 2 Switches and 1 × 1 Modulators Using a ${\bf Ge_2}{\bf Sb_2}{\bf Te_5} $ Self-Holding Layer. *J. Light. Technol.* **2015,** *33,* 1805–1813.

Liedel, C. Sustainable Battery Materials from Biomass. *ChemSusChem*. **2020,** *13,* 2110–2141.

Liew, S. Y.; Juan, J. C.; Lai, C. W.; Pan, G.-T.; Yang, T. C.-K.; Lee, T. K. An Eco-friendly Water-soluble Graphene-incorporated Agar Gel Electrolyte for Magnesium-Air Batteries. *Ionics* **2019,** *25,* 1291–1301.

Liu, N.; Huo, K.; McDowell, M. T.; Zhao, J.; Cui, Y. Rice Husks as a Sustainable Source of Nanostructured Silicon for High Performance Li-ion Battery Anodes. *Sci. Rep.* **2013,** *3.*

Liu, T.; Jean Pierre, M.; Li, H.; Wu, W.; Tu, M.; Wang, Q.; Ma, H. Nitrogen and Phosphorus Doped Activated Carbon Catalyst Prepared from Shrimp Shell and Its Application in MFC Air Cathode. *Chem. Select* **2020,** *5,* 2690–2695.

Liu, W.; Feng, K.; Zhang, Y.; Yu, T.; Han, L.; Lui, G.; Li, M.; Chiu, G.; Fung, P.; Yu, A. Hair-based Flexible Knittable Supercapacitor with Wide Operating Voltage and Ultra-high Rate Capability. *Nano Energy* **2017,** *34,* 491–499.

Liu, X.; Zhang, S.; Wen, X.; Chen, X.; Wen, Y.; Shi, X.; Mijowska, E. High Yield Conversion of Biowaste Coffee Grounds into Hierarchical Porous Carbon for Superior Capacitive Energy Storage. *Sci. Rep.* **2020,** *10,* 3518.

Lu, D.; Xiao, C.; Xu, S. Starch-based Completely Biodegradable Polymer Materials. *Express Polym. Lett.* **2009,** *3,* 366–375.

Ma, L.; Bi, Z.; Xue, Y.; Zhang, W.; Huang, Q.; Zhang, L.; Huang, Y. Bacterial Cellulose: An Encouraging Eco-friendly Nano-candidate for Energy Storage and Energy Conversion. *J. Mater. Chem. A* **2020,** *8,* 5812–5842.

Mensah-Darkwa, K.; Zequine, C.; Kahol, P. K.; Gupta, R. K. Supercapacitor Energy Storage Device Using Biowastes: A Sustainable Approach to Green Energy. *Sustainability* **2019,** *11,* 414.

Mujib, S. B.; Vessalli, B.; Bizzo, W. A.; Mazon, T.; Singh, G. Cassava-and Bamboo-Derived Carbons with Higher Degree of Graphitization for Energy Storage. *Nanomater. Energy* **2020,** *9,* 54–65.

Muzaffar, A.; Ahamed, M. B.; Deshmukh, K.; Thirumalai, J. A Review on Recent Advances in Hybrid Supercapacitors: Design, Fabrication and Applications. *Renew. Sust. Energ. Rev.* **2019,** *101,* 123–145.

Nomura, T.; Tanii, S.; Ishikawa, M.; Tokumoto, H.; Konishi, Y. Synthesis of Hollow Zirconia Particles Using Wet Bacterial Templates. *Adv. Powder Technol.* **2013,** *24,* 1013–1016.

Osherov, N.; May, G. S. The Molecular Mechanisms of Conidial Germination. *FEMS Microbiol. Lett.* **2001,** *199,* 153–160.

Park, M. S.; Lim, Y. G.; Hwang, S. M.; Kim, J. H.; Kim, J. S.; Dou, S. X.; Cho, J.; Kim, Y. J. Scalable Integration of Li5FeO4 Towards Robust, High-performance Lithium-ion Hybrid Capacitors. *ChemSusChem* **2014,** *7,* 3138–3144.

Pei, Z.; Li, H.; Huang, Y.; Xue, Q.; Huang, Y.; Zhu, M.; Wang, Z.; Zhi, C. Texturing In Situ: N,S-enriched Hierarchically Porous Carbon as a Highly Active Reversible Oxygen Electrocatalyst. *Energy Environ. Sci.* **2017,** *10,* 742–749.

Plackett, D.; Hansen, N. Nonxylan Hemicelluloses as a Source of Renewable Materials. In *Polysaccharide Building Blocks: A Sustainable Approach to the Development of Renewable Biomaterials*, 2012; p 387.

Qu, K.; You, Y.; Qi, H.; Shi, C.; Sun, Z.; Huang, Z.; Yuan, B.; Guo, Z. Fungus Bran-Derived Porous N-doped Carbon–Zinc Manganese Oxide Nanocomposite Positive Electrodes Toward High-performance Asymmetric Supercapacitors. *J. Phys. Chem. C* **2020,** *124,* 15713–15722.

Radloff, C.; Vaia, R. A.; Brunton, J.; Bouwer, G. T.; Ward, V. K. Metal Nanoshell Assembly on a Virus Bioscaffold. *Nano Lett.* **2005,** *5,* 1187–1191.

Ramamurthy, P. C.; Singh, S.; Kapoor, D.; Parihar, P.; Samuel, J.; Prasad, R.; Kumar, A.; Singh, J. Microbial Biotechnological Approaches: Renewable Bioprocessing for the Future Energy Systems. *Microb. Cell Factories* **2021,** *20,* 55.

Rebentrost, P.; Mohseni, M.; Kassal, I.; Lloyd, S.; Aspuru-Guzik, A. Environment-Assisted Quantum Transport. *New J. Phys.* **2009,** *11,* 033003.

Ren, L.; Guo, L.; Wark, M.; Hou, Y. Self-integration of Aligned Cobalt Nanoparticles into Silica Nanotubes. *Appl. Phys. Lett.* **2005,** *87,* 212503.

Rinaudo, M. Chitin and Chitosan: Properties and Applications. *Prog. Polym. Sci.* **2006,** *31,* 603–632.

Royston, E.; Ghosh, A.; Kofinas, P.; Harris, M. T.; Culver, J. N. Self-assembly of Virus-structured High Surface Area Nanomaterials and their Application as Battery Electrodes. *Langmuir* **2008,** *24,* 906–912.

Santos, V.; Marques, N.; Maia, P.; Lima, M.; Franco, L.; Campos-Takaki, G. M. Seafood Waste as Attractive Source of Chitin and Chitosan Production and their Applications. *Int. J. Mol. Sci.* **2020,** *21,* 4290.

Shackley, S.; Carter, S.; Knowles, T.; Middelink, E.; Haefele, S.; Sohi, S.; Cross, A.; Haszeldine, S. Sustainable Gasification–biochar Systems? A Case-study of Rice-husk Gasification in Cambodia, Part I: Context, Chemical Properties, Environmental and Health and Safety Issues. *Energy Policy* **2012,** *42,* 49–58.

Shaheen, I.; Ahmad, K. S.; Zequine, C.; Gupta, R. K.; Thomas, A. G.; Malik, M. A. Modified Sol-gel Synthesis of Co3O4 Nanoparticles Using Organic Template for Electrochemical Energy Storage. *Energy* **2021,** *218,* 119502.

Shaheen, I.; Ahmad, K. S.; Zequine, C.; Gupta, R. K.; Thomas, A.; Malik, M. A. Organic Template-assisted Green Synthesis of CoMoO 4 Nanomaterials for the Investigation of Energy Storage Properties. *RSC Adv.* **2020,** *10,* 8115–8129.

Shang, L.; Yu, H.; Huang, X.; Bian, T.; Shi, R.; Zhao, Y.; Waterhouse, G. I. N.; Wu, L.-Z.; Tung, C.-H.; Zhang, T. Well-Dispersed ZIF-Derived Co,N-Co-doped Carbon Nanoframes through Mesoporous-Silica-Protected Calcination as Efficient Oxygen Reduction Electrocatalysts. *Adv. Mater.* **2016,** *28,* 1668–1674.

Shao, H.; Huang, B.; Liu, N.; Wang, W.; Zhang, H.; Wang, A.; Wang, F.; Huang, Y. Modified Separators Coated with a Ca (OH) 2–Carbon Framework Derived from Crab Shells for Lithium–Sulfur Batteries. *J. Mater. Chem. A* **2016,** *4,* 16627–16634.

Shenton, W.; Douglas, T.; Young, M.; Stubbs, G.; Mann, S. Inorganic–Organic Nanotube Composites from Template Mineralization of Tobacco Mosaic Virus. *Adv. Mater.* **1999,** *11,* 253–256.

Shim, H.-W.; Jin, Y.-H.; Seo, S.-D.; Lee, S.-H.; Kim, D.-W. Highly Reversible Lithium Storage in Bacillus Subtilis-directed Porous Co3O4 Nanostructures. *ACS Nano* **2011,** *5,* 443–449.

Shinde, S. S.; Lee, C.-H.; Sami, A.; Kim, D.-H.; Lee, S.-U.; Lee, J.-H. Scalable 3-D Carbon Nitride Sponge as an Efficient Metal-Free Bifunctional Oxygen Electrocatalyst for Rechargeable Zn–Air Batteries. *ACS Nano* **2017,** *11,* 347–357.

Sidhu, S. S. Engineering M13 for Phage Display. *Biomol. Eng.* **2001,** *18,* 57–63.

Song, H.; Xu, S.; Li, Y.; Dai, J.; Gong, A.; Zhu, M.; Zhu, C.; Chen, C.; Chen, Y.; Yao, Y.; Liu, B.; Song, J.; Pastel, G.; Hu, L. Hierarchically Porous, Ultrathick, "Breathable" Wood-Derived Cathode for Lithium-Oxygen Batteries. *Adv. Energy Mater.* **2018,** *8,* 1701203.

Sotiropoulou, S.; Sierra-Sastre, Y.; Mark, S. S.; Batt, C. A. Biotemplated Nanostructured Materials. *Chem. Mate.* **2008,** *20,* 821–834.

Stephen, A. M.; Phillips, G. O. *Food Polysaccharides and Their Applications*; CRC Press, 2016.

Sudhakar, Y.; Selvakumar, M.; Bhat, D. K. *Biopolymer Electrolytes: Fundamentals and Applications in Energy Storage*; Elsevier, 2018.

Sugunan, A.; Melin, P.; Schnürer, J.; Hilborn, J. G.; Dutta, J. Nutrition-driven Assembly of Colloidal Nanoparticles: Growing Fungi Assemble Gold Nanoparticles as Microwires. *Adv. Mater.* **2007,** *19,* 77–81.

Tang, Z.; Pei, Z.; Wang, Z.; Li, H.; Zeng, J.; Ruan, Z.; Huang, Y.; Zhu, M.; Xue, Q.; Yu, J.; Zhi, C. Highly Anisotropic, Multichannel Wood Carbon with Optimized Heteroatom Doping for Supercapacitor and Oxygen Reduction Reaction. *Carbon* **2018,** *130,* 532–543.

Wang, Y.; Lin, X.; Liu, T.; Chen, H.; Chen, S.; Jiang, Z.; Liu, J.; Huang, J.; Liu, M. Wood-derived Hierarchically Porous Electrodes for High-performance All-solid-state Supercapacitors. *Adv. Func. Mater.* **2018,** *28,* 1806207.

Wang, Z.-D.; Liu, Q.; Liu, H.-H.; Li, S.; Zhang, L.; Zhao, Y.-K.; Zhu, X.-Q. Prevalence of Cryptosporidium, Microsporidia and Isospora Infection in HIV-infected People: A Global Systematic Review and Meta-analysis. *Parasit. Vectors* **2018,** *11,* 1–19.

Wen, A. M.; Steinmetz, N. F. Design of Virus-based Nanomaterials for Medicine, Biotechnology, and Energy. *Chem. Soc. Rev.* **2016,** *45,* 4074–4126.

Xia, Y.; Xiao, Z.; Dou, X.; Huang, H.; Lu, X.; Yan, R.; Gan, Y.; Zhu, W.; Tu, J.; Zhang, W.; Tao, X. Green and Facile Fabrication of Hollow Porous MnO/C Microspheres from Microalgaes for Lithium-Ion Batteries. *ACS Nano* **2013,** *7,* 7083–7092.

Xie, L.-S.; Yu, S.-X.; Yang, H.-J.; Yang, J.; Ni, J.-L.; Wang, J.-L. Hierarchical Porous Carbon Derived from Animal Bone as Matric to Encapsulated Selenium for High Performance Li–Se battery. *Rare Metals* **2017,** *36,* 434–441.

Xu, J.; Tan, Z.; Zeng, W.; Chen, G.; Wu, S.; Zhao, Y.; Ni, K.; Tao, Z.; Ikram, M.; Ji, H.; Zhu, Y. A Hierarchical Carbon Derived from Sponge-Templated Activation of Graphene Oxide for High-Performance Supercapacitor Electrodes. *Adv. Mater.* **2016,** *28,* 5222–5228.

Yadav, M.; Goswami, P.; Paritosh, K.; Kumar, M.; Pareek, N.; Vivekanand, V. Seafood Waste: A Source for Preparation of Commercially Employable Chitin/Chitosan Materials. *Bioresour. Bioprocess.* **2019,** *6,* 1–20.

Yao, H.-B.; Fang, H.-Y.; Wang, X.-H.; Yu, S.-H. Hierarchical Assembly of Micro-/Nano-building Blocks: Bio-inspired Rigid Structural Functional Materials. *Chem. Soc. Rev.* **2011,** *40,* 3764–3785.

Zhang, S.; Li, H.; Wang, S.; Liu, Y.; Chen, H.; Lu, Z.-X. Bacteria-assisted Synthesis of Nanosheet-assembled TiO2 Hierarchical Architectures for Constructing TiO2-based Composites for Photocatalytic and Electrocatalytic Applications. *ACS Appl. Mater. Interfaces* **2019,** *11,* 37004–37012.

Zhang, X.; Jiang, W. J.; Mauger, A.; Qilu; Gendron, F.; Julien, C. M. Minimization of the Cation Mixing in Li1+x(NMC)1−xO2 as Cathode Material. *J. Power Sour.* **2010,** *195,* 1292–1301.

Zhang, X.; Yang, Y.; Zhou, Z. Towards Practical Lithium-metal Anodes.. *Chem. Soc. Rev.* **2020,** *49,* 3040–3071.

Zhang, X.; Zhang, X.; He, W.; Yue, Y.; Liu, H.; Ma, J. Biocarbon-Coated LiFePO 4 Nucleus Nanoparticles Enhancing Electrochemical Performances. *Chem. Commun.* **2012,** *48,* 10093–10095.

Zhao, B.; Shao, Q.; Hao, L.; Zhang, L.; Liu, Z.; Zhang, B.; Ge, S.; Guo, Z.; Yeast-template Synthesized Fe-doped Cerium Oxide Hollow Microspheres for Visible Photodegradation of Acid Orange 7. *J. Colloid Interface Sci.* **2018,** *511,* 39–47.

Zhao, Y.; Qiang, C.; Wang, X.; Chen, Y.; Deng, J.; Jiang, C.; Sun, X.; Chen, H.; Li, J.; Piao, W. New Alleles for Chlorophyll Content and Stay-green Traits Revealed by a Genome Wide Association Study in Rice (Oryza sativa). *Sci. Rep.* **2019,** *9,* 1–11.

Zheng, F.-Y.; Li, R.; Ge, S.; Xu, W.-R.; Zhang, Y. Nitrogen and Phosphorus Co-doped Carbon Networks Derived from Shrimp Shells as an Efficient Oxygen Reduction Catalyst for Microbial Fuel Cells. *J. Power Sour.* **2020,** *446,* 227356.

Zheng, J. M.; Li, J.; Zhang, Z. R.; Guo, X. J.; Yang, Y. The Effects of TiO2 Coating on the Electrochemical Performance of Li[Li0.2Mn0.54Ni0.13Co0.13]O2 Cathode Material for Lithium-ion Battery. *Solid State Ion.* **2008,** *179,* 1794–1799.

Zhou, H.; Fan, T.; Zhang, D. Hydrothermal Synthesis of ZnO Hollow Spheres Using Spherobacterium as Biotemplates. *Microporous Mesoporous Mater.* **2007,** *100,* 322–327.

Zhou, H.; Fan, T.; Zhang, D.; Guo, Q.; Ogawa, H. Novel Bacteria-templated Sonochemical Route for the In Situ One-step Synthesis of ZnS Hollow Nanostructures. *Chem. Mate.* **2007,** *19,* 2144–2146.

Zhu, Y.; Huang, H.; Zhou, W.; Li, G.; Liang, X.; Guo, J.; Tang, S. Low Temperature Reduction of Graphene Oxide Film by Ammonia Solution and Its Application for High-performance Supercapacitors. *J. Mater. Sci.: Mater. Electron.* **2017,** *28,* 10098–10105.

Index

H

I

L

M

N

W

Z